The Practical Handbook of Eating Difficulties

A comprehensive guide from personal and professional perspectives

Edited by
James Downs, Mark Hopfenbeck, Hannah Lewis, Isla Parker and Nicole Schnackenberg

Pavilion

The Practical Handbook of Eating Difficulties

A comprehensive guide from personal and professional perspectives

Published by:
Pavilion Publishing and Media Ltd
Blue Sky Offices, 25 Cecil Pashley Way
Shoreham by Sea, West Sussex
BN43 5FF

Tel: 01273 434 943
Email: info@pavpub.com
Web: www.pavpub.com

Published 2022

A catalogue record for this book is available from the British Library.

ISBN: 978-1-913414-68-9

Pavilion Publishing and Media is a leading publisher of books, training materials and digital content in mental health, social care and allied fields. Pavilion and its imprints offer must-have knowledge and innovative learning solutions underpinned by sound research and professional values.

Cover art by Lorna Collins
Editors: Isla Parker, Mark Hopfenbeck, James Downs, Hannah Lewis & Nicole Schnackenberg
Production editor: Mike Benge, Pavilion Publishing and Media Ltd
Cover design: Emma Dawe, Pavilion Publishing and Media Ltd
Page layout and typesetting: Emma Dawe, Pavilion Publishing and Media Ltd
Printing: Ashford Press

Contents

Foreword

By Beat

The compelling need for additional research, more effective treatments, and better access to care for people with disordered eating has been made clearer than ever in recent years. In the UK, 1.25 million people are estimated to have a diagnosable eating disorder (Beat, 2020). The sharp rise in hospital admissions for people with eating disorders in the last few years shows that this is a growing problem – admissions more than doubled (from 10,318 to 22,001) in the four years between 2016 and 2020 (NHS, 2021). Despite this, NHS waiting lists for specialist care continue to grow at a concerning rate (Beat, 2021). The pressures on services have been further compounded by the Covid-19 pandemic and resultant lockdown measures (Robertson *et al*, 2021). Beat saw a 200-300% increase in people seeking help through our Helpline over around 12 months. Never before have eating disorder services been so pressed. Never before has the need for research and treatment been more urgent.

Early intervention has, in recent years, been highlighted as a key concern for researchers (Rosello *et al*, 2021). The early or 'subthreshold' stages (i.e. when symptoms do not meet full diagnostic criteria for an eating disorder as defined by the DSM-5 or ICD-11) have been identified as a critical period for preventing the progression of an eating disorder (Spettigue *et al*, 2020). However, stigma directed towards those experiencing disordered eating not believed to be 'serious enough' to warrant support (Boero & Pascoe, 2012), could present a barrier to seeking help. Considering these factors, amongst others, it is high time for a comprehensive guide such as this handbook, which takes a broad, dimensional (rather than categorical) look at the subject. Instead of considering diagnosable eating disorders alone, the editors have created a volume which seeks to thoughtfully represent a fuller range of experiences and the diverse ways they are described, understood and responded to.

With its deliberate use of non-clinical language, *The Practical Handbook of Eating Difficulties* affirms a validating message that all difficulties around eating are worthy of help, understanding and support, irrespective of whether or not these difficulties have been diagnosed or meet the criteria for a diagnosable eating disorder. In this regard, the guide both takes a step forward towards early intervention, and creates a freer space for the drawing together of multiple perspectives, both clinical and personal. The book has a thoroughly multidisciplinary approach, bringing together an array of perspectives that range from dentists and teachers to policy-makers and paediatricians; researchers and dance therapists to people with experience of living with and caring for loved ones with disordered eating. The subject matter of the chapters is widely varied, too. Topics covered are as diverse as Mentalization-Based Treatment; the role of the GP; disordered eating in the LGBTQ+ community; lived experience perspectives; and guidance on help-seeking.

The strengths of this handbook are many – in the breadth of questions it opens; in providing a place for different perspectives and roles within the field to encounter and learn from one another; and in its practical nature. The use of "Learning Points" has allowed contributing authors to offer a range of ways for readers to extend and embed their learning. From self-reflection exercises and critical thinking tools, to practical ways of putting therapeutic techniques into practice, the theoretical content of the book is brought to life in imaginative and helpful ways. Ideas which may be new or challenging to the reader are always offered in a spirit of curiosity and encouragement, and not to the exclusion of other ways of seeing or experiencing things.

The Practical Handbook for Eating Difficulties is an original, thought-provoking and accessible guide. It is well worth reading for anyone with an interest in this area, be that from a personal or professional perspective, or simply as part of a society in which this is an increasing concern. Whether you are a person with lived experience, a carer for someone who is struggling, a policy-maker or researcher, a healthcare or educational professional, or are broadly interested in the role of eating in relation to health, this book is for you.

References

Beat (2020) *Statistics for Journalists* [online]. Available at: www.beateatingdisorders.org.uk/mediacentre/eating-disorder-statistics/ (accessed November 2021)

Beat (2021) *NHS loses momentum on eating disorder waiting times targets* [online]. Available at: www.beateatingdisorders.org.uk/news/eating-disorders-news/nhs-loses-momentum-on-eating-disorderwaiting-times-targets/ (accessed November 2021)

Boero N & Pascoe CJ (2012) Pro-anorexia Communities and Online Interaction: Bringing the Proana Body Online. *Body & Society* **18** (2) 27–57. https://doi.org/10.1177/1357034X12440827

Le Grange D & Loeb KL (2007) Early identification and treatment of eating disorders: prodrome to syndrome. *Early Intervention in Psychiatry* **1** (1) 27–39. https://doi.org/10.1111/j.1751-7893.2007.00007.x

NHS (2021) *Hospital Admissions for Eating Disorders* [online]. Available at: https://digital.nhs.uk/data-and-information/find-data-and-publications/supplementary-information/2019-supplementary-information-files/hospital-admissions-for-eating-disorders (accessed November 2021)

Robertson M, Duffy F, Newman E, Prieto Bravo C, Ates HH & Sharpe H (2021) Exploring changes in body image, eating and exercise during the COVID-19 lockdown: A UK survey. *Appetite* **159** 105062. https://doi.org/10.1016/j.appet.2020.105062

Rosello R, Gledhill J, Yi I, Watkins B, Harvey L, Hosking A, Viner, R. and Nicholls, D. (2021), Early intervention in child and adolescent eating disorders: The role of a parenting group. *Eur Eat Disorders Rev* **29** 519-526. https://doi.org/10.1002/erv.2798

Spettigue W, Aldaqqaq Z, Isserlin L, Bishop B, Norris ML, Valois D & Obeid N (2020) A Brief Modified Family-Based Treatment Intervention for Youth With Mild Eating Disorders: A Case Series. *Frontiers in Psychiatry* **11** (March), 1–8. https://doi.org/10.3389/fpsyt.2020.00105

Turnbridge S (2020) Eating disorder charity sees 70% increase in calls for help during lockdown. Huffington Post. Available at: www.huffingtonpost.co.uk/entry/eating-disorder-coronavirus-lockdown-beat_uk_5f0c605ac5b6480493d2fe80 (accessed November 2021).

About the contributors

Editors

Mark Hopfenbeck

Mark Hopfenbeck is social anthropologist specialising in health and social policy, an assistant professor at the Norwegian University of Science and Technology (NTNU), visiting fellow at London South Bank University (LSBU) and individual partner at the Collaborating Centre for Values-based Practice in Health and Social Care, St Catherine's College, Oxford University. At NTNU he teaches mindfulness, is a member of the Relational Welfare and Wellbeing research group and is involved in the development of a reflective group approach to support inmates' wellbeing and reduce isolation within prisons. For the past 15 years he has been teaching and supporting the implementation of the Open Dialogue approach in mental health care. He is one of the co-editors of *The Practical Handbook of Hearing Voices*.

James Downs

James Downs is a writer, mental health campaigner and expert by experience in eating difficulties. He recently completed a Masters in Psychology and Education at the University of Cambridge and holds various roles at the Royal College of Psychiatrists and NHS England aimed at improving support for those experiencing mental health problems and eating difficulties. James also represents several UK mental health charities and works as a Lived Experience Designer for Mind. As well as being a yoga and barre teacher, he has written extensively about his own experiences – from textbook chapters to blog posts – with the hope that those who read his work find comfort, affirmation and hope.

Hannah Lewis

Hannah Lewis is a PhD researcher at Queen Mary, University of London, where she studies culturally inclusive prevention strategies for eating disorders and body dysmorphic disorder – both of which she has lived experience of. Prior to this, Hannah worked in a senior role for a national mental health charity across their research, policy and practice areas. Here, Hannah championed co-production at a national level, as well as influenced the mental health transformation in schools' agenda, but her biggest achievement is working with national public health agencies to acknowledge the harm of traditional 'obesity' messaging for people with mental health and eating difficulties. Alongside her studies, Hannah still works with charities where she delivers mental health and resilience training in schools, facilitates research and co-production, and leads on a peer-delivered group-CBT project for the BDD Foundation. In her spare time (of which there is very little!) Hannah is a dancer with the School of Strut, a body positive dance school which aims to reject diet culture and promote female empowerment.

Isla Parker

Isla Parker is a pen name. Isla is a freelance editor and writer who promotes the understanding of health issues and wellbeing. She undertook a degree in English, and found it interesting to study how literature explores illness. This led to Isla writing a novel about anorexia for teenagers called *Size Zero?*, which is loosely based on her own experience. Isla has co-edited *The Practical Handbook of Hearing Voices* and *The Practical Handbook of Dementia* for the publisher PCCS Books. In her free time Isla enjoys playing the piano. She also takes part in an online writing group that has introduced her to writers from different countries.

Nicole Schnackenberg

Dr Nicole Schnackenberg is a child, community and educational psychologist, yoga teacher and yoga therapist. She has lived experience of eating struggle. Nicole divides her time between working as an educational psychologist in Southend, Essex, and her position as a trustee of the Body Dysmorphic Disorder Foundation. She is also a director of the Yoga in Healthcare Alliance and a trustee of the Give Back Yoga Foundation UK. Nicole has authored books on food and body image struggles: *False Bodies, True Selves: Moving Beyond Appearance-Focused Identity Struggles and Returning to the True Self* and *Bodies Arising: Fall in Love with your Body and Remember your Divine Essence*. She co-authored *The Parent's Guide to Body Dysmorphic Disorder* and co-edited, *Reflections on Body Dysmorphic Disorder: Stories of Courage, Determination and Hope*.

Authors

Adrienne Adams

Adrienne Adams (RGN.RMN. RP.MSC of Systemic Family Psychotherapy) commenced her nursing career in 1989. Firstly training as a general nurse in the Whittington Hospital North London, specialising in oncology, before embarking on a higher diploma in mental health nursing in 1994. Adrienne gained her mental health experience in the Maudsley Hospital, London, for two years specialising in care of the elderly. In 1996 she returned to Ireland and worked as a staff nurse in St Stevens Hospital Cork before joining the West Cork Mental Health Services in 1997. In 2000, Adrienne was involved in setting up the first Primary care Liaison Mental Health Nursing post in Ireland. She successfully developed this post to an Advance Nurse Practitioner post in Mental Health in Primary Care. Currently she is involved in setting up the First Open Dialogue Clinic in Bantry, West Cork, with her colleague Iseult Twamley, Senior Psychologist. Her interest in Open Dialogue comes from work as a systemic therapist and from personal experience of a family member struggling with mental health issues. She completed a three-year study program in Open Dialogue Practitioner course Train the Trainer in the UK in 2018. She has been involved in supervision and training both in Ireland and the UK since completing her practitioner course.

Sarah Alicea

Sarah Alicea is a Senior Diabetes Dietitian at Barts Trust, London. She worked as a T1DE specialist on NHS England's ComPASSION project and has co-authored national guidelines for best practice in diabetes in primary care and T1DE. Sarah is a Diabetes UK Clinical Champion 2021-2023 and Events Organiser for the British Dietetic Association diabetes specialist group.

Esther Altmann

Esther Altmann (PhD) is a psychologist in private practice in New York City and is the Director of Pastoral Education at Yeshivat Maharat Rabbinical School. Dr Altmann is an eating disorders consultant to schools and institutions, and helped develop a treatment program for Orthodox Jewish women. Dr Altmann writes and lectures on mental health topics and specializes in psychotherapy with adolescents, young adults, couples and families.

Yvette Arthur

Dr Yvette Arthur is a Chartered Clinical Psychologist, currently working in a Psychosis service and private practice. She is the secretary for the National Spirituality and Mental Health Forum and BPS Spirituality lead. She is passionate about community psychology, mental health among people from minority backgrounds, and highlighting the positive relationship between faith and mental health. She has conducted various pieces of research around ethnicity, faith and mental health, including her doctoral thesis entitled 'Narratives of Christian and Muslim qualified and trainee clinical psychologists working in the NHS'. She is a visiting lecturer at the University of East London, University of Surrey, Royal Holloway, and King's College London, delivering lectures on working with religion and spirituality in therapy, social inequalities in psychosis presentations, and diversity and inclusion. She also supports Clinical Psychology doctoral programs on addressing issues around diversity and inclusion within the curriculum, and facilitating diversity reflective practice for trainees.

Simon Atkins

Simon Atkins is a family doctor, writer and medical journalist. He presented the four-part BBC3 television series 'Make Me a Baby' and has appeared on local and national radio discussing health issues. He is the author of eight books on a wide range of health topics including *Dementia For Dummies* and *First Steps to a Healthy Heart*. He has been a columnist for The Guardian and has contributed to The Observer Magazine, FHM, GQ, Take a break, The BMJ and Men's Health.

Sara Betteridge

Dr Sara Betteridge is a Counselling Psychologist and Family Therapist with over 20 years' experience working in adult mental health settings. Her specialities are working with faith/religion/spirituality in therapy and using the systemic approach of Open Dialogue to inform any work which involves holding a space for herself and others. Sara was part of the first cohort of people in the UK to receive training in Open Dialogue and travelled to Finland to complete a Master's in teaching Open Dialogue in 2016. She currently has an independent practice offering individual and family therapy, individual and group supervision, training and consultation. Among many other endeavours, after working for a year in an adult inpatient eating disorder unit she now works with an eating disorder charity continuing to offer family therapy to those affected.

Jennifer Bibb

Jennifer Bibb (PhD) is a Senior Music Therapist and Research Fellow at the University of Melbourne in Australia. She has been a music therapist in mental health care and eating disorders for over 10 years. Her research focuses on the role of music therapy in improving treatment outcomes for people with eating difficulties as well as the use of music listening during mental health recovery. She is committed to conducting research that translates into practice and that privileges lived experience perspectives.

Geraldine Bishop

Geraldine Bishop is a counselling psychologist in training with a specific interest in working with eating difficulties. Geraldine has a 1st class joint honours degree in psychology and counselling, and her key areas of interest are eating difficulties, addiction and trauma. Working with the emotional impact of eating difficulties is something that she feels passionate about and falls closely in line with her position as a trainee psychologist. Throughout her journey, she has been privileged to work therapeutically with a number of individuals experiencing eating difficulties and she is now in the process of finalising her research into the lived experiences of bulimia nervosa. Areas in which she has worked include domestic abuse services, eating disorder services, mental health charities, crisis prevention services, drug and alcohol rehabilitation, rape crisis and sexual abuse support services and bereavement counselling services.

Timothy Brewerton

Timothy D Brewerton (MD, DLFAPA, FAED, DFAACAP, CEDS-S) is an experienced clinician, researcher, teacher, mentor, writer, editor and advocate, as well as a recognized leader in the eating difficulties field. He is Affiliate Professor of Psychiatry and Behavioral Sciences at the Medical University of South Carolina in Charleston, South Carolina, where he is in private practice. He is: Distinguished

Life Fellow of the American Psychiatric Association; Distinguished Fellow of the American Academy of Child and Adolescent Psychiatry; Founding Fellow of the Academy of Eating Disorders; the Eating Disorders Research Society (EDRS), and former president of EDRS and the South Carolina Psychiatric Association, and Certified Eating Disorder Specialist Supervisor. He has achieved board certifications in general, child-adolescent and forensic psychiatry, as well as addiction medicine. He has authored over 170 articles and book chapters and has edited/co-edited two books. Dr Brewerton currently serves as the Director of Clinical Outcomes and Research for Monte Nido and Affiliates. He has been instrumental in exploring the overlaps between trauma, post-traumatic stress disorders and eating disorders, as well as promoting integrated treatment approaches for eating and related comorbid disorders.

Sarah Brewster

Sarah Brewster (BSc, MBBS, MRCP) commenced her medical career in 2004, studying medicine and also intercalating a BSc in Diabetes and Endocrinology at Guys, Kings and St Thomas' (GKT) Medical School in London. After qualifying in 2010, Sarah spent her first four years as a junior doctor at the Royal Bournemouth Hospital (now part of University Hospitals Dorset NHS Foundation Trust) where she completed her foundation years and core medical training, achieving membership to the Royal College of Physicians in 2013. After her initial time at the Royal Bournemouth Hospital, Sarah went on to specialize in diabetes and endocrinology in the Wessex Deanery and worked across a number of its various trusts including Poole Hospital (also now part of University Hospitals Dorset NHS Foundation Trust) and Salisbury Hospital. More recently she devoted her time to a PhD with the University of Southampton, supported by Southern Health NHS Foundation Trust, looking at the role community pharmacies have in the delivery of care to those with diabetes identified as 'hardly reached' and who are at greatest risk of complications from the condition. In November 2022, after returning from maternity leave, Sarah looks forward to starting her consultant post with the West Hampshire Community Diabetes Service.

Amanda Bye

Dr Amanda Bye is a Research Associate in the Department of Psychological Medicine at the Institute of Psychiatry, Psychology and Neuroscience, King's College London. Amanda completed her PhD at UCL Great Ormond Street Institute of Child Health. Her doctoral research explored the challenges of identifying and managing pregnant and postnatal women with eating disorders in maternity and health visiting services, from the perspectives of women with lived experience and health professionals. The findings led to a collaborative project with the co-authors of this chapter to co-produce web-based training on eating disorders for health professionals caring for pregnant and postnatal women. This project was supported by The Health Foundation and King's Improvement Science, part of the Centre for Implementation Science within the National Institute for Health Research (NIHR) Applied Research Collaboration South London (NIHR ARC South London) at King's College Hospital NHS Foundation Trust.

Simon Chapman

Dr Simon Chapman is a children's doctor with a background in diabetes and endocrinology. Since 2010 he has led the medical management of eating disorders at the Maudsley Child and Adolescent Eating Disorders Service (MCCAED). He is a joint lead of Junior MaRSiPAN, a national group aiming to guide best practice on the medical management of eating disorders in children and young people. He is also a founding trustee of the British Eating Disorders Society.

Nuha Chowdhury

Nuha Chowdhury is a Royal College of Psychiatrists-accredited Peer Support Worker at East London NHS foundation Trust. She has a decade of lived experience of an eating disorder. She now uses her experience to help others with eating difficulties and mental illness to move forward in their recovery. She also uses her experience to co-produce and facilitate various forms of training around eating disorders and mental illness, and engages with broader work to improve mental health services.

Lorna Collins

Lorna Collins is an artist, filmmaker, writer, journalist and Research Fellow in medical sociology at University College London. Her research trajectory examines themes around arts and health. This started during her PhD, where she was a triple scholar at Jesus College, Cambridge University. Lorna has written articles in several newspapers and journals. She spoke about her life story and research in a TEDx Talk ('How Creativity Revived Me').

Brian Cook

Dr Brian Cook has developed an original line of research examining the etiological role, management and therapeutic potential of exercise in eating disorders. His education at the Universities of Rhode Island and Florida and a NIMH post-doctoral fellowship at the Neuropsychiatric Research Institute in Fargo, ND allowed him to train under experts in the eating disorder field. This has resulted in presenting research at international conferences (e.g., Eating Disorders Research Society, the Academy for Eating Disorders), chairing conference paper sessions, publications in leading journals (e.g., International Journal of Eating Disorders) and book chapters, and a keynote address at the IAEPD 2017 Symposium. He is a sought-after presenter, author and consultant for exercise, eating disorders, behavioural medicine and behavioural addictions.

Catherine Cook-Cottone

Catherine Cook-Cottone (PhD, C-IAYT) is a Licensed Psychologist, Certified Yoga Therapist, and Professor at SUNY at Buffalo. She is creator and director of the Mindful Counseling Advanced Certificate program and co-founder and president of Yogis in Service, Inc., a not-for-profit organization that creates access to yoga. Catherine's research specializes in embodied self- regulation (i.e., yoga, mindfulness and mindful self-care) and psychosocial disorders (e.g., eating disorders, substance use and trauma). Her research has been funded by the National Science Foundation, UNICEF, lululemon athletic, and the Give Back Yoga Foundation. Catherine has written ten books and over 85 peer-reviewed articles and book chapters. She has served as a consultant for the UN Foundation, Africa Yoga Project, and the Recon and Sniper Foundation. She is co-founder of Yogis in Service. In 2018, she was awarded the American Psychological Association's Citizen Psychologist Presidential Citation. She is co-editor in chief of *Eating Disorder: Journal of Treatment and Prevention* and author of *Embodiment and the Treatment of Eating Disorders: The body as a resource in recovery* (W.W. Norton) and *Mindfulness and Yoga for Self-regulation* (Springer).

Kate Daigle

Kate Daigle is a licensed professional counselor and Certified Eating Disorders Specialist residing in Denver, Colorado, USA. She has had her private practice since 2010 and has experience working with populations dealing with body image, eating disorder issues in addition to a sub-specialty of working with women also struggling with infertility and postpartum challenges. In 2019, she published her first book: *The Clinical Guide to Fertility, Motherhood and Eating Disorders*, and has spoken nationally as well as contributed to several other publications on the topic of eating disorders and fertility. She loves teaching her daughter the joys of gardening and spending time with her family on her downtime. Learn more about Kate at www.katedaiglecounseling.com.

Jasmine Daisy

Jasmine Daisy has written her chapter from the perspective of a sibling as her brother was diagnosed with anorexia nervosa in 2016 after being admitted to general hospital. He was in an inpatients unit for seven months before coming home to continue his recovery. He has now moved out of the family home, and Jasmine is currently at university studying Marine Biology in Cornwall.

Jennifer Danby

Jennifer is a Systemic Family Psychotherapist working in a lifespan eating disorder service in London. She has over 10 years of experience working in the field of eating disorders and has extensive experience working closely with families, particularly parents, in enabling them to support their loved ones experiencing eating difficulties. Jennifer is an Advanced Therapist, Supervisor and Trainer in Emotion-Focused Family Therapy (EFFT) which is an innovative treatment model that strongly advocates and supports the active involvement of caregivers in overcoming mental health and behavioural difficulties. Jennifer is one of the founding Board Members for the International Institute for Emotion-Focused Family Therapy. Jennifer is also involved in research into different treatment approaches for anorexia nervosa.

Yngvild Sørebø Danielsen

Yngvild Sørebø Danielsen, (PhD/clinical psychologist) is currently employed as Associate Professor at the University of Bergen, Norway. She is conducting research about treatment of eating disorders and severe obesity, and has written a textbook on family-based treatment of severe obesity in children. She is teaching and supervising psychology students, as well as practicing as a clinical psychologist. She also has experience from working in mental health care for children and youth, and at a specialized eating disorder unit. She has specialized training in treating eating disorders and obesity, clinical psychological work with children and youth and emotion-focused therapy.

Madelaine de Valle

Madelaine de Valle (BPsychHons) is a provisionally registered psychologist and PhD candidate in Clinical Psychology at Flinders University in South Australia, being supervised by Matthew Flinders Distinguished Professor Tracey Wade. Her research and clinical interests include perfectionism, body image, and eating disorders, and her PhD thesis concerns the relationship between social media use and risk factors for eating disorders. She received the Australian Psychological Society Prize for academic excellence in psychology in 2017 for her Honours research, which investigated online cognitive behaviour therapy for perfectionism and has been published in a peer-reviewed journal.

Russell Delderfield

Russell's PhD is in male eating disorders, which he completed as a mature student, after time away from academia. He is the author of the book *Male Eating Disorders: Experiences of Food, Body and Self*. He has experience as a charity trustee and delivers training to medical and health professionals in male eating disorders. Russell has also written chapters and articles on eating disorders in men, the university experience of men with eating issues, and strategies for counsellors when supporting men with eating disorders. He works at the University of Bradford, UK, and has diverse expertise, including researcher mental health, person-centredness in doctoral education, and reflective practice. In the latter topic, he authored the latest edition of the book *Reflective Practice: Writing and Professional Development* with Dr Gillie Bolton. You can follow him on Twitter (@MaleEDResearch) or see his research website: www.bradford.ac.uk/eating-disorders-in-men/.

Dr Abigail Easter

Dr Abigail Easter is a Senior Lecturer in Maternal and Newborn Health in the Department of Women and Children's Health, School of Life Course Science, at King's College London and Deputy Lead for the Maternity and Perinatal Mental Health research theme of the NIHR Applied Research Collaboration (ARC) South London. Dr Easter completed her PhD in maternal eating disorders, and the effects on pregnancy, birth, and motherhood. Her current research focuses on maternal morbidity and mortality among women experiencing mental health problems and bridging the gap between maternity and mental healthcare services to inform care of women with multi-morbidity.

Bethany Elms

Dr Bethany Elms is an Educational Psychologist who undertook her doctorate at Cardiff University. She currently works in Hertfordshire Educational Psychology Service, where she supports schools, families, and young people with additional needs. She has a special interest in mental health, particularly eating disorders. Her thesis explored the role of educational psychologists working with schools supporting young people with eating disorders and their families. Bethany grew up in Kenya, in a small area on the outskirts of Nairobi called Karen. She undertook her education in Kenya until the age of 16, where she then attended a boarding school in England. Bethany completed her undergraduate degree in psychology at Royal Holloway University of London, then worked in a range of educational settings in Kenya and England before starting her training at Cardiff University.

Esther Estey

Esther Estey (PhD, RYT-200) is a certified yoga and meditation teacher and psychologist. She earned her PhD at the University at Buffalo and has Master of Arts degrees in counseling and human resources/executive leadership. Her research, teaching, training and clinical work focus on factors that cultivate self-regulation, resilience and positive embodiment. As an adjunct professor, Estey has taught on the treatment of trauma and abuse, mindfulness in clinical practice, and contemplative approaches for greater health and peak performance. Clinically, she has provided bilingual, mindfulness-based psychotherapy for diverse populations with co-occurring, severe psychiatric and medical conditions in community as well as military settings. She completed her clinical internship at Stanford University Medical School/VA Palo Alto Health Care System and is a postdoctoral fellow at Harvard Medical School/Cambridge Health Alliance. Estey has a private practice specializing in integrated treatment of traumatic stress and associated disturbances in mind and body.

Carla Figueiredo

Dr Carla Figueiredo is a Consultant Psychiatrist working with the Dorset All Age Eating Disorders Service since 2010. She has led on Mental Health for the NHS England funded Wessex ComPASSION Pilot Study, looking into the assessment and management of people with Type 1 Diabetes and an eating disorder.

Mary Franklin-Smith

Mary Franklin-Smith is a HCPC registered Sesame Drama and Movement Therapist, having trained at the Royal Central School of Speech and Drama in London. She worked for over 17 years in specialist NHS mental health services before taking her own leap of faith to fully fly with her own business, "Light of Mind" (www.lightofmind.co.uk). She learned and witnessed so much working as the CAMHS Lead Therapist in a prison and as a senior leader at the West Yorkshire Adult Eating Disorder Service, she remains forever grateful for these enriching and humbling experiences. She continues to offer therapy, training, consultation and supervision to a range of NHS patients and health and social care clinical staff. She has made several radio, podcast and TV appearances speaking about different aspects of mental health, research and innovation. Her work takes her across the globe offering bespoke Light of Mind services in business, education and theatres. She has a range of clients from all walks of life. She regularly presents at local, national and international conferences and universities. Her research interests include: embodied group therapy, innate health and use of tele therapies and multi/social media. She is co-author of several academic papers and is in the process of writing a book about innate health and disordered eating with a colleague. She lives In West Yorkshire with her husband, three children and two dogs.

Sarah Fuller

Sarah Fuller is a registered Dietitian who has worked with children and young people with eating disorders in specialist eating disorder units, paediatric wards and as part of her local CAMHS service. Sarah is an active researcher who has published several papers relating to eating disorders, and is currently working at Imperial College London for her research. @chattydietitian

Alaa Galadari

Alaa Galadari is a psychiatrist at Sheikh Khalifa Medical City, the largest psychiatric facility in the United Arab Emirates. She is interested in academic psychiatry and has published in peer reviewed journals. She is currently a member of the Emirates Society for Child & Adolescent Mental Health, Emirates Medical Association.

Ifigeneia Giannopoulou

Dr Ifigeneia Giannopoulou is a Senior Lecturer in Exercise, Nutrition and Health Sciences in the University of Brighton. She comes from a diverse background of educational and research experiences in Europe and America. She holds a BSc in Exercise Science from the University of Athens, Greece; an MscEdu in Exercise Science from Northern Illinois University in America; and a PhD in Exercise Physiology/Science Education from Syracuse University, USA. She was previously a lecturer in Applied Physiology at Strathclyde University in Glasgow and a lecturer in Exercise Physiology/Sports Nutrition at the University of Athens. Ifigeneia also holds a practitioner's diploma on Eating Disorders by the National Centre of Eating Disorders, UK, and is a certified MB-EAT instructor in Mindful Eating by the Mindful Eating Training Institute, USA. Ifigeneia teaches a variety of courses in exercise and health, nutrition for health, exercise testing and prescription for athletes and clinical populations both in the BSc and MSc level. Her research interests lie in the area of exercise, health, nutrition and applied psychology and has a number of research publications investigating the effects of lifestyle interventions on obesity and related comorbidities such as diabetes and cardiovascular disease. More recently her research is focused on mental health, and particularly on disordered eating and eating disorders in the general population and athletic individuals.

Ken Goss

Dr Ken Goss (D. Clin. Psy), is a Consultant Clinical Psychologist and Head of Coventry Eating Disorders Service in the UK. He has over 25 years' experience of working with people with eating difficulties. He has published a number of academic papers and book chapters on the role of shame and compassion in eating disorders. He leads an on-going research program exploring these issues and their relationship with therapeutic practice and outcomes. Ken is a regular speaker at national and international conferences. He has worked closely with Professor Paul Gilbert (OBE), the originator of Compassion Focused Therapy, for over 30 years. He is a Board Member of, and trainer for, the Compassionate Mind Foundation (www.compassionatemind.co.uk). Ken has pioneered the use of Compassion Focused Therapy for Eating Disorders (CFT-E) and is the author of *The Compassionate Mind-Guide to Ending Overeating: Using Compassion-Focused Therapy to Overcome Bingeing & Disordered Eating* (New Harbinger Publications, 2011). If you are interested in collaborative research, training or supervision, Ken can be contacted at k.goss@sky.com.

Andrew Green

Andrew Green is an occupational therapist by profession with 35 years' experience in mental health and neuropsychiatry. Being attached to a sleep clinic, he began in 1999 to work with people with insomnia and increasingly specialized in sleep problems, working with a team of leading sleep specialists, and seeing patients with the whole range of sleep disorders. To support that work he did specialized training – including short courses on sleep medicine and cognitive behaviour for insomnia and regularly attended conferences and meetings on sleep. He has been involved in research on insomnia and has written several articles on sleep. He also co-edited two books on sleep (writing about half the content of one of them). He now has a private practice specialising in insomnia and does online work as a sleep coach with clients around the world as well as running training sessions for health professionals who want to help their patients manage their sleep difficulties.

Frances Grey

Frances' son was diagnosed with anorexia nervosa when he was 13, when he went into an eating disorder unit for seven months. Since then, he has been in recovery, returned to school eventually, went to college and is now 18 and living independently. Frances has completed a psychology degree, changed career and is currently working as an Assistant Psychologist in the Eating Disorders Team locally. She is applying for further post-doctoral training as a clinical or counselling psychologist. I run a carers group and Carers Skills Workshops at work and volunteer for BEAT as an ECHO coach.

Jess Griffiths

Jess Griffiths (MBACP) trained as an eating disorders therapist and practitioner after recovering from her own eating disorder. Jess co-chairs the Parliamentary Health Service Ombudsman's delivery group that was formed after the publication of *Ignoring the Alarms* and works alongside NHS England as a consultant for adult eating disorder treatment. Jess directed the charity I*EAT from 2009-2015 and now works as the Clinical Lead for Beat. Through her role with Beat, Jess has been commissioned by Health Education England to write an eating disorder training package for medical students and doctors. Jess has worked alongside the Royal College of Psychiatrists as a lead reviewer, accreditation committee member and advisory group member for adult eating disorder inpatient units. She is passionate about early intervention in eating disorders and has provided training and higher education lectures for healthcare professionals around the UK.

Nick Hawkes

Dr Nick Hawkes (he/him) works with the compassionate and skilled multi-disciplinary team, charity and NHS partners and the diverse population of Bedfordshire and Luton, UK, to address the challenges of severe and complex adult eating disorders. Nick is Consultant Clinical Psychologist and Head of Service at ELFT NHS Trust. Nick has worked in eating disorders for many years, as well as in obesity, bariatric, trauma and veteran mental health services. Nick also teaches and supports research at the University of Hertfordshire and University College London. He obtained his Doctorate in Clinical Psychology with the University of East London and CBT Diploma with the Oxford Cognitive Therapy Centre. Nick is a current committee member and past Chair of the British Psychological Society Faculty for Eating Disorders, and is a founder and deputy Chair of Trustees of the British Eating Disorder Society. Nick has previously served as Associate Editor of *The Cognitive Behaviour Therapist* (BABCP/CUP), and on the Scientific Committees of the BABCP and the European and World CBT Congresses.

Catherine Haynes

Dr Cath Haynes is a Clinical Psychologist who has over ten years' experience in providing Compassion Focused Therapy to clients with eating disorders. She has worked with Dr Ken Goss to develop the CFT-E approach in a clinical setting and is involved in CFT supervision and training.

Andrea Higgins

Andrea has had 35 years of experience as a practising educational psychologist, having trained originally in Manchester. During her career she has worked in both England and Wales and has undertaken many roles including 12 years as a Principal Educational Psychologist. In recent years, until her retirement in the summer of July 2021, Andrea has been the Program Director for the Cardiff doctoral training program for educational psychologists. Andrea is passionate about working collaboratively with schools to improve the educational experiences of children and young people and has been the author of several documents on whole-school approaches.

Rachel Jenkins

Rachel Jenkins is a PhD student at Durham University, with a speciality in Medical Law and Ethics. Rachel graduated with an LLM and LLB from The University of Bristol and is now continuing her research into the law pertaining to eating disorders with funding from the Economic and Social Research Council. Her keen academic and personal interest in disordered eating has informed her research into the socio-cultural and legal aspects of treating eating disorders.

Clive Kelly

Dr Clive Kelly is a Consultant Physician at James Cook University Hospital (JCUH) and holds academic positions at several UK Universities. He graduated with a Distinction at MBBS from Newcastle University on his 23rd birthday and trained in Exeter and the West Midlands before returning north to complete his MD in Respiratory Immunology and obtain his FRCP. He has worked in the North East England for most of his consultant career, combining a full-time clinical role with much teaching at both under- and post-graduate level. His father, a psychiatrist, fostered his interest in the psychology of illness and practice of holistic medicine, areas which have contributed significantly to his 150 peer-reviewed publications. Having worked on all five major continents, in recent years Clive has developed clinical and humanitarian services in Asia and East Africa where he has helped chronicle evidence of a rising incidence of mental health issues in the young, including a variety of eating disorders. His insight into the diagnosis and management of chronic illness lends itself to a broad approach to supporting those with neurodiversity and associated comorbidity who often demonstrate an overlap of psychological and physical manifestations. He is President of the Association of North-east Physicians and Secretary of the British Rheumatoid Interstitial Lung group.

Ameerah Khadaroo

Dr Ameerah Khadaroo is a Lecturer in Psychology, Chartered Psychologist and Early Career Researcher at UAL. Ameerah lectures on the Psychology of Fashion undergraduate and postgraduate courses at the London College of Fashion. Before joining LCF, she completed a PhD in Psychology at the University of Warwick. Ameerah has contributed to the press, academic journals and conferences in her main areas of expertise; notably developmental psychology, well-being, fashion and identity, parenting, qualitative research methods and mixed methods. She has a growing interest in exploring fashion from a developmental psychological perspective, particularly with a focus on fashion, wellbeing and identity among young people.

Mia Kurtti

Mia Kurtti is a nurse MSc and a trainer and supervisor in Family Therapy and Open Dialogue. She has been working in mental health services as a nurse in Western Lapland, Finland, since 2002, with individuals and their networks. During the last decade she has been a trainer on several international Open Dialogue/ Collaborative training programs. Crucial part of her work during recent years has been developing the role of peer specialists in Western Lapland healthcare district, together with peer specialist trainer and other colleagues. One of Mia's aims in training processes is to open and expand the dialogue in a way that increases people's own creativity and resourcefulness. In her role as a trainer she is keen to emphasize and invite people who work in mental health settings to explore their own life narratives and the impact that these stories have on their current professional practice.

Antonia Lagou

Antonia is an Eating Disorder Service Manager and a strong advocate for peer support in the eating disorder community. With personal experience of delivering peer support to individuals of all ages through her work with First Steps ED, a local charity in the East Midlands, alongside coordinating a peer support service driven by experts by experience, she has an enthusiasm and passion to empower sufferers to take control of their recovery journey. Antonia has worked in the third sector since 2015, specifically in the eating disorder context. She was involved in the launch of an eating disorder service specifically for university students in the East Midlands, and has progressed forwards to manage a number of services available to individuals nationwide through Beat. She continues to volunteer for First Steps ED, delivering peer support to young people as well as training professionals.

Judy Laing

Judy Laing is a Professor of Mental Health Law, Rights & Policy at the University of Bristol Law School. She teaches mental health law to undergraduate and postgraduate students and has a long-standing research interest in mental health law and human rights. She has published extensively in these areas and is also a member of the Editorial Board for two health law journals – the *International Journal of Law & Psychiatry* and the *Medical Law Review.* She is currently undertaking a Parliamentary Academic Fellowship in the Social Policy section of the House of Commons Library working on a project on mental health law reform.

Georgie Lazzari

Georgie is a mental health blogger, campaigner and an ambassador for First Steps ED – the Midland's leading mental health and specialist eating disorder organisation. Having worked in marketing and communications for over ten years, Georgie wanted to focus her career and strengths on helping to make a difference to the lives of people impacted by eating disorders and the associated mental health difficulties. She is currently studying for a qualification in Counselling ahead of undertaking a mental health peer support role in the near future.

She also dedicates her time to raising awareness by writing for her own and other well-known mental health blog sites, facilitating support groups, part-taking in research projects, speaking at training events, creating educational resources and working as an Expert Patient for the Derbyshire Healthcare Foundation Trust.

Elina Löhönen

Elina Löhönen is a psychologist and a trainer in Family and Couple Therapy and Open Dialogue. She has been working in mental health field for over two decades. In Western Lapland health care district she has been developing the practice in adolescence and child psychiatry and during the last years she has also been working as an administrative lead for psychologists. Her inspiration to work comes from working with families and networks and supporting their agency through dialogical practice in crisis.

Grace Lucas

Grace Lucas is an academic and yoga teacher. She was diagnosed with anorexia nervosa at age 18. Ten years later, she wrote a bestselling account of her experiences *Thin* (Penguin, 2007) and spoke widely in media, educational and medical settings about her diagnosis and recovery. After the birth of her two children, Grace returned to academia completing a Masters and PhD in medical humanities exploring the role of bodies and narratives in accounts of mental illness. Grace now works as a lecturer in Mental Health and Society at City, University of London. Her research interests centre on the relationship between embodiment and mental health and wellbeing.

Danielle Mills

Danielle has worked in mental health all her professional life and has experience at working in the statutory, voluntary and private sectors, with disordered eating being her specialist area of practice. Danielle experienced her own difficulties with disordered eating and was in inpatient treatment for some time before continuing her recovery in the community. Danielle has experience setting up and running a service for young people affected by eating difficulties and disorders. During this period, Danielle qualified as a counsellor and is an accredited member of the BACP. After three years in this role, Danielle left to study a PhD at the University of Nottingham, completing an ethnographic study looking at young men and their perspectives of health and healthy bodies. Danielle was also Chair of the Board of Trustees for another eating disorders charity for two years. During this period Danielle also completed training in EFP with LEAP and The Herd Institute with which she is now a senior practitioner and faculty member, respectively. Danielle also runs a community interest company, Pony Partnerships CIC, providing equine facilitated therapies to children and young people. Danielle also runs UK training in EFL and EFP.

Victoria Mountford

Dr Victoria Mountford (BA(Hons), DClinPsy) is a Consultant Clinical Psychologist. She combines her clinical work with research and teaching. She has 20 years' experience of working with individuals with eating disorders and body image concerns and their families. She is a BABCP accredited practitioner, supervisor and trainer. She was part of the founding team who developed FREED, the first early intervention eating disorder service in the UK. She has published widely, including three books – *Cognitive Behaviour Therapy for the Eating Disorders: A Comprehensive Treatment Guide* (2007), *Beating Your Eating Disorder: A Cognitive-Behavioural Self Help Guide for Adult Sufferers and their Carers* (2010) and *Brief Cognitive Behavioural Therapy for Non-Underweight Patients: CBT-T for Eating Disorders* (2019). Her research interests include early intervention, body image and cognitive behaviour therapy. Victoria was joint recipient of the Academy for Eating Disorders Outstanding Clinician Award 2020.

Nicola Murdoch

Nicola Murdoch (BDS(Bris) MSc(Leeds) MFDS RCS (Eng) FFGDP(UK)) is a General Dental Practitioner who qualified from the University of Bristol. Following an Oral Surgery position in Cambridge she returned to General Dental Practice in 2005. She has been awarded Membership of the Faculty of Dental Surgery and Fellowship of the Faculty of General Dental Practice by the Royal College of Surgeons of England. In 2014 she completed an MSc in Restorative Dentistry from the University of Leeds with Distinction. Nicola has examined for the Royal College of Surgeons of England and taught undergraduate students at the University of Bristol. She appraises dentists throughout the Thames Valley for Health Education England. As well as providing General Dentistry, her particular interests are the treatment of tooth wear and aesthetic dentistry. She often treats multi-disciplinary cases in conjunction with Specialist Dentists. Nicola has a minimally invasive, caring and holistic approach to dentistry and treats patients of all ages, especially those who may be apprehensive. She enjoys improving her patients' confidence by helping them to achieve healthy and bright smiles.

Dasha Nicholls

Dr Dasha Nicholls is Clinical Reader in Child Psychiatry in the Division of Psychiatry at Imperial College London, Honorary Consultant Child and Adolescent Psychiatrist in the Children and Young People's (CYP) Eating Disorders Service in Central and North West London NHS Foundation Trust, and Clinical and Strategic Director for National Audits and Research at the Royal College of Psychiatrists. She is a member of the Beat Clinical Advisory board. Until moving to Imperial in 2018, Dr Nicholls co-led the Feeding and Eating Disorders service at Great Ormond Street Hospital. She is past-President of the Academy for Eating Disorders and was Chair of the Eating Disorders Faculty (2015-19).

Nancy Nsiah

Dr Nancy Nsiah is a Highly Specialist Clinical Psychologist who is deeply committed to nurturing culturally sensitive and anti-racist practices. She enjoys delivering creative workshops and presentations around these themes across both the NHS and private organisations. Dr Nsiah serves on advisory committees for a Clinical Psychology doctoral program focusing on decolonising the curriculum and centering equality and diversity work within training. Inspired by her Christian faith and Ghanian heritage, Dr Nsiah identifies as a storyteller and values compassion, inclusive collaboration and cultural humility as central to her justice and therapeutic work. Within her NHS role, Dr Nsiah leads a family clinic, supporting children and young people within families who have been impacted by a diagnosis of cancer.

Ivana Osenk

Dr Ivana Osenk (BPsychHons, PhD ClinPsych) is a registered psychologist and clinical registrar who completed her PhD in the area of perfectionism in 2021 at Flinders University in South Australia under the supervision of Matthew Flinders Distinguished Professor Tracey Wade. Her clinical and research expertise lie in the area of eating disorders, perfectionism and investigating the differences between pursuing perfection versus excellence, and she has published a number of peer-reviewed publications. In 2018 she was awarded the Telethon Kids Institute Fraser Mustard Scholarship for her PhD thesis which investigated the efficacy of a universal school-based prevention program for combatting perfectionism in adolescents.

Helen Partridge

Dr Helen Partridge is a Consultant in Diabetes at University Hospitals Dorset and visiting fellow at Bournemouth University. She is the clinical lead for the diabetes insulin pump service and the COmpASSION project providing care for people living with type 1 diabetes and an eating disorder. Dr Partridge is also lead for the award-winning Bertieonline providing a free digital platform offering structured education to people with type 1 diabetes. Her specialist interests are in the psychology of living with type 1 diabetes and technology for diabetes having undertaken a fellowship in advanced diabetes technologies at University of Toronto

Shira Pollack

Shira Pollack is a PhD student in counseling psychology at the University of Buffalo. Her research and clinical work focuses on positive psychology interventions (self-care, self-compassion, gratitude) and emotion-driven behaviors in young adults (procrastination, substance use, disordered eating). Shira has provided individual and group psychotherapy to college students at the university counseling center. Currently, she is a psychologist-in-training at a partial hospitalization program for eating disorder treatment.

Lilian Prince

Lilian Prince is a recent BSc graduate of Psychology from Plymouth University, with a focus on Child Psychology and Eating Disorders. Lilian took a particular interest in the eating disorder modules, after two of her close family friends were diagnosed with anorexia within a matter of months of one another. Seeing how this diagnosis affected both friends and their families, acted only to strengthen her interest. Lilian chose to further this interest by focusing her dissertation on the use of dance and movement therapy in the treatment of eating disorders. Lilian is currently working as a nursery-school teacher in her hometown in Surrey and following her own advice on the benefits of creativity for mental health by designing and making her own clothes and costumes.

Andrew Radford

Andrew Radford has been Chief Executive of Beat, the UK's eating disorder charity, since 2015. Previously he worked in a variety of roles for UNICEF UK, starting with 10 years leading an accreditation-based program to improve NHS support for new mothers' feeding decisions, followed by short stints as Communications and Fundraising Director before a final period as Strategy and Innovation Director, leaving in 2011 to become Chief Executive of children's advocacy charity Voice. Before that he worked for a small NGO researching and campaigning on the marketing activities of the infant feeding industry. He originally graduated in Modern Languages before realising he didn't like working as a translator.

Rachel Raw

Dr Rachael Raw is an academic foundation doctor, also at JCUH. Originally graduating with a First-Class honours degree in Applied Psychology from Durham University, Rachael was later awarded a Medical Research Council Scholarship (MRC) to study for a PHD in Cognitive Neuroscience at the University of Leeds. After gaining her PHD in 2012, Rachael won an MRC Centenary Post-Doctoral Fellowship and two grants from the Leeds Teaching Hospital Charitable Foundation that allowed her to conduct independent research into the effects of stroke on cognition and motor control. In 2020, Rachael also graduated from medical school, gaining an MBBS in Medicine and Surgery from Newcastle University. Throughout her academic career, Rachael has published her work in peer-reviewed psychology and neuroscience journals and has presented at local and international conferences. While her prior work has focused on older adult psychology and health, Rachael has a personal interest in Eating Conditions and feels strongly about improving the provision of practical resources for people trying to live with these difficulties.

Guro Rekkedal

Guro Årdal Rekkedal has been working as a clinical psychologist at a specialized Department for Eating Disorders since 2013. She is specialized in Cognitive Behavioral Therapy (CBT) and Emotional Focused Therapy (EFT). Rekkedal finished her PhD in 2013 on the topic depression and cognitive functioning. She has published several papers in international peer-reviewed journals. Rekkedal is currently focusing on research concerning factors contributing to drop out from eating disorder treatment. She is member of the steering group of the National Quality register for Eating Disorders in Norway (NORSPIS).

Paul Robinson

Dr Paul Robinson is an associate professor at University College London and a consultant psychiatrist at Orri UK. He was formerly consultant psychiatrist at the Royal Free Hospital and at St Ann's Hospital eating disorders service where he wrote the books *Community treatment of Eating Disorders*, *Severe and Enduring Eating Disorders* and co-edited *Critical care for anorexia nervosa*. He has developed Mentalization Based Therapy for eating disorders and co-written a book, *Hunger*, on this subject. He produced the first version of MARSIPAN, guidance for the management of patients with severe anorexia nervosa and continues to work on the revisions. He launched the first Masters' course in Eating Disorders and Clinical Nutrition at UCL.

Reid Robinson

Reid Robison, MD, is a board-certified psychiatrist and eating disorder specialist. Dr Robison is Chief Medical Officer of Novamind, co-founder of Cedar Psychiatry, and serves as the Medical Director for the Center for Change, a leading Eating Disorder center. Dr Robison has led over 100 clinical trials in psychiatry, including a study of group-based, ketamine-assisted psychotherapy for eating disorders in a residential setting, and emotion-focused, ketamine-assisted psychotherapy for anorexia nervosa. He is currently the coordinating investigator for the MAPS-sponsored MDMA-assisted psychotherapy study of anorexia nervosa and binge eating disorder. Dr Robison is also an adjunct professor at both the University of Utah and Brigham Young University and is the founder of the Polizzi Free Clinic, a free mental health clinic for uninsured individuals in Salt Lake City, Utah.

Jekaterina Rogaten

Dr Jekaterina Rogaten is a Course Leader for the MSc Applied Psychology in Fashion program and Teaching and Learning co-ordinator at the Fashion Business School, University of the Arts London. Her teaching expertise is in positive psychology and well-being in fashion industry. Her research is centred on creativity, flow, motivation, metacognition and optimal human functioning. In addition, she is also interested in the evaluation of learning environments and how people develop new knowledge whether it is acquired in the formal educational settings or incidentally.

Emily Rothwell

Emily Rothwell is currently a trainee clinical psychologist at Lancaster University. Prior to this, she initially joined Beat as an Ambassador, where she used her personal experiences of recovery from an eating disorder to support and educate others. Following the completion of her MSc by Research, which investigated the acceptability of a digital treatment for those affected by binge eating difficulties, Emily joined Beat as a staff member in 2017. During her three years at Beat, Emily undertook various roles including Senior Helpline Advisor and Clinical Advisor. Emily is now a trustee for Beat, a position that she feels privileged to hold.

Prabhleen Sandhu

Dr Prabhleen Sandhu is a Clinical Psychologist who currently works in paediatric health and child and adolescent mental wellbeing. The principles of Prabhleen's faith – Sikhism – richly inform her values both in therapeutic work, teaching and delivering workshops. She is an advocate who has a keen interest in gender equality and reducing gender stereotyping, as well as incorporating culture and religion in therapy. Prabhleen is passionate about breaking down barriers and addressing stigma associated with mental health difficulties, especially within minority ethnic communities, and has first-hand experience of challenges relating to ethnic diversity in the workplace. She is passionate about supporting interventions that are inclusive of an individual's needs. Outside of clinical practice, Prabhleen volunteers with a variety of South Asian mental health charities raising awareness of mental wellbeing and increasing access to services.

Finn Skarderud

Finn Skårderud (MD, PhD) is a Norwegian professor, psychiatrist and author. He is adjunct professor in Eating Disorders at University of Southern Denmark, Odense, and also adjunct professor at University of Agder, Norway, and Norwegian School of Sport Sciences, Oslo. He is an internationally acknowledged expert in eating disorders. He is a co-founder and in the leadership of the Norwegian Institute for Mentalizing. He runs a private practice. Together with Bente Sommerfeldt, co-authoring this book chapter, he founded in 2014 the Norwegian Institute for Eating Disorders. This is a non-profit foundation, striving be an innovative centre of excellence for treatment, research, education and training. Skårderud has produced 20 books, more than 150 book chapters, about 100 scientific papers and numerous articles and essays and podcasts. He has also produced or contributed to many radio and television programs and podcasts within the fields art, literature, film, psychiatry, psychology and culture.

Lawrence Smith

Lawrence is an actor and singer, currently based in London. Born and raised in the Scottish Highlands, Lawrence went on to study classical singing at the *Royal Conservatoire of Scotland*, followed by a master's degree in musical theatre at the *Royal Academy of Music*. Since graduating, Lawrence has performed for *Shakespeare's Globe*, *The Old Vic* and the *National Theatre of Scotland*, as well as playing the lead in the 2019 UK tour of *Avenue Q*. Over the years, Lawrence has experienced various mental health challenges. As a Type 1 diabetic, Lawrence has been involved in the research and awareness raising of the particular challenges that face Type 1 diabetics with an eating disorder.

Wendy Solomons

Dr Wendy Solomons (PhD) is a Clinical Psychologist and Academic Lead of the Doctorate in Clinical Psychology program at the University of Hertfordshire, UK. She completed her professional training at University College London, and has worked in the NHS and related professional training programs for over 25 years. Her clinical, research and teaching interests focus on the interplay of physical and 'mental' health across the lifespan, with particular attention to the impact of social contexts and inequalities. Her PhD and subsequent research consider ways in which critical and constructionist research methods can add to our understanding, especially to processes of transition, marginalisation and identity construction. She feels energised by moves in co-production of research, teaching and service development, and how this can bring change to the 'status quo'.

Bente Sommerfeldt

Bente Sommerfeldt is a specialist in adult clinical psychology with over 15 years' experience in eating disorders. Together with Finn Skårderud, co-authoring this book chapter, she founded in 2014 the Norwegian Institute for Eating Disorders. This is a non-profit foundation, striving be an innovative centre of excellence for treatment, research, education and training. She is currently professional director at the institute. She is in the leadership of the Norwegian Institute of Mentalizing. She has extensive experience in providing and supervising mentalization based therapy and MBT-ED in Scandinavia. She is a PhD student at the University of Oslo, Institute of psychology with a special interest in eating disorder and motherhood.

Justin Thomas

Justin Thomas is chair of the department, and professor of experimental psychology at Zayed University in the United Arab Emirates (UAE). Justin is also a chartered health psychologist with the British Psychological Society and a credentialed mindfulness instructor. Justin has long standing research interests in body image disturbance and eating difficulties. He has lived and worked in the UAE for more than a decade and has a firsthand knowledge of working with Muslims who are experiencing eating difficulties. He has published over 50 peer-review research articles and is the author of *Psychological Well-being in the Gulf States: The New Arabia Felix*.

Cathy Thorley

Cathy Thorley qualified as a trainer in Dialogic Practice after completing a two year course in Helsinki. She is the lead family therapist and Clinical Lead for Peer Supported Open Dialogue (POD) within adult mental health services in North East London NHS Foundation Trust. She also set up and managed an England wide non-crisis NHS Open Dialogue style service working with families and networks. Cathy is a tutor on the Peer Supported Open Dialogue post graduate training. She also holds reflective spaces and supervises teams using a systemic and dialogical approach with different staff groups within and outside the NHS. She has facilitated Open Dialogue workshops nationally and internationally. Cathy is also an Association of Family Therapy accredited supervisor and an EMDR consultant. In the past, Cathy worked as a family therapist in an adolescent unit where many of the adolescents were admitted due to having an eating difficulty. She currently supervises family therapists in eating disorder settings who are working within the NHS and independently. Cathy is especially interested in the area of eating difficulties as she has an adult son who is living with an eating difficulty who has experienced community and inpatient services.

Iseult Twamley

Dr Iseult Twamley is a Clinical Psychologist. Since 2012 she has been Clinical Lead of the Cork Open Dialogue Implementation, Ireland, implementing Open Dialogue as part of the Adult Mental Health Service. She has trained and supervised Open Dialogue in the UK, Australia, Israel, Italy and the Netherlands. As a family member and trauma survivor herself, Iseult is passionate about collaborative and co-productive approaches to mental health. She credits her involvement with the Hearing Voices Network as challenging her previous 'education' and ethics and continues to seek opportunities to hear and learn from non-professional sources of wisdom.

Tracey Wade

Tracey Wade (BScHons, MClinPsych, PhD) is a Matthew Flinders Distinguished Professor of Psychology at Flinders University. She is currently an Associate Editor for the *International Journal of Eating Disorders*. In 2015 she was elected a Fellow of the Academy of the Social Sciences in Australia, and in 2019 she was the recipient of the Australia and New Zealand Academy of Eating Disorders Distinguished Achievement Award and appointed a Fellow of the Australian Psychological Society.

She is the director of the Flinders University Services for Eating Disorders and conducts research across a range of clinical settings as well as in schools, with over 200 peer-reviewed publications. She has co-authored three books describing evidence-based therapy approaches for perfectionism and eating disorders.

Sophia Webber

Sophia Webber, half Japanese and half English, was born in Japan, which is the country with which she connects to most. She is currently doing the Ib program at Le Regent College in Switzerland. Before this Sophia was living in Malaysia, and the cultural differences between Switzerland and Malaysia have at times caused a lot of struggle, mentally. However, Sophia is now able to say that she has pushed through those times and is able to see the beauty and wonders in Switzerland, and has developed a passion for running and football. Both Sophia's parents are very hard workers and have given her many beautiful opportunities. Although her eating disorder was a very low moment in her life, she is now able to appreciate many things more and has also been able to discover life's passions, for example learning new things and playing sports every day. Sophia aspires to go to a university in England and keep living her life to the full.

Christina Wilson

Christina Wilson is the mother of three children and a poet. She has over two decades of lived experience of eating difficulties, which she has used in her work to support others and raise awareness. She has over ten years' experience of working in the voluntary sector, working for mental health charities Leeds Mind, Project 6 and The Cellar Trust, where she was the perinatal lead and Crisis and Complex Support Lead. Christina worked on the co-production of the web-based training on eating disorders for health professionals and has spoken at conferences and training events around the UK, including the Institute of Health Visiting and Storytelling for Health. Christina is passionate about the therapeutic benefits of creative writing and facilitates therapeutic writing groups. She has a PGCert from Metanoia in Creative Writing for Therapeutic Purposes, an MA in Creative Writing, and is currently doing her doctoral research on creative writing and inclusivity.

Annie Zimmermann

Annie Zimmerman (PhD) is researcher and psychotherapist with a specialism in disordered eating and obesity. She completed her PhD on obesity and decision making in 2018 and has since worked as a post-doctoral researcher at King's College London. She also works clinically as a psychotherapist in her private practice in London. Annie writes both fiction books and non-fiction articles about our relationships with food, eating difficulties and mental health.

Introduction

We all require nutritional sustenance for our physical bodies to survive and thrive. Food, however, is not only a means for physical survival. Indeed, emotional and social survival are vital also. Thus, food is a conduit for connection, socialization, celebration and self/other nurturance. We all, therefore, have a relationship with the nutrition we take in and assimilate, and indeed with the body thereby sustained. For some people, for a complex variety of reasons, the relationship experienced with food and the body can become strained and complicated. This may lead to such actions as regularly taking in more food than the body requires; restricting one's intake of food; purging food away; eating only certain types of food; using insulin in self-injurious ways (i.e. where eating struggles and diabetes overlap) and many other kinds of experiences. These actions very often emerge alongside emotional distress, including in the form of nervous system dysregulation, and/or pervasive feelings of self-loathing and shame.

Approximately 1.25 million people in the UK and 9% of the population worldwide are experiencing an eating difficulty which meets the criteria for a diagnosable eating disorder. Of these, about one quarter identify as male (Beat, 2020; Arcelus et al, 2011). Many more experience eating difficulties which may not be diagnosed as an 'eating disorder', such as in the case of restrictive eating within sensory processing difficulties and autism spectrum conditions, as explored in Kelly & Raw's chapter on eating difficulties within autism (Chapter 20).

People of any age can be affected, with reports of people as young as six and as old as 70 experiencing eating difficulties (Beat, 2020). The majority of eating difficulties emerge in adolescence, with the prevalence of diagnosable eating disorders among adolescents (age 16-20) twice that of children (age 11-15) or young adults (age 21-24) (Wood et al, 2019). It is vital, therefore, not to rely on common misconceptions and stereotypes, including related to age and gender, when considering who needs help and support, otherwise many who are struggling with eating difficulties may be missed. Eating difficulties can affect almost anyone and, as chapters such as Easter et al's Chapter 24 on pregnancy attest to, can emerge and exist within a variety of life stages and transitions.

It is also necessary to acknowledge that eating difficulties can not only occur at any age, they can also occur at any weight (e.g. Whitelaw et al, 2018). As referred to in the chapter on the role of the GP by Atkins (Chapter 16) GPs can overemphasise the relevance of a person reaching a particularly low body mass index (BMI) before making a diagnosis, which has led to people being deemed 'not thin enough' and being told to wait until their weight reaches a dangerously low level before seeking a referral for specialist services.

Sadly, and importantly, deleterious physical ramifications of eating difficulties can and do occur at any weight. This book, alongside numerous other endeavours, advocates for early intervention and prevention and support for all people experiencing eating difficulties, including compassionate physical healthcare and monitoring. Supporting the physical health of those experiencing eating difficulties is explored in numerous chapters in this book, including in Atkin's chapter on support within primary care (Chapter 16) and Murdoch's chapter on dental care (Chapter 23). The chapter on the role of sleep by Green & Zimmerman is another important contribution in this regard (Chapter 13).

Too often, experiences of the care of eating difficulties can feel 'siloed' into fragmented parts – physical health here, mental health there, general practice here, specialist care over there. Sometimes a gulf exists between the person helping and the person being helped, as well as a hierarchy of knowledge whereby some voices and approaches to treatment are privileged over others. The hope for this book was to bring together an array of perspectives on how eating difficulties can be experienced, understood, lived with, and recovered from. We believe that embracing this multiplicity of voices and perspectives on eating difficulties has created a unique book that will bear much usefulness and relevance.

This book will appeal and have application for people with lived experience of eating difficulties and their loved ones and supporters; mental health professionals from a wide range of disciplines and perspectives; educational professionals working in schools, colleges, universities and alternative provisions; policy makers; and anyone with an interest in what it means to experience emotional pain within one's relationship with food and eating. There are chapters directly addressing the nuances of working with children and young people, including Chapman's chapter written for paediatricians (Chapter 19) and Elms & Higgins chapter on how schools can support young people (Chapter 43).

The use of the word 'difficulties' over 'disorders' for the title of the book was a conscious and deliberate decision. While mental health diagnoses in the current dominant socio-political and cultural paradigm often facilitate access to specialist support and can be validating in terms of offering a 'name' for one's distress, they can also be experienced as disempowering and damning, and espouse a medical-model view of eating difficulties, 'within person'. You will, however, find in some chapters of this book the use the term eating 'disorders', or diagnostic categories such as anorexia nervosa and bulimia nervosa, when reporting findings from research studies that have used these categories or where mental health diagnoses are being explicitly discussed and when it felt important for people with lived experience to express their experience as such. There are also occasions where more medicalized or technical language has been used to reflect the language used in certain policy initiatives and theoretical frameworks, such as in Laing & Jenkin's chapter on the law (Chapter 14) and Skarderud & Sommerfeldt's chapter on Mentalization-based treatments (MBT) (Chapter 32).

Another way of viewing emotional distress, and one which we have endeavoured to highlight throughout this volume, is that it takes place, and Arises from, a particular interpersonal and systemic context. This includes how power has operated in a person's life, what threat this power differential has posed to them, and the meaning they and others have made of this (Johnstone *et al*, 2018). From this perspective, eating difficulties can be conceived of as understandable and adaptive responses to life circumstances – not disorders but attempts at order. Not about being in control for control's sake, but about exercising control over aspects of one's life in order to gain or retain a sense of agency and safety. Not self-destructive acts, but sense-making acts that can give voice to a person's experiences in a way which is often impossible to ignore.

The concept for this book was to create a 'Practical Handbook' that would provide concise and accessible information in a format that is both easy to read and to assimilate. We have thus endeavoured to create a book which feels, and can be used as, truly practical in nature, providing opportunities for self-reflection and useful suggestions for readers from a range of backgrounds. The reader may choose to read the book in its entirety from cover-to-cover, or to 'dip' into sections or individual chapters – all of which can be read as stand-alone pieces. These pages should offer you a range of practical and readily applicable approaches and ideas, including Key Learning Points for each area. The Learning Points offered in each chapter provide an opportunity for the reader to pause and reflect on important aspects relevant to the topic covered. The reader may like to use these Learning Points as a springboard for reflection and further exploration. Some readers might find it helpful to read a particular chapter in its entirety in the first instance, and later return to check in on the Learning Points to refresh their memory, apply a particular idea or share a key aspect with others such as loved ones or colleagues in the context of supervision, training etc.

The book has been divided into five sections to support navigation. Part one is a good place to begin as it brings together a range of personal perspectives on, and experiences of, 'Understanding Eating Difficulties' in their various forms, including the perspectives of parents and siblings. Part two then delves into the nuances of 'Providing Healthcare', including both inpatient and outpatient care and how to seek support through the NHS in the UK; leading onto Part Three, which explores ways of 'Supporting People': a particularly useful section for loved ones and those working therapeutically with this population. Lazzari & Lagou's chapter on peer support within this section (Chapter 47) may be particularly helpful for friends, school contemporaries and colleagues. We hope therapists from a range of disciplines will find Part Four supportive to their professional practice as it is here that various 'Therapies for Eating Difficulties' are delved into, including dramatherapy, equine therapy, compassion-focused therapy, dialectical behavioural therapy (DBT), narrative therapy and a range of other evidence-based therapeutic approaches. These are explored through the lens of research and both professional and expert-by-lived-experience perspectives. Finally, Part Five offers a range of 'Creative Approaches', with chapters written both by experts-by-lived-experience and therapists, through such varied avenues as art, music, creative writing, dance and yoga.

This book should support people from different personal and professional backgrounds to understand each other's roles and perspectives, and thereby work better and more effectively together. If you come from a particular professional background, you might want to start with a chapter written by someone in a similar role as you. Or you may want to consider other professionals you work with and read about their perspectives of working to support those with eating difficulties. Perhaps you are curious about an aspect of eating difficulties you are unfamiliar with, or a therapeutic approach you haven't heard much about. And of course, eating difficulties are experiences people live with, and so reading any of the varied sections and chapters about living with and recovering from eating difficulties will be, we believe, invaluable.

The reader may find that some of the content within these pages touches a nerve, or offers a perspective which is jarring or painfully illuminating. It may be helpful to turn to Goss & Haynes's chapter on compassion-focused therapy (Chapter 28) and Estey, Pollack & Cook-Cottone's chapter on incorporating mindful self-care (Chapter 34) in this case; to seek connection with a supportive other; and/or to pause and engage in even a small act of self-validation and self-care. There are numerous charitable organizations which can offer support, which are listed at the end of a number of chapters.

Any book is necessarily limited by such aspects as word counts, availability of chapter authors, time constraints and much else besides. While we have done our utmost to include a diversity of voices within this volume, we regret that many perspectives and topics are missing. You will find an array of voices within these pages, all of whom have some connection to the experience of eating difficulties in their various forms. It was clear to us from the outset of this project that the voices of those with lived experience of eating difficulties and their loved ones – the 'experts by lived experience' – would take centre-stage with an endeavour to include voices from a diversity of genders, cultures and demographics. To have given voice to all those who would have offered tremendous value and insight within this book, however, would have required hundreds of chapters! Thus, there are necessarily 'missing' voices and perspectives. If you do not find your experience or perspective represented within these pages, please both accept our apologies and know that we had hoped with this book to recognize all perspectives and experiences as equally valid, important and necessary to be shared and heard. Perhaps you will consider creating a Volume Two with us!

Ideally, this book would have been equally weighted with all possible iterations of eating difficulties, of which there are many, yet the reality is that we have ended up with more chapters on restrictive eating than other expressions. We also recognize that many co-occurring experiences have been missed, for example dedicated chapters related to substance use, hyper- and hypo- nervous system arousal, familial breakdown etc. We would also like to have included more experiences and perspectives of those who identify as being from a Black, Asian, or ethnic minority background: importantly and concerningly, NHS digital data indicates that hospital admissions for eating difficulties are increasing most rapidly among these groups (NHS Digital Data, 5th October 2020).

Naturally, this book has been written at a particular time, within a particular socio-political context, by authors and editors whose perspectives can only come through the lens of their (limited) understanding and experience. We recognize, as editors, that we have our personal and collective 'blindspots' which will undoubtedly have impacted on this volume in ways beneath the level of our conscious awareness. Thus, what we offer is certainly not a practical volume on eating difficulties which is complete in any way but which, nevertheless, we hope offers much useful information on an area which continues to be under-researched and regularly misunderstood.

We owe a tremendous debt of gratitude to the many contributing authors, to Pavilion Publishing who have appreciated and supported this book's value from its conception, and to the UK's leading eating difficulties charity, BEAT, who have written a compelling foreword. Our thanks also extend to you, the reader, for taking the time to explore this important subject of eating difficulties further through these pages. It is our sincere hope that anyone reading this book will recognize and appreciate the multiplicity of experiences that eating difficulties represent. We also wish for this book to contribute to endeavours to dismantle stereotypical views of eating difficulties with the voices of lived experience, and to both recognize and value the many and varied ways in which recovery can be supported for each individual.

This book is an attempt and an invitation to recognize all experiences of eating difficulties as equally valid and worthy of care and support. Its most important, and perhaps ambitious, aim is to offer those with personal experiences of eating difficulties – who may be struggling themselves or supporting someone else – some comfort, affirmation, empowerment, sense of agency and hope.

References

Arcelus J, Mitchell AJ, Wales J & Nielsen S (2011) Mortality rates in patients with anorexia nervosa and other eating disorders: a meta-analysis of 36 studies. *Archives of general psychiatry* **68** (7) 724-731.

BEAT (2020) *How many people have an eating disorder in the UK?* [online]. Available at: https://www.beateatingdisorders.org.uk/media-centre/eating-disorder-statistics/ (accessed August 2021).

Johnstone L, Boyle M, Cromby J, Dillon J, Harper D, Kinderman P & Read J (2018) *The Power Threat Meaning Framework: Towards the identification of patterns in emotional distress, unusual experiences and troubled or troubling behaviour, as an alternative to functional psychiatric diagnosis*. Leicester: British Psychological Society.

NHS Digital Data (2020) *Hospital admissions for eating disorders by gender and ethnicity* [online]. Available at https://digital.nhs.uk/data-and-information/supplementary-information/2020/hospital-admissions-for-eating-disorders-by-gender-and-ethnicity (accessed August 2021).

Public Administration and Constitutional Affairs Committee (PACAC) (2019) *Ignoring the Alarms follow-up: Too many avoidable deaths from eating disorders* [online]. Available at: https://publications.parliament.uk/pa/cm201719/cmselect/cmpubadm/855/85502.htm (accessed August 2021).

Whitelaw M, Lee KJ, Gilbertson H & Sawyer SM (2018) Predictors of complications in anorexia nervosa and atypical anorexia nervosa: degree of underweight or extent and recency of weight loss? *Journal of Adolescent Health* **63** (6) 717-723.

Wood S, Marchant A, Allsopp M, Wilkinson K, Bethel J, Jones H & John A (2019) Epidemiology of eating disorders in primary care in children and young people: a clinical practice research Datalink study in England. *BMJ open* **9** (8) e026691.

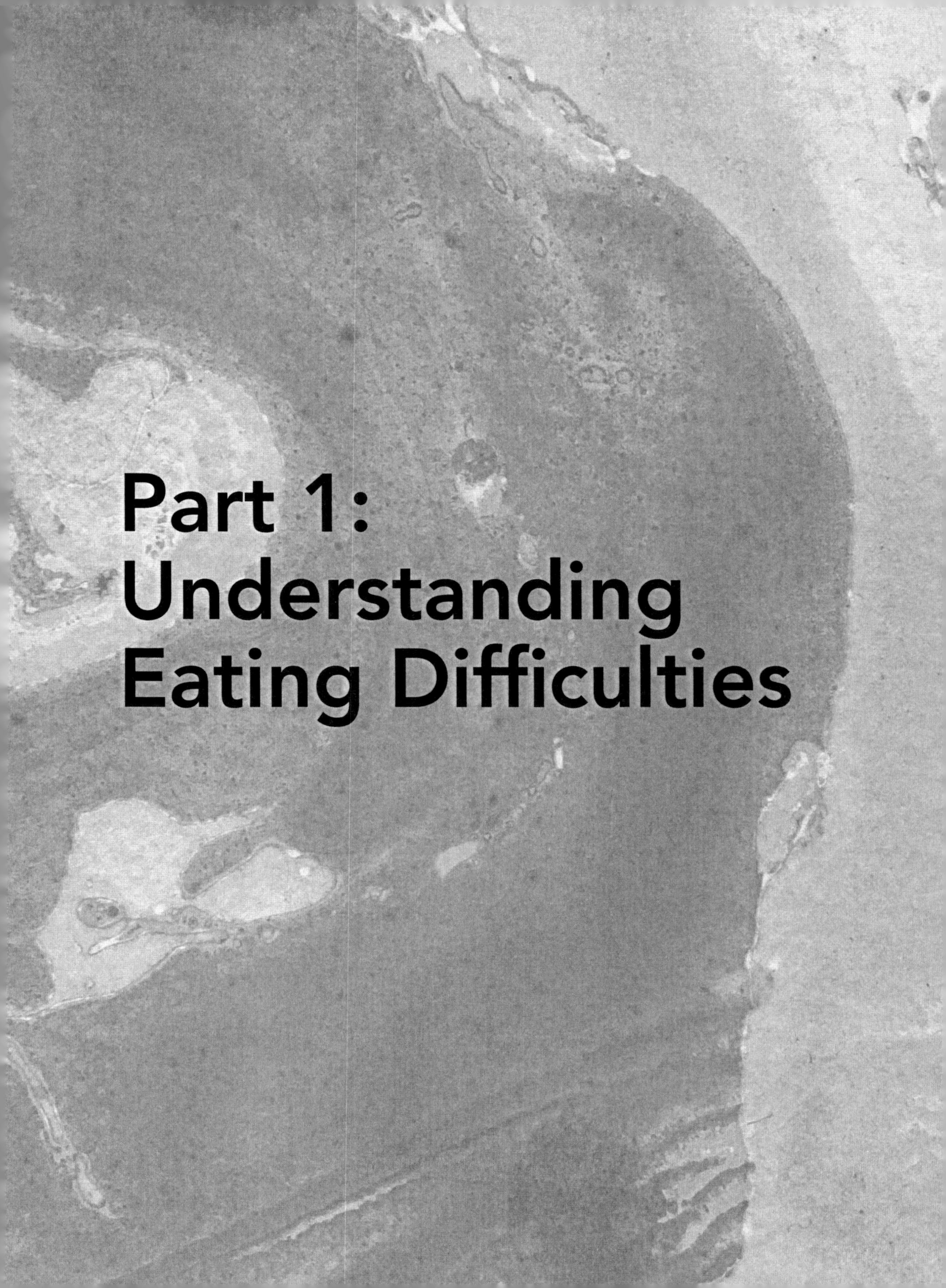

Part 1: Understanding Eating Difficulties

1. The recovery rollercoaster: a young person's story

By Sophia Webber

Suffering from an eating disorder can be life threatening. Food, exercise and looking a certain way was what I would think about for most of the day. But things get to a point at which you cannot continue any longer. There was no option but to recover. At the start it is the most frightening thing, but soon after, all these fears become a success. Recovery is not going to come easy, but it is also not that hard. Once you start, you won't look back; you can't look back. You are going to feel the positive effects and question how you ever lived with an eating disorder. In this chapter, I discuss how I overcame the most dreadful mindset, and became a happy, strong girl without anorexia.

Recovery was a bit like teaching yourself how to ride a bike. At first it takes many attempts to try and push yourself to recover. But once you have found a way to get better, you swiftly keep going.

Some people may think that as soon as you leave the hospital or treatment clinic you have recovered, but in fact the opposite is actually true. The most important thing for recovery is 'mindset'. Without the mindset, and acknowledging the fact that you have an eating disorder, recovery is impossible. I experienced spending time in hospital on two occasions; it was definitely not pleasant! I cried non-stop, begging to go home. You would have thought that after the first time in hospital, I would try to recover and stop myself from going into hospital again, but no, I lost that battle to recover. My eating disorder took over.

The 7th September 2019, at 3:05 pm, was the moment that I stepped foot on the pavement outside of the hospital – that's when I knew. I knew that I would not be coming back here; I needed to get better. Football was my motivation. I always aspired to be an amazing footballer. But remaining a sick, frail girl with no muscle whatsoever meant that there was no way that I could be good at football. So during my stay in hospital I would watch endless football videos, which taught me that being strong is so much more important than dieting. Instead of scrolling through Instagram and seeing a lot of diet culture pages, I started following people who were very body positive.

Katie Noel and her podcast 'Take the cake' taught me that recovery was possible[1]. It also helped me to read books like Helena Grace Donald's *Learning to Love the Girl in the Mirror* (2017), as it made me understand that resting is okay. I had a burning desire for doing well in my future. Maybe that was part of my eating disorder screaming that I had to do well, but it certainly started the journey of my recovery. Although I never went back to the hospital and I did manage to gain weight, my journey with an eating disorder continued. I knew that recovery was not going to be linear, but I didn't think that it would be this hard either. I constantly kept putting myself down, and calling myself horrible words such as a 'failure', and telling myself I had 'no use in the world'.

Soon enough I was diagnosed with depression. After you start to put on weight and finally seem to be doing well, it is quite common for an eating disorder to turn into depression. Although I was not certain why I got depression, part of me believes that it's because of the loss of control that I felt, since I could not control my weight. It felt as though I was left with nothing. This period of recovery was possibly the worst that I had ever felt in my life. I had no friends, and nothing I did seemed to be any fun. I felt constantly isolated, and if I didn't follow my schedule for every second of the day, I would restrict what I ate.

I remember that on my birthday I went to my room to study or exercise, giving myself just a 30-minute break to shower, eat dinner and open my presents. Instead of making positive memories, I was making a death trap for myself. There does come a point though when you can't keep living like this. I had two options, either remain as I was and eventually get to a point where I couldn't live, or open up and get help. Luckily, I chose the second option.

Although a person may look much healthier than before, inside they may be suffering to a great extent. The number of comments that I heard, telling me how much healthier I looked, and how I seemed to be so much better, were quite triggering. No-one ever seemed to understand that inside I felt worse than I did before. It also made me feel like I should stop trying, as I was already in a healthy state. The number of comparisons that I was making with others were also getting out of hand. Before it was just other people's looks that I would compare myself to, but then it all took a turn and I was comparing grades, athletic abilities, and even my hair. Whenever a girl walked past me in the street, in my head I would be thinking, 'Oh, I wish I had her legs', or, 'Oh, I wish my face looked like that'. In fact, that's all I could think about.

1 Katie Noel's 'Take the cake'. https://soundcloud.com/user-801674213 (accessed November 2021).

After hours of treatment and opening up about how I felt, and watching endless YouTube videos on self-love, I actually started to do things that I enjoyed, instead of forcing myself to do these things. I finally started to feel a sense of joy. During your eating disorder, you don't understand what being happy truly is. You get fully consumed by the eating disorder, to the point that the only thing that you can focus on is losing weight. So it was a bit of a shock when I first laughed and had proper 'fun'. I remember this day so vividly: it was during December, and three of my friends invited me to go on the Ferris wheel with them, and that night I did not stop laughing.

Learning point 1

- Have you ever gone through something that took several tries to finally get the correct outcome?
- Have you been told that you look very happy or healthy, and inside you were clearly struggling?
- Is making comparisons a common occurrence in your life?
- Were you able to push through and not return to any of your old habits?

Some of my major struggles

During my journey to recovery, some of the discomforts that I felt were unbelievably horrible. My guilty feelings mixed with hatred towards myself, left me in tears for hours on end. If I had one big meal, I had a huge urge to throw up the food that I had eaten. But of course I managed to focus on something else which helped stop me. One huge tip that I recommend for anyone having the urge to throw up after a meal is to take a walk outside and listen to some music. This made me feel like I ruled the world. My favourite song is 'Confident' by Demi Lovato. Another tip would be to focus on the negative side-effects of purging. By doing this, I managed to stay purge free, and I don't plan on ever purging again. Opening up about having depression was very difficult, as there is some sort of stigma around mental health; I felt ashamed and a bit embarrassed. I thought people would judge me, and call me all sorts of names, although your friends may not understand anything about depression or eating disorders, or even any kind of mental health. The most important thing is to tell them what's going on, so that they can make you feel a whole lot better. During my depression I distanced myself from all of my friends, without giving them an explanation. I should have told them that I was struggling and that I needed some space, as not only would my friends have felt better about themselves, but they also could have offered me more support. Reaching out for help is the most vital step to achieve recovery from any mental health issue. I remember when I finally had the right mindset to recover from my mental health issues, but I was so reluctant to reach out for help that I let my mental health issues get even worse as a result of trying to handle it all myself. I would experience a lot of stress and anxiety, as I constantly felt that I was a failure, and that there was no point even trying to recover because nothing I could do would be correct. It may be very scary trying to reach out, but just know that nobody will judge you, especially if they are your loved ones. They will be as supportive as possible.

Trying to recover with social media, friends and even family bringing up the most dreadful topic, was very hard. Negative body image and diet talk. These have got to be some of the most triggering topics, along with seeing your friends dieting. Healthy eating is excellent, but moderation and balance are certainly key to staying well. The problem with society now is that people believe that in order to lose weight you have to eat as little as possible. A lot of other teenagers believed this in my school. During lunchtimes, I remember just looking around and seeing quite a few people with just a bowl of salad, or two apples, and when I was trying to recover this put me off eating. The worst possible comment I got was when I got quite a few pieces of bread, with a big bowl of tuna, and someone said to me, 'You're gonna eat all that?' This instantly made me feel bad about my body. People will probably make these comments, and we can't stop them, but we can control how it's going to affect us. All people have different calorific needs, and now when someone comments on my food, I repeat to myself that I am on a different journey to everyone else, and so yes, I am going to eat all of this.

Learning point 2

- When was the last time you reached out for help?
- Who do you think of when you want to go talk to someone?
- What makes you feel better?
- Have you ever been asked, 'Are you going to eat all that?', or said to someone, 'That's all you're going to eat?' How do you think that this makes someone else feel?

The fear of recovery

Before I had the mindset to recover, I never truly thought that recovery would in fact lead me to a much happier life. I had wanted to recover for a while, but several questions kept leading me to put a pause on my recovery. Before I ate I would always think to myself 'no one will like me if I recover', but no one liked me when I was sick. I was alone and I got absolutely no romantic attention. I was boring, and people were scared to hang around me because I was always so stressed and I always looked so upset. Another major question I would ask myself was 'Am I going to grow big?' Rebecca Leung's TED talk discusses exactly why we should challenge these questions. Rebecca argues that 'rejection is temporary, but regrettably lasts with us forever'[2]. This TED talk resembled exactly how I felt. When I was trapped in anorexia, it was my comfort zone, and I knew exactly what to expect. Pushing ourselves out of our comfort zone is a phrase that I hear so often. I have mixed feelings about this. During my eating disorder, and when teachers would give us talks as to how we should 'challenge ourselves' and 'push ourselves', I remember always taking this the wrong way. So every time I heard one of these talks, I would harm myself even more. I would think to myself, 'Oh gosh, I needed to challenge myself more in my running. Maybe I need to run for an extra hour', or 'I need to wake up earlier, if everyone else is challenging themselves. Maybe I need to wake up at 4am instead'. These extremes were a way of coping for me. I always had to be the best, or the one that pushed herself the most. Pushing yourself or going out of your comfort zone is great for someone that maybe wants to try riding a bicycle but has always been too scared. Or in my case, by choosing my 'recovery'. I also have to be careful when using this phrase, because people with eating disorders always have to be perfect or the best, and this can push us to extremes.

I am now at a stage of life where I can balance going out and having fun, with exercise and study. I still strive to be the best version of myself that I can be, but I'm much more caring towards myself. August and September 2020 were some of the best months of my life. Every weekend I would go out with my friends, and realise how much I had really missed out. I thought of all the times that I had been invited out for dinner but rejected my friends because I was scared of the unknown calories and messing up my schedule. This made me appreciate going out with my friends even more.

I know that saying this may sound a bit weird, but I want to say 'thank you' to my eating disorder. It helped me to become very self-driven, and have a huge amount of self-discipline. These are two aspects which have been very useful for my studies and my athletic abilities. I don't think that I am fully recovered yet, but again, I don't really know what a full recovery truly is. I am able to eat pretty much all foods, although sometimes a ray of guilt will sweep over me, and the urge to exercise daily is still there, but I am certainly not trying to lose weight, and I am happy with my body. I get excited to go out on the beach with my friends now, whereas before I hated the idea of me in a swimsuit. Being happy with my body only started to happen when I was at a healthy weight. Now when I look in the mirror and see my body, I feel very confident.

2 Please see Rebecca Leung's TED Talk '"What if" I actually recovered'. www.ted.com/talks/rebecca_leung_what_if_i_actually_recovered (accessed November 2021)

Learning point 3

- Have you thought that something awful would happen if you did a certain thing?
- Is there a time when you took 'pushing yourself' to an extreme?
- Has a very negative thing that happened in your life taught you something?
- Do you believe that you can fully recover?

Recovery was the first step to actually living. During anorexia I was basically a prisoner. I did everything anorexia told me to do, and I became so self-absorbed that I only cared about my success. I am not going to say that recovery is easy, because it's not. It took me several tries to actually go in the right direction, but it's definitely all worth it. I hated the fact that I had to miss lessons to go to therapy, or the constant bloating that I felt after each meal, but all these struggles meant that I was one step closer to being fully comfortable with myself. Being comfortable with myself was not just having a good body image; it was also allowing myself to have days when I didn't wear makeup. Now I am proud to say that I don't wear any makeup to school. I have learnt that we all have imperfections. When I have had these little successes, I make sure that I reward myself. Recovering from anorexia is very different from person to person. Every journey is unique, but trust me, you do get to the point where you actually enjoy something for the first time; anorexia will then just be a phase of your life.

2. The journey through anorexia: a father's perspective

By Rory Webber (father to Sophia, who authored the previous chapter)

I will remember a particular day clearly for the rest of my life. I was having a lovely time skiing in the mountains when I received a call from my wife that Sophia, our daughter, had collapsed. An ambulance was on its way. When I saw her lying on the bed unconscious, I started to cry. I felt hopeless. Seeing Sophia lying there was heart-breaking. I remember following the ambulance down to the hospital thinking, 'Why?'. How could my daughter, who was so good at everything, be in such a poor state of health? She was a very keen runner, an avid footballer and always trained hard. I remember feeling incredulous as to how she had ended up in in this state.

Looking back, I wonder if I should have seen the warning signs a lot earlier. But being busy and knowing nothing of eating disorders, I perhaps buried my head in the sand and convinced myself that nothing was wrong. Back in November, Sophia had started to become very selective about her eating and talked about becoming a vegetarian or vegan. I listened but did not pay too much attention to it. She was running every morning for about an hour, was doing weights for about an hour and played football in the evenings for the local club. She was waking up earlier and earlier in the morning to fit all this in. I remember her booking an online Japanese lesson for 3am in the morning because there was no other time to take it.

Sophia became more intense and would become agitated if I offered her advice around doing less training and perhaps enjoying the odd lie in. On Christmas day 2018 we had a lovely, large meal and I remember Sophia saying beforehand that this would be her last big meal because she needed to train hard and lose weight. Again, I largely ignored these obvious signs, believing everything was fine. We returned from our Christmas holiday and Sophia seemed more reserved and stopped mixing with her friends. Instead, she concentrated on her studies, her fitness and her football. She did not want to go out in the evenings with her friends any longer. I remember that she even took up an evening French class (quite possibly to give her an excuse to avoid going out with friends). Looking back, these were all signals that something was not quite right.

Learning point 1

It is vital to follow your instincts as a parent. If you are worried that your child's eating habits, fitness regime and socialisation patterns have suddenly changed, it is important to take early action and to seek a professional opinion/support.

Going downhill rapidly

Sophia started to eat less and less. I noticed her weight loss but, again, thought she was in control. I now realise she had far too much control over her eating habits and was highly obsessive. One weekend in late January, Sophia went to the local town with a couple of friends. As her parents, we were happy about this because Sophia had been withdrawing from everyone. The next day, her good friend's mother spoke to my wife and myself and said Anna (the friend) was very worried because Sophia had not eaten anything for the entire day. We thanked the mother for passing this information on and spoke with Sophia. She made a plausible excuse and, again, we did not follow this up. I began to become concerned, however, as I noticed how thin Sophia looked and that she seemed to lack energy. Regardless, she continued to push herself with her running, studies and football. A small part of me perhaps admired her dedication and her strong will. I was worried but did not have any idea that Sophia was sinking into anorexia, and very rapidly. I remember speaking to my wife about how little Sophia was eating. My wife said everything would be fine and she would cook Sophia her favourite foods. I agreed and thought this was a good plan of action. Over the next few days, Sophia began to truly starve herself and I noticed she would have just a small segment of apple for breakfast. We did not monitor what she was eating at lunch because she was at school, but looking back on it, I am sure she was regularly skipping lunch or perhaps going to the bathroom to dispose of the food.

I remember speaking to Sophia at length on the 1st February as she was preparing to go to her French lesson. She looked terrible. Her school uniform now seemed too big for her and she could barely stand up. I spoke with her and said we were very worried about her condition. I asked her if she had been vomiting after meals and she admitted to doing this a few times. I asked her why she had lost so much weight and why her energy levels were now so low. I remember her answer clearly when I asked her how she felt. She answered, 'I feel empty'. I asked if she felt empty in her stomach and she replied, 'Yes, and I also feel empty in the mind'. I suggested she stay at home and rest, but she insisted on going to her French lesson. I tried to insist that she stayed at home, but her will was so strong that she won again. I remember speaking with my wife that evening and sharing my fear that things were going very wrong.

Admission to hospital

The day I was skiing and Sophia collapsed was the day that changed many things and taught us a huge amount as parents. Sophia was admitted to hospital, unconscious. It was distressing to see her lying there with her pupils rolled to the back of her eyes. We spoke to the doctors who were excellent and tried to keep us calm. They took blood tests and various other things. My wife and I were sitting with Sophia, who was on a drip. Sophia woke up after an hour or two and immediately started asking when we could go home. Again, looking back on it, I was incredibly naïve. I said we might be there at the hospital for a few hours and that she would have to be patient. Sophia became anxious, saying she needed to be back at school. We tried to calm her down and insisted that she would be home soon enough. We sat with her and tried to make her realise she was doing herself some serious damage.

At this stage, I still had no idea Sophia was experiencing anorexia. I genuinely thought she had exhausted herself through exercise and a lack of eating and that all we needed to do was to fill her up with food and everything would be fine. I suppose this was true in some way, yet I had no idea how difficult this would prove to be.

The doctor returned and asked to speak with my wife and me. He said in no uncertain terms that Sophia had caused herself a lot of damage. He said that her potassium levels were dangerously low, and that this particular hospital was quite possibly not able to support her. They told us that she may have to be moved to a hospital in Geneva and put into an induced coma. This was both startling and unnerving. How could this be? The doctor said they would conduct further tests to determine what action would need to be taken. We thanked him in a total state of shock. It was simply too much for us to process.

An hour or two later, we had the very welcome news that Sophia would not need to be transferred to Geneva and was in a stable condition. We asked how long she would have to stay in hospital and were told it was not clear, but that she would not be home soon. After a day or two of visits, I asked when Sophia could leave the hospital and the answer was a surprise. The doctors said she would be in hospital for as long as it took and that this was quite often about six weeks. This is also when they slipped in the word 'anorexia'. I was taken aback and remember wondering if all this fuss was necessary. I still believed Sophia would come home, realise she had made a mistake with her eating habits, and all would be fine in our family again.

Learning point 2

A period of denial is quite common for parents when they first hear their child is struggling with an eating difficulty like anorexia. It can take time to full comprehend, and to get over the shock of the seriousness of the situation.

Learning about anorexia as parents, and ongoing treatment

When we were in the hospital and Sophia was lying unconscious, I was still not aware she was suffering from anorexia. It might be blatantly clear for many people and for the medical staff, but I did not realise this at first. I did not really know what anorexia was. At this point, I wish I had been made to realise the seriousness of the situation. I wish a doctor had explained clearly that Sophia was suffering with anorexia, what anorexia was, that the hospital was the best option and that a long stay would be beneficial. It would also have been useful to have been told not to listen to Sophia's requests to come home.

Over the next week or two we came to terms with Sophia's illness and did a lot of reading about anorexia. The doctors made it clear that anorexia was a very serious illness, and one which could take Sophia a very long time to get over.

Sophia was allowed out of the hospital after about two weeks as she had put on enough weight. I soon noticed a pattern – that Sophia was able to lose weight at an alarming rate and also able to put weight on for a reason, such as to get herself out of hospital. Sophia had no intention of maintaining the weight when out of hospital. In hospital, she was told not to exercise (not even walking up or down the stairs) and to refrain from exercise for three months once out of the hospital. Even in the hospital, she would ask my wife or I to take her out for a short walk. She would then insist on running. When we said she should not do this, she would say things to us like, 'You hate me, you don't want me to be happy, I will kill myself if I can't run' etc.

The hospital made some clear guidelines and told Sophia in no uncertain terms that she would be re-admitted to the hospital if she did not follow them. She was told to maintain a weight of 45kg. Sophia, however, was very good at finding ways around these rules. Her doctor, I have to say, was not very good at first. He would ask Sophia to weigh herself and tell him how much she weighed. This was of course easy for Sophia – she simply lied about her weight. At no point did the doctor make it clear to Sophia that her illness was serious and that if her weight or heartrate fell below expectations, she would be re-admitted to the hospital. He did tell her, however, that her iron levels and blood sugar levels were very low, but did not act on these findings. He also failed to answer emails from the psychologist. Later, Sophia told me that she found it easy to get around the doctor. She was told not to exercise by the hospital, but the doctor said she was fine to exercise and to play football, so Sophia was able to use this as ammunition when we told her not to exercise. Sophia was also seeing a psychologist who was excellent at giving good advice. I remember sharing with the psychologist that I thought things were getting better, but she responded that this was far from over and that Sophia had a high chance of relapsing.

Learning point 3

Joined-up care is paramount; GPs should communicate regularly with other involved professionals such as psychologists to ensure the child or young person is closely monitored and supported in the best way possible.

Eventually we changed doctors. The second doctor saw Sophia for the first time and said plainly that she needed to be re-admitted to the hospital. Her heartrate was dangerously low and her weight was now a full 5kg below the agreed weight (45kg) and a full 15 kg below the average weight for a 15-year-old girl of the same height. She was also still exercising far too much.

I look back on this time and recognize that changing Sophia's doctor was one of the best decisions we made. I can honestly say that having the correct doctor and psychologist is one of the most important aspects of recovery. While Sophia was in hospital the second time, we believed the recovery might truly begin. The second stay in hospital was very difficult. Sophia kept telling me that she would kill herself. She told me in an email or to my face about 20 times per day that she hated me and did not need me. It was all very heart-breaking.

The gradual road to recovery

Sophia came out of the hospital after a few weeks and had to visit the doctor on a weekly basis to be weighed. She hated the doctor but, I have to say, having a doctor who was consistent with his expectations and rules was of huge importance. The doctor raised the target weight every few weeks and Sophia would follow his instructions, fearing as she did being re-admitted to hospital.

Sophia is still a very precise eater who will not eat most things. My wife has been amazing at cooking everything she desires and, after 18 months, I feel we have made significant progress. We are not out of the woods yet and still need to be vigilant. Yet, with the help of the psychologist, the doctor and lots of love from her parents, there is light at the end of the tunnel.

Family dinners are still a rarity, but this is possibly due to our jobs as much as Sophia's difficulties. Sophia continues to be very precise and generally has to eat at 6.30pm on the dot each evening. My wife prepares her food and does so with love and understanding. Sophia continues to have check-ups at the doctors regularly.

I feel we are lucky in that Sophia now eats well at mealtimes. She generally chooses what she wants to eat, which tends to include a lot of salmon, chicken and vegetables. She eats three good meals a day now and I think having choice has helped her. We certainly do not count calories, but I imagine Sophia has some idea of the calories in her food. Sophia now seems to enjoy what she is eating and we often notice her taking a little extra food which is very pleasing.

Final reflections

I still do not know why Sophia developed anorexia. There is no family history of mental illness. My wife and I both enjoy eating and have never encouraged dieting or any such thing. My daughter is very sporty, and I took it for granted that she would realise she needed to eat a lot. We feel blessed that Sophia received such excellent treatment here in Switzerland. The clinicians were strict, patient, and had an excellent support structure in place. They would not let Sophia leave the hospital until she had a doctor and a psychologist in place. They also suggested a nutritionist. I remember thinking what a nuisance it was having to sort everything out but, in retrospect, it was vital. In many ways, I look back and feel that a good six months of recovery time was wasted because the first doctor did not pay enough attention to putting strict rules into place for Sophia. Having the correct support has helped immeasurably.

I know we are not yet in the clear, and I think I will always have a slight worry that Sophia might stop eating again. I pray that she will continue on the path to wellness and am immensely proud of her dedication to getting better.

3. Anorexia: a sibling's story

By Jasmine Daisy

Our story

Liam was diagnosed with anorexia nervosa in early 2017, and soon after he was admitted to the general hospital with bradycardia. I had an instinct that on this morning he was not going to come home from his appointment, so I got into bed with him for what seemed like a goodbye. It felt as if my family was slipping away, my heart sank in the knowledge that he may not be home that evening. I then went to school and when I came home he wasn't there – instead, he spent most of that year in an inpatient's hospital. At the general hospital he still refused to eat, so he was put on a naso-gastric feeding tube. I guess this was easier, as he did not have to make the effort to eat anything. At this stage he was unrecognisable, I'm not sure if he even recognized himself. The lack of food caused him to faint in the shower at hospital. This removed any independence that he had from then on, as he needed permanent supervision from our mum and the nurses at the hospital during his stay.

Liam had started displaying noticeable changes in behaviour months before this, such as offering to cook – little did we know this was to monitor the ingredients – and to exercise more than ever. However, at the time (for a reason that I cannot understand now), this didn't seem an obvious sign of anorexia. He was extremely sporty, so his decision to eat a healthier diet and increase the amount of exercise that he was doing seemed almost natural.

In hindsight, I think that I noticed quite early on that Liam was different and was potentially developing an unhealthy obsession with healthy eating. Without telling anyone, I was researching these changes in behaviour, but it is difficult to act on a hunch like this as in my mind anorexia seemed so terrifying that I didn't want to believe that my brother could really be showing signs of that.

Inpatients' unit

After two weeks in the general hospital, Liam was transferred to an inpatient's unit further away from home. Yet, while everything in our family was changing, nothing else stopped to allow me to absorb what was happening. During Liam's stay in the inpatient's unit I did not attend many of the appointments, although my mum did go at every possible opportunity. She would go alone to these appointments as I was studying for my GCSEs, and my dad would get easily frustrated. He was supposed to come home in the summer of 2017. So as to make this transition easier for Liam (and for me) I went away to Cornwall for six weeks. However, he stayed in the hospital. I'm not sure how much of a decision that was for him, or if it was fuelled by his fear of being discharged and going back to where it had all begun. In the end, he stayed in the hospital for much longer than the average patient, and during his stay he began to push us away by not coming to the phone or reaching out to speak to us. Eventually, we reached the point where we would go down to visit Liam and he would not come into the visitor's room. We would go to family-therapy sessions and he would refuse to attend them. When he did attend the sessions or agree to see us, he was usually angry, and he would blame us for his hospitalization and the anorexia diagnosis. This blame has continued until today, and it has caused a huge rift in our family, especially between him and my mum.

The aftermath

In an attempt to prepare for Liam's return home, my mum and I watched videos about how to act at mealtimes in order to be as helpful as possible. There were references to what type of animal you should act like: for example, you should nudge like a dolphin, rather than bury your head in the sand like an ostrich. However, we found that for us the best method was to distract him from eating by playing games at mealtimes. Despite this, life following his return from the inpatient's unit seemed to get consistently harder. Somehow, despite him being closer, I felt more helpless, as if he was more of a risk to himself at home. I think that one of the hardest parts for me once Liam was home was fitting into my role as the sibling, rather than being a parent. During the time that he was in hospital I had become almost a team with my mum, after seeing how upset she was, and abandoning this role was difficult for me. I became a kind of in-between person, where I often had to choose whether to collude with my brother or try to parent him. On many occasions the way I handled things was not successful, such as the first snack that I 'supervised' him eating, when we were alone together. I insisted that he finished his snack, as I thought that this was right, but in response he proceeded to go to the toilet and vomited it back up. I think that after this my brother and I both appreciated that I had no authority over his eating, so my position became someone that he could confide in. Liam would often ask me to lie to my mum about whether he had eaten or not, and I often had to choose between doing the right thing (telling her) or maintaining my position of confidence with him, so as to keep a line of communication open.

Liam had developed a fierce hatred for our house, family and life at home. When he lost his temper, it was as if a monster had possessed him. His eyes would glaze over, his voice would become a hiss, and immediately you would feel only fear. At times like this it was like talking directly to the anorexia, rather than to him. Following this, he would forget or misremember these events, which led him to think that we were lying. He would also continuously bang his head against the wall, throw his things around his room, and occasionally burst into tears. Moments like this imprinted on my mind, and ever since it is as if I have actually been experiencing grief. It is a strange form of grief, because physically my brother is still here, but mentally and spiritually he has been replaced by someone else that I have had to familiArise myself with. You cannot say to people that your sibling has died, but sometimes you feel as if those are the necessary words. It is like his soul is gone.

Impact on family relationships

Before Liam's anorexia nervosa I would have described my family as being close. However, the battle my brother has been fighting in his mind became a battle against our family, and it continues to be just this. It goes in phases. There are days when Liam will talk and confide in me, and days where he will ignore me completely. It is actually easier when he ignores me. My mum has the hardest task of enforcing the rules to try to prevent him from getting more ill, so that he can focus on his recovery. But Liam blames my mum, as he thinks that it is her fault that we got here in the first place. There have been times when Liam has been out of control. He has tried to leave the house late at night, screaming and breaking everything. On one particular occasion we had to call the police. I think that it was at this moment that our family truly divided; even the memory of this event is different for us and him.

Even now, our family life centres around the mood that Liam is in that day. He often decides the role that my father can have, which is to be either a saint, or completely irrelevant.

More recently, my mum decided to attempt an 'it takes a village' approach, as keeping his anorexia within our family seemed to be moving us backwards. This involved having his friends or any family friends help by having dinner for him or just simply starting conversations so that he knows that he is loved. Mostly this has been successful, as friends or more distant family seem to be able to have normal conversations with Liam. This is great, and I am thankful that he is still well enough to hold normal conversations with some people. However, it can be frustrating knowing that this is possible and yet he doesn't make the same effort with my family and me.

I think that my relationship with Liam suffered most when I was studying for my A-levels, and he would hide my flashcards and revision resources anywhere so that I could not work. I would take all of my things to my mum's friend's house and revise there for most of the day. I found this difficult as I was trying to do as much as I could to help him to recover and succeed, but he just did not want the same for me. I tried not to let this affect our relationship and the role that I had, but I often got frustrated and accused him of taking things, which resulted in me distancing myself from him.

Generally, the scary thing that I have come to realise is how much potential there is for the fight with anorexia to continue to affect our family life. Since 2010, we have been living with a stepfamily, but there have been multiple times when my mum has suggested moving out in an attempt to improve my brother's condition. I do wonder whether at some level this would cause more upset and sadness than there is already. I don't know if these thoughts are acceptable, but I wonder whether this kind of act may feed the anorexia, resulting in him never wanting to move back.

Over the years I have seen Liam transform into someone that I did not know before. However, alongside this my mum has changed a great deal, too. In my opinion, both of them have lost the ability to be truly and undeniably happy. I think that learning this has been one of the things that has had the greatest impact on me, as they are the two people that I love the most in the world.

Being the in-between person

As mentioned above, my role became that of communicator. I think that this may be because Liam felt more comfortable speaking to me, mainly as I was not trying to enforce rules such as meal plans. As well as this, I understood more about his academic stress and the other pressures that he faced at school from his peers. However, this was a difficult role because many of the things that he told me made me worried about his wellbeing. When he confides in me properly, I feel stuck between the right and wrong. I love my brother and want him to continue to have trust in me, but underneath this I know that someone in a position of authority needs to know his thoughts and feelings during his recovery. If I decide to share what Liam says, it is obvious that I am the one who has shared it, which breaks his trust so I have to work hard to gain it again. This cycle can sometimes feel never ending.

Having this role made it difficult for me to feel completely comfortable leaving home because I was unsure whether he would talk to anyone else in this way and I didn't want him to become completely isolated. When I come home, I feel on the backfoot as everything can change so quickly with this illness. Fortunately, I have found that any attempt to keep in contact with Liam while I'm away has helped. He never answers his phone, especially text messages, which makes this increasingly difficult. So instead, I make him things such as postcards, letters or little gifts, as this makes me feel as connected to him as I can, while also moving on with my own life.

Moving on with your own life

Since the very beginning I have found it difficult to separate my life from everything happening at home. Before Liam was hospitalized, I had to write a speech for my English GCSE and I could not think of any topic other than body image. As I wrote the speech, I realised that all I could talk about was the differences that I could see in my brother, such as his anxiety, reduced confidence, his refusal to take his t-shirt off at the beach, among other behavioural changes. I think that from this moment onwards I realised that I would never truly be able to move on properly without his safety being in the back of my mind. This was proven when, in my first year of university, he called to say that he was struggling, and I took the 7.5-hour journey home the following day, only for him to refuse to speak to me. Yet still, sometimes when I am away, and I laugh a lot or feel happy, it is followed by a wave of guilt – I know that Liam is probably not experiencing the same, so why should I?

Beyond my brother, I have struggled to engage in the inevitable conversations that come with being a young woman. Dieting, detox drinks, meal replacements, wanting to be two sizes smaller… the list goes on. I shut down in conversations like this, I get a rush of fear, anger and sadness all at once, and I become speechless. I think that this hypersensitivity that I have developed around the topic will stay with me for the foreseeable future. Not only is it a day-to-day occurrence in real life, but it also comes in other forms, such as every older romance movie when a man just cannot love a 'fat' size-10 woman.

I am now 20 and I have not weighed myself since I was 16. The idea of seeing a number that is not 'normal' scares me; I know how dangerous knowing this can be. There have been many occasions since where I have looked at a plate of food and got nervous, and then looked at myself in a mirror and been unhappy. I get worried about whether this could be the beginnings of what affected my brother so badly. I think this is a result of food becoming such a taboo topic in our household that much of the enjoyment I used to get from eating, especially when I have meals with him, is gone.

What I have found to be most effective is allowing myself to have time away. Ultimately, the sibling experiences all of the arguments and tense mealtimes too, and learning to acknowledge this doesn't make you selfish. I find that when I get very wrapped up in everything, it is helpful to get out of the house and see a friend or boyfriend, or just to go walking with upbeat music or an unrelated podcast.

How to be a sibling of someone with anorexia

Even four years on I don't know that there is a rule book for living with anorexia. As a sibling, I think the most important part is to learn how to detach yourself from the situation without letting the guilt taking over. However, I think that it is undeniable that sibling solidarity is crucial to keeping a brother or sister on track with their eating, as often the sibling is seen as a friend, rather than the enemy or enforcer. Remind your sibling that you do not blame them, and that you still love them for being themselves. Remind yourself that it is okay to feel overlooked sometimes and it is not anyone's fault that this is happening to your family. Although it may often seem unlikely, everything will be okay; it may just take more time than anticipated.

Do not feel obliged to 'stay strong'. I went to therapy in the early years, which was extremely helpful for me. Initially I felt guilty because I was not the one battling with my own mind, but now I look back and I am glad that I went to therapy sessions – I now recognize that we are all joined in the fight against anorexia.

Further reading

A website about how to take care of yourself as the sibling/ family member can be found at: www.anorexiabulimiacare.org.uk/family-and-friends/siblings

A DVD about which animal to be when eating with your family member with an eating disorder can be found here: https://newmaudsleycarers-kent.co.uk/the-succeed-dvd/

4. My journey through anorexia and bulimia over three decades

By Isla Parker

Summary

This chapter explores how my anorexia was triggered when I was 13 years old, and the treatment that I received in a specialist unit in London for adolescents with eating disorders. This was nearly 30 years ago. At the time I kept a diary that formed the basis for my recently published semi-fictional novel *Size Zero?*. During my late teens and 20s I experienced episodes of bulimia, but I did my best to keep it a secret. In this chapter I describe how writing and therapy helped me to express myself, so that I could recover.

My teenage years with anorexia

When I was 12 I was roughly five kilos overweight – my granny called it 'puppy fat', and she said that 'I would grow out of it'. I attended a large comprehensive school in Surrey where I struggled to fit in, so when I attracted unwanted attention for coming top in my favourite subjects such as English and History, some of the boys in my class would pick on my weight issue, as well as calling me "a boffin" or "whale", which I found very upsetting.

My classmate Gemma gave me a food diary for my birthday, in which she wrote some diet tips for losing weight. Encouraged by the food diary, I started to lose weight. Initially I just cut out crisps and chocolate, but then I stopped eating butter, mayonnaise, and anything fatty. The diet accelerated and eventually I couldn't eat anything apart from melon and fat free yoghurt.

I was unhappy at home as well, which didn't help. My parents separated when I was two years old, and all contact soon stopped with my father and his family. I grew up wondering who my father was. Sometimes I reminded my mum of my dad, who she hated, which didn't help our relationship. My mum, brother and I lived with my grandparents until I was seven years old. As a young teenager, I went back to my grandparents' house after school. I resented having to do chores and finish my homework. I wished that I could spend more time doing fun outdoors activities like climbing trees or running. My brother and I had our evening meal at my grandparents' house, then my granny gave me a lift back to my mum's house. By this time, my mum had stopped teaching the piano (after working all day as a secretary), and all she wanted to do was sit downstairs in front of the telly with my step-dad, eating their dinner and enjoying a bottle of wine. I would watch telly or play computer games upstairs. I wasn't allowed to play my cello because it would make too much noise.

Learning point 1

- Did you experience any peer pressure to diet?
- Have you ever tried to keep a food diary, in which you express your feelings about food and eating?

Things got better when I turned 13 and lost some weight. I went to a disco at the local youth club and met a boy. He had spikey blonde hair and was tall. I liked how he was easy to chat to, and that he was musical like I was. Nick and I soon started dating. Nick often invited me round to his house after school, and there we would write songs together. Like me, he had a step-dad, but his step-dad was different to mine in the respect that he would talk to me about my interests, and include me in family meals. I still struggled to eat, but I did try. Nick's mum would drive Nick and me up to their stables, and she encouraged me to ride their pony. I enjoyed learning how to trot and canter.

As I lost weight I stopped being teased at school. Unfortunately though, the diet had taken such a grip on me that I lied to my friends and family about how much I was eating. Sometimes I would hide food in small plastic bags at mealtimes, which I would throw away in the bin concealed beneath rubbish or behind bushes. My granny did notice my weight loss, and she was concerned enough to arrange for my mum to take me to see a GP. I didn't like the GP weighing me, or showing me two meal plans that included calorific puddings. I couldn't talk about how stressed I felt by how my music was being hot-housed. In one afternoon I took two grade 7s on the piano and cello, and gained Merit in both exams. I didn't like all of the emphasis being on exams; I would have preferred to have played the cello in a more creative way.

My weight loss escalated in France, when my mum and step-dad took me on holiday in the Dordogne. One day we were canoeing down the river and I was putting extra effort into the rowing. We stopped for a baguette lunch, but all I would eat was melon. It was when we were back near the tent that I passed out. It was at that point that my mum phoned a GP in England, and the decision was taken to cut short our holiday.

Back in England I was taken to see a psychiatrist, and within a week I had been referred to a specialist eating disorders clinic in London. My distress at being weighed is captured in the following scene from my novel *Size Zero?*:

> "The doctor took a big bunch of keys out of her pocket, but she knew the right one straightaway. I followed her into a square room that had nothing in it except for a desk and a chair. Looming in front of the window were some scales, with a white bar hanging over the top of a black platform. A big mirror reflected the scales. To me the room felt claustrophobic.
>
> 'Can you take off your clothes?' Penny said. 'Leave just your bra and knickers on.'
>
> This was embarrassing. 'I don't want to get weighed,' I said.
>
> Penny turned round, with a slight smile on her face, and lowered her clipboard. 'Why's that, Suzy?'
>
> 'I don't like people seeing my weight.'
>
> 'Well, you don't have to look.'
>
> I stared at her.
>
> 'We need to know what the position is. Come on.'
>
> My fingers fumbled with the button of my skirt, and then I pulled it over my head and dumped it onto a chair. As I balanced precariously, pulling off my tights and shoes, I was scared of what the scales might say. I didn't pick up the tights.
>
> 'Onto the scales, please.'
>
> I stepped up, and as I watched her chubby fingers move the counter along the bar, I regretted doing it.
>
> *The bar stretched nearly as wide as my arms would be if they were stretched out. The bar stretches and stretches and becomes an aeroplane's wings to fly me out of here. I crash through the open window and, hearing the noise, Mum and Dr Avery together downstairs go running out into the garden. 'Suzy, come back! You need help!' they shout.*
>
> *'No, I'm fine', I shout. I smile and wave. Then my plane starts climbing into the air.*

'You've lost another kilo since Dr Avery weighed you last week,' said Penny.

I was smiling. The push-ups and other exercises in my room had paid off. Even the avocados I'd eaten hadn't made me gain.

'Do you know what this means?' asked Penny, carefully studying my face.

Slowly the consequences dawned on me, as I recalled what Dr Avery had said: that if I didn't start to gain weight, I might be hospitalised. My stomach knotted tighter, so that its hollowness became a cramp. 'You can't admit me,' I said, barely able to speak the words.

Penny said, 'I'm afraid I've got no choice. You're very underweight, and you've lost more since last week. Do you understand how serious this is? We can't let this dieting go on, as it's very dangerous.'

'But I'm not anorexic. I can eat.'

'So why have you lost more… hm? Knowing this could happen?'

I couldn't think of a good answer.

'You can get down from the scales now,' she said.

My clothes felt like a shield when I put them back on, though I couldn't get what she'd said out of my mind.

'Do you think you look fat?' she asked.

I caught sight of myself in the mirror, and mumbled, 'Yes'. I was staring at my tummy.

Penny had moved towards me, so that she was nearly parallel now. 'But you're very underweight. Can't you see that? Look, I'm much bigger than you are.'

I stared at her body next to mine."

I weighed 39 kilos and I was five foot five inches tall. I was admitted that day to the clinic for two-and-a-half months. Thirty years later I wonder if this admission to the clinic could have been avoided. Sadly, my granny had limited knowledge of anorexia, and her reaction a few months earlier had been to cook my favourite foods and watch everything that I ate. It felt as if she was spying on me at mealtimes. It would have been helpful if my granny had taken me to see the GP (instead of my mum), as I got on with her better. Anorexia was not well understood at this time, and my granny did not think to ask for me to be referred to an eating disorders outpatients' clinic, to have specialist input from a counsellor, a dietitian, and an eating disorders nurse.

Learning point 2

- How do you see yourself in the mirror? What feelings does it evoke?
- What strategies do you have for eating when you are under pressure?

When I entered the clinic I was surrounded by several other teenagers who had suffered from anorexia for longer than I had. As a result, I was now exposed to the tricks that they had learnt for outwitting the doctor! For example, some of them hid cereal and ate it before weigh-ins, when they would consume large amounts of water, so that the scales gave a false reading. I also learnt from one of the teenagers how to make myself sick.

I would sit at the table being watched by the doctor as I ate. If I did not eat, she told me that I would have to be tube-fed. Eating fish and chips, even chocolate fudge cake, suddenly seemed to be better alternatives.

I was only allowed to speak to my mum on the telephone for scheduled calls. At that time there was no internet connection either – only letters and stamps. I felt very cut off from my boyfriend, Nick, my other friends, and my grandparents, so I turned to my diary to express my feelings. I had to share a bedroom with another teenage girl, and I was aware that staff searched through our belongings to check that we did not make ourselves sick or hide food, so I hid my diary beneath a piece of loose fabric inside my cello case.

The doctor did encourage me to attend sessions with a male psychotherapist. I didn't like his tweed suit. He sat in silence until I spoke, so I would spend most of the 50 minutes not saying anything. The sessions took place twice a week and I dreaded them. Never once was I offered a different therapist. I was so unhappy that I ran away from the clinic on two occasions; the second time I was brought back by the police.

When I was finally discharged, I had reached my target weight of 52 kilos, but my obsessional thinking about food had not changed. Everything that I ate was ready-meals that were calorie counted, and I did not relax around food. I also dreaded returning to my school. As it turned out, the other teenagers were welcoming, but during my time in the clinic I had changed in such a way that I found it hard to relate to others because of what I had been through.

My adult life with bulimia

My problem with bulimia was not constant over the next 15 years. It would flare up at times of stress. The rest of the time I would try to restrict what I ate, but my weight remained within the normal range. I never sought any help for my eating disorder when I studied at university doing post-graduate degrees over the next few years and worked as an English tutor. I didn't want help, as I still wanted to be able to binge. The bulimia did put a strain on close relationships, and I lost a boyfriend because he did not like the secrecy of it. There were also medical consequences. I needed to make trips to the dentist; I had two fillings on two different occasions. Occasionally I used to pass out after I had been vomiting, or I had a hot shower.

It was not until my early 30s when I passed out in the bathroom after vomiting and knocked my head against the wall that I became genuinely frightened. I did tell my GP and she referred me to a psychiatrist, who then referred me to Cotswold House eating disorders unit in Oxford for outpatients' sessions. I found some of the cognitive strategies that I was taught to be helpful, and I followed the meal plans that I was given. But I didn't like being weighed.

My GP also referred me to a psychodynamic psychotherapist that she recommended[1]. Fortunately, the new therapist was good at giving me a sense of safe boundaries, where I felt that I could share my eating disorder with her, and my painful memories from the past. She brought more cognitive approaches into therapy for managing thoughts about restricting and my obsession with calorie counting, which were useful. My therapist helped me to see why my difficult early attachment pattern had affected later relationships. I was able to develop new interests (such as joining a writing group, and studying for a Master's degree in Medical Humanities), and I made friends. Gradually my life became fulfilling, and bingeing and restricting shrank in their importance. It is now ten years later, and while I still deal with difficult thoughts about my weight and shape at times, I remain a normal weight and I rarely binge.

Learning point 3

- Have you found it helpful to read any specialist books about anorexia or bulimia? Why would you recommend this book to others?
- When you are struggling with your eating disorder, do you confide in any health professionals? What do you feel comfortable sharing with them?

1 Therapists are listed on the BACP website. Please see: www.bacp.co.uk

References

Butler G, Grey N & Hope T (2007) *Manage your mind: the mental fitness guide*. Oxford: Oxford University Press.

Dawson D (2001) *Anorexia and bulimia: a parent's guide to recognising eating disorders and taking control*. London: Random House.

Austin R (2021) *Size Zero?* UK: Amazon.

5. Lived experiences of bulimia nervosa: findings from a qualitative study

By Geraldine Bishop

Summary

This chapter will explore the lived experiences of individuals experiencing bulimia nervosa, focusing specifically on the emotional impact of this eating difficulty. The content of this chapter are a reflection from a qualitative study conducted exploring individual experiences of bulimia nervosa. The chapter will draw upon the various therapeutic interventions used to treat bulimia and highlight the importance of addressing the emotional aspect of this eating difficulty. It is key for families, practitioners and for individuals themselves experiencing bulimia to gain an understanding of the ways in which it affects one's life physically and mentally, in the understanding of these aspects of bulimia one can identify an effective way of allowing the individual to overcome the eating difficulty, working with both cognitions and emotions. The chapter will provide contemporary research findings in relation to lived experiences of bulimia, whilst exploring why one way of working with bulimia may be effective for one individual and not for the other, which will lead on to the role of individual differences in eating difficulties. Co-morbidities associated with bulimia nervosa will be discussed and aspects of the journey to recovery will be highlighted.

Learning point 1

- Take a moment to think about how you view bulimia.
- What are your experiences of individuals with bulimia?
- How has this shaped how you understand the eating difficulty?

Underlying feelings associated with bulimia

The role of control

This piece of research demonstrated the existence of shame and inner conflict in individuals with bulimia, as well as highlighting control, or a lack thereof, as a major theme in these people's lives. This common feeling of 'loss of control' underlies many attempts to gain control through bulimia. Feeling a loss of control was present in many domains within the lives of the participants such as education, intimate relationships, family relationships and mental health co-morbidities such as depression and anxiety. Underlying feelings of being controlled was common, with some discussing their experiences of being controlled by mothers and other participants sharing their experiences of controlling partners.

A number of participants talked about loss of control as an original factor present at the onset of their bulimia. One participant talked about the cycle of chasing the position of being in control and yet finding herself feeling completely out of control and instead being controlled by her bulimia. Being able to control what she would and wouldn't consume gave her a sense of controlling at least one aspect of her life.

Secrecy and guilt

Individuals experiencing bulimia often struggle with finding support due to it being a 'hidden difficulty' because bulimia is not always visible, and it can be very difficult for the individual engaging with these behaviours to bring the issue to light. Participants discussed a number of ways in which they would hide their behaviours, including disguising laxatives, leaving the family home to purge, hiding binge foods in unexpected places and using music to disguise sounds of purging. These secretive behaviours often led to feelings of guilt, which in turn seemed to discourage people from seeking support. Many participants talked about feeling separate from their loved ones due to the honesty they had to employ in order to be able to engage with bulimic behaviours.

Learning point 2

- Before you continue reading, think about your own personal experiences of feelings such as guilt and shame. What's your understanding of inner conflict? Have you experienced this?
- What do you feel may be useful in supporting a person experiencing shame?
- Take a moment to write down some possible first steps in support seeking.
- Who would be the first person you would turn to? What are the professional services available in your area?
- Take a look at those first steps, what are the challenges that come with these? How would you address the challenges?

The emotional impact of bulimia

Hearing the accounts of individuals with lived experiences of bulimia, it was evident that considering and attempting to understand the emotional impact is of great importance for professionals and the family and friends of the person.

A sense of feeling misunderstood

A number of participants expressed that they did not feel understood by those around them and only felt comfortable talking to others that may be able to relate to their experiences. When focusing on support seeking, the recovery journey and professional interventions, a large number of participants unfortunately felt that they were being pathologized. It seems that there may be a need to move away from the typical medical model of 'pathologising' bulimia and take a step towards becoming curious about how we as professionals can empower individuals and encourage recovery. It was evident that the majority of my participants simply wanted to feel heard and to work on the underlying, deeper-rooted psychological issues they were experiencing, which seemed difficult when being offered a limited number of therapy sessions and which they reported focused mostly on how much they weighed and what they had eaten that week.

A sense of feeling trapped

The feeling of being 'trapped by bulimia' was extremely common and reoccurring throughout the analysis. One participant stated, 'Once you're in it, it feels too late, you're trapped', and this experience of feeling imprisoned was closely linked to the secretive aspect of bulimia.

The feeling of being trapped by bulimia highlighted the desire to be free of feeling controlled and free of shame-inducing thoughts. One participant shared the feeling of being 'freed' when discussing the emotions associated with recovery. The importance of acceptance was strongly associated with this, and was emphasized by the participant's account of working towards accepting their true self and gaining an understanding of the reasons bulimia may have presented itself initially.

A battle with the self

It is common for people with bulimia to be critical of themselves, often talking about the 'critical voice' that would leave them harbouring guilt, feeling ashamed of their behaviours and depressed about the existence of their eating difficulty. In addition to this, it was common for the participants to feel misunderstood, and unfortunately it seemed that many felt misunderstood by professionals, with the emotional impact of this eating difficulty often not being fully addressed leading to a felt sense of loneliness.

Learning point 3

- Take a moment to think if you can recall a time where you have felt misunderstood? How did you process this?
- How did it affect your actions and behaviours?
- Are you in a position where you are able to ask a person with bulimia what they feel they need emotionally?
- Are you able to provide this for them? If not, is there someone else who can?
- If you are experiencing bulimia, what is it that you need emotionally? Think about how you can access this and the things you can do to enhance your own emotional wellbeing.
- Think about how your emotions may drive some of your behaviours.
- Can you pinpoint one emotion you experience?
- How does this impact on your actions?
- Is there a healthier way of managing the feeling?

Conditions associated with bulimia nervosa

Bulimia is often associated with co-morbidities such as anxiety disorders, depression, substance abuse, obsessive compulsive disorder, and personality disorders. There are a number of commonalities between psychiatric conditions and bulimia, some of which include trauma, low mood and impulsivity. Hudson *et al* (2007) argue that a crucial step in the management of bulimia is to identify and address the psychiatric co-morbidities as these are suggested to decrease levels of psychosocial functioning.

In addition to this, suicidal ideation, suicide attempts and suicide are dangerous co-morbidities found in individuals presenting with bulimia, yet successful treatment of bulimia can often resolve depressive and anxiety disorders (Patel *et al*, 2018).

In addition to the psychiatric co-morbidities associated with eating difficulties, it is important to highlight the range of medical complications that are linked to an eating disorder diagnosis, such as endocrine system dysfunction, cardiovascular diseases, anaemia and electrolytes disturbances. The severity of the medical complications is typically dependent on the speed and severity of weight loss, the age of patients, duration of the difficulty and with bulimia and the intensity of purging (Dalle & Calugi, 2007).

Treatment and support for individuals experiencing bulimia nervosa

It is important to remember that eating disorders are often not about the food itself but about what is happening for a person emotionally. It is therefore essential that treatment for bulimia is able to address the underlying thoughts and feelings that contribute to the bulimic behaviours.

Enhanced cognitive behavioural therapy (CBT-E) is currently the first-line treatment model for adults experiencing bulimia nervosa (Fairburn, 2003). Cognitive behavioural therapy for eating disorders is designed to challenge problematic thoughts and attitudes around weight and body shape, formulate coping mechanisms for resisting binge and purging behaviours, and replace the individual's dieting with normal eating habits (Fairburn *et al*, 2009). It seems that at present the use of family-based treatment is increasing (Hurst *et al*, 2015). A variety of interventions have been formulated during recent years with group psychotherapies (Ball & Mitchell, 2004), multi-dimensional approaches, family therapies (Folse & Krawzak, 2013) and feminist psychotherapies (Maine & Bunnell, 2008) being practiced with this client group.

A number of participants had sought therapy to aid them in the process of recovery. The majority had experience of CBT-E, yet only one shared that she had found it helpful due to the challenge of attempting to change behaviours and learn new management techniques within a limited amount of therapy sessions. It became apparent from my participants' accounts that they did not feel CBT-E addressed the deep-seated emotions of shame, anger and sadness that were present as a result of their engagement with bingeing and purging cycles.

Learning point 4

- What are your understandings of these different therapeutic approaches?
- Which type of therapy do you feel may be most suitable to address bulimia?
- Take a moment to reflect on what you feel may arise emotionally for a person with bulimia?

A recovery journey

As recovery appears for some to be an ongoing process, it is important to work towards the person accepting themselves and to not rush the process but rather to take the time that is needed, which depends on the individual and their personal experiences of bulimia. Since a common behaviour for an individual living with bulimia is to compare themselves to others, it is important that this is discouraged in recovery and that one is able to work towards accepting the time it may take to recover and to engage with the emotional journey that takes place alongside this, as opposed to dissociating from the underlying feelings that may Arise. While support seeking is difficult for a person with bulimia, it seems that professionals, family members, partners and friends have a role to play in making this accessible. It is important for a person with bulimia to feel heard and understood, as a sense of feeling supported seems to be a key aspect in a successful recovery.

Learning point 5

- What is your understanding of acceptance?
- Do you accept yourself for who you really are? If so, what has helped you feel able to do this? If you struggle with this, what do you feel stops you from accepting yourself? What steps can you take to work towards self-acceptance?
- Are you in a position where you are able to support a person in feeling accepted? How may you do this?
- Are you in a role where you have the opportunity to support someone in recovery from bulimia? What do you now feel you need to do for this? If you identify with bulimia, are you able to reflect on your feelings towards recovery?

Conclusions

Throughout this chapter, we have looked at the lived experiences of individuals with bulimia nervosa. This has included looking at the underlying difficulties associated with bulimia as well as current approaches utilized to work with this eating difficulty.

While CBT is currently the first line treatment approach, CBT is a short-term therapeutic intervention which is often offered with a limited number of sessions. From this research, it was evident that there are deeper-seated emotions to be worked with throughout the recovery of bulimia nervosa, and that a longer-term therapeutic intervention such as trauma focused, relational or an integrative approach may indeed be more effective.

While behaviours can be a core issue for individuals experiencing bulimia, there may be a requirement to work on processing the underlying roots of their bulimia, an approach that works with the interpretation of mental and emotional processes prior to addressing behaviours. It could be argued that this would be particularly effective if combined with a framework that steps back from pathologising individuals with eating difficulties and towards empowering them through their journey in recovery, regardless of where one may be on this journey.

Reflection points

- Are you able to revisit your initial views of bulimia, the ones you identified when starting this chapter?
- Have any of these changed?
- Do you feel more informed in relation to the emotional impact of bulimia after reading this chapter?

References

Ball, J., & Mitchell, P. (2004). A Randomized Controlled Study of Cognitive Behaviour Therapy and Behavioural Family Therapy for Anorexia Nervosa Patients. *Eating Disorders*, **12**(4), 303-314.

Dalle, R., & Calugi, S. (2007). Eating disorder not otherwise specified in an inpatient unit: the impact of altering the DSM-IV criteria for anorexia and bulimia nervosa. *European Eating Disorders Review*, **15**(5), 340-349.

Devlin, M. J. and Walsh, T. (1995) Medication treatment for eating disorders. *Journal of Mental Health*, **4**: 459– 469.

E. Garfinkel (Eds.), Handbook of psychotherapy for anorexia nervosa and bulimia (pp. 160–192). New York: Guilford.

Fairburn, C. G., Cooper, Z., Doll, H. A., O'Connor, M. E., Bohn, K., Hawker, D. M. et al. (2009) Transdiagnostic cognitive-behavioural therapy for patients with eating disorders: a two-site trial with 60-week follow-up. *American Journal of Psychiatry*, **166**: 311– 319.

Folse, V., & Krawzak, K. (2013). Family Experience with Eating Disorders Scale: A Systematic Way to Engage the Family in Treatment. *Perspectives in Psychiatric Care*, **6** (1).

Hudson, J., Hiripi, E., Pope, H., & Kessler, R. (2007). The Prevalence and Correlates of Eating Disorders in the National Comorbidity Survey Replication. *Biological Psychiatry*, **61**(3), 348-358.

Hurst, K., Read, S., & Holtham, T. (2015). Bulimia nervosa in adolescents: a new therapeutic frontier. *Journal of Family Therapy*, **39**(4), 563-579.

Maine, M., & Bunnell, D. (2008). How do the Principles of the Feminist, Relational Model Apply to Treatment of Men with Eating Disorders and Related Issues? *Eating Disorders*, **16**(2), 187-192.

Patel, R., Olten, B., Patel, P., Shah, K., & Mansuri, Z. (2018). Hospitalization Outcomes and Comorbidities of Bulimia Nervosa: A Nationwide Inpatient Study. *Cureus*, **10**(5).

Salvy, S. J. and McCargar, L. (2002). Nutritional interventions for individuals with bulimia nervosa. *Eating and Weight Disorders*, **7**: 258– 267.

6. Boys and men living with eating difficulties

By Dr Russell Delderfield

Summary

Written by a researcher with personal experience of male eating difficulties, this chapter acknowledges what is already known about boys and men with eating problems, while focussing on those issues specific to this group. Key myths are raised and challenged. The complications arising from being male with eating problems are presented. These issues include the predominance of receiving an atypical diagnosis (this means that the boy or man does not fit a clear diagnosis, even if they have many of the symptoms) and our narrow understanding of eating problems being about restriction. Men are more likely to experience muscularity-related eating difficulties or problems with excess and overeating. Finally, I will outline what might be expected from treatment.

For over a decade, my research has centred on male disordered eating. I did not begin researching this area by accident – I am a man with an eating disorder. My difficulties with food began when I was 14 years old. When I first tried to access information and services there was very little help and all the medical leaflets and texts were about girls and women. I felt like an oddity of some sort, but my exhausting cycle of bingeing and purging finally had a name. It was a relief to see a GP (Delderfield, 2018).

My aim here is to offer some insight into eating and body problems as found in boys and men. I use medical terms only when necessary, as my hope is to illustrate that many men may have experienced these difficulties, with or without a formal diagnosis. Where I share male experiences, these are not identifiable individuals, but instead they are composites of several people's lives, so as to highlight issues that are particular to the male experience.

Myths and misconceptions

Recently, I feel as if we have seen a shift, where more men have been able to be open about their difficulties with food and their bodies[1]. A sportsperson, Freddie

1 www.bbc.co.uk/news/newsbeat-54343453

Flintoff, presented a documentary about male eating disorders; Christopher Ecclestone, a well-known actor in the UK and beyond, shared his own struggles with anorexia[2]; and Ed Sheeran, a famous singer-songwriter, gave an interview about his difficulties with bingeing on food[3]. When men speak out there is hope that another boy or man may realise that he is not alone, and may find their first steps to getting help and support.

Nevertheless, misconceptions abound about boys, men and eating problems. One myth that it is crucial to dispel is that we do not know very much about boys and men with eating issues. This is no longer the case – the last 20 years have not been unproductive. Arguably, the issue is that our knowledge has stalled somewhat. As clinical and medical studies continue, we are missing something crucial in the improvement of services and treatments, which is listening more to the voices of men who live with eating difficulties.

I have not gone into detail here relating to male sexuality and eating difficulties, as this is covered in Chapter 7. However, there is a further myth to challenge, namely that the majority of boys or men with eating difficulties are gay or bisexual. In my own research, that has not been the case. Most of the men whose stories I have studied identify as straight (that is, they are attracted to the opposite sex). It is true that many teenage boys and adult men who end up interacting with services sometimes have underlying issues with their sexuality, or already identify as gay or bisexual. A renowned disordered-eating specialist once warned that associating these issues with one group of men due to outdated understandings of sexuality, masculinity and femininity, may be damaging to both sexual minority men and heterosexual men (Morgan, 2008). Not all gay or bisexual men will end up with eating problems. It is also the case that not all straight men escape such concerns, and therefore it is not helpful to promote a message that these issues 'do not exist' in straight men, or that services are not for them (Morgan, 2008). Eating issues do not discriminate based on gender or on sexuality.

> *"Paul was studying for a chemistry degree and loved playing rugby when he realised he only allowed himself to eat when he had trained or played a match. His concentration in labs and classes was patchy, and his girlfriend expressed her concerns about how 'moody' he had suddenly become. After suffering an injury during a match, he became secretly terrified of gaining weight. This made his food avoidance worse and by the time his partner persuaded him to see a doctor he was living on a single bowl of cereal a day."*

2 www.theguardian.com/culture/2019/sep/16/christopher-eccleston-reveals-he-is-lifelong-anorexic

3 www.standard.co.uk/showbiz/celebrity-news/ed-sheeran-binge-food-alcohol-sick-anxiety-a4509586.html

So, we know that the three most common eating difficulty diagnoses (anorexia nervosa, bulimia nervosa, and binge-eating disorder) apply to men as well as women. MaleVoicED (2021), the UK male eating disorders charity, provides a good overview of the symptoms of these eating difficulties[4]. Medically, we know there are certain similarities between men and women when it comes to the development of eating difficulties and their severity (Zayas *et al*, 2018), in which case, why is this chapter on boys and men even needed?

The same but different...

Put simply, not everything we know is the same, irrespective of biological sex or gender. And one critical difference is that boys and men are often disadvantaged when it comes to getting help.

Key differences are:

- Boys and men still have less chance of developing disordered eating than women. This could well change in our lifetime, but until now this is the case. Nine to ten per cent of all cases are said to be men. This can become as high as 25% of all cases who end up needing treatment and therefore end up in health service figures (Delderfield, 2018). Unfortunately, we continue to lack accurate information on this, and figures shown in the media and elsewhere are often estimates.
- While osteoporosis occurs in both men and women who restrict their food intake, this bone-weakness is worse in men, even if they have had their eating issues for less time (Delderfield, 2018).
- In eating difficulties that involve bingeing then compensating (with other behaviours intended to 'undo' the binge), men are more likely to use laxatives or engage in obsessive exercise as a response to their binges, rather than vomiting.
- When men do get help for eating (and related) issues, their quality of life after they have been discharged is worse than for women. This means recovery seems to be partial with more relapse and less freedom from eating difficulties.
- Avoidant Restrictive Food Intake Disorder (ARFID) appears to be increasing in children, and boys appear susceptible. This is characterised by severe restriction in textures and types of food, with great distress being evident if someone's tolerated foods are not available. MaleVoicED (2021) provides helpful, succinct information about this.
- Stereotypes continue about boys and men – they are expected to have hearty appetites; they are said to be 'growing boys' and are fed more, even though many no longer need many additional calories for manual jobs in manufacturing or mining (Contois, 2020).

4 www.malevoiced.com/arfid

- Eating difficulties relating to overeating (bingeing) are more likely in men, and account for more cases than issues related to restricting food intake.
- Boys and men are more likely to be missed altogether or mis-diagnosed when they do decide to seek help, or their family takes them for a medical assessment (Cohn & Lemberg, 2014).

If the higher mortality rates were not alarming enough, that last point is a significant cause for concern – it is the critical difference that I referred to earlier. Summoning the courage to access help or tell someone what is happening is tough. The shame and stigma associated with eating difficulties is already known to be a barrier to accessing/accepting help. Imagine, then, that someone is dismissed or told that their eating issues are something else entirely.

Anorexia tends to receive significant attention. This is understandable, of course, as once the body mass of a male child or adult drops drastically, it can become physically obvious (more so in men, arguably, who are not 'valued' by society for slenderness). It also becomes quickly dangerous, meaning that treatment may be more immediate. Despite neat categories being given as medical diagnoses, most men, however, do not match the various criteria for the three eating difficulties mentioned above. It is common, therefore, for men to be deemed 'atypical'. This means that the boy or man does not fit a clear diagnosis, even if they have many of the symptoms. This can cause confusion and further distress. It can also potentially complicate access to treatment, as a clear-cut diagnosis often comes with a recognized treatment. This may have implications for drugs that might be prescribed, and the types of therapies that could accompany a type of disordered eating (see 'Treatment' below).

Learning point 1

- What was your understanding of male eating difficulties prior to reading the list above?
- Why might boys and men be mis-diagnosed or not even given a diagnosis at all?
- To what extent do you think that eating issues in boys are the same as those in adult men?

Muscularity-oriented disordered eating (MODE)

There is a move to recognize that men's eating difficulties may stem from a preference for, and an obsession with, building a more muscular body. This has recently led to the term 'muscularity-oriented disordered eating' (MODE). One of the ways that male eating and body problems might be atypical becomes clear when we look at prevalent trends around the male body. While my phrase 'the brain of a banker, the body of a warrior' may sound like a slogan and is a sweeping generalization, it captures the way that society often perceives men's bodies and could be fuelling eating difficulties (Delderfield, 2018). By way of explanation, more than ever before in recent history, many men spend their paid time in static jobs that require brainpower, but do not require bodily strength. Many physically demanding jobs have diminished or vanished altogether – the nation's men are not all working on the land to provide for their loved ones anymore. Yet, just as a man is less likely to have an exercised, labour-hardened body, we seem to prize visual displays of masculinity that can be shown outwardly, through a visibly muscled body of the kind frequently found on cinema screens and across social media. It is not enough to be fit – we must look it, even when we are fully dressed (Martschukat, 2021).

A couple of decades ago, the term 'bigorexia' was coined (Pope *et al*, 2000). Its clinical name is 'muscle dysmorphia'. It is characterized by a consuming obsession with muscle, its quality, appearance and maintenance. This is not merely a recreational interest in going to the gym, working out and attaining fitness with muscular strength and endurance (MSE). Men with this issue have far-reaching, compulsive habits that take over their lives. They often feel that they are not good enough because they are not big or defined enough. The link with eating difficulties is present as obsessing about nutrition, muscle-building supplements, and exacting dietary regimes, meaning that the man becomes increasingly socially isolated. In essence, food becomes fuel for muscle, and no amount of muscle is ever quite enough. The man cannot conceive of a life where the building and maintenance of muscle is second to other relationships or commitments. As such, there is a conscious effort by many researchers and clinicians to have this set of damaging behaviours classified within disordered eating as MODE (Murray *et al*, 2017; Murray *et al*, 2018).

> *"Evan began weightlifting as he had been bullied for being so small at primary school. By the time he was a teenager he loved the compliments from family and friends about how fit he was and how 'buff' he looked, but he had specific measurements of his major muscle groups that he needed to reach. Over time, friends got used to his automatic response to social invitations being 'I've got training'. He became irrationally angry if his carefully planned intake was disrupted, such as when his elder brother ate his meal-prepped protein, leaving him with nothing."*

This is of genuine concern, as researchers investigating children's toys have suggested that even young children now think 'muscles are best' and that they equate to strength and value (Baghurst *et al*, 2018), to a point of disparaging lesser physiques. Of further concern is the unrealistic muscle mass we now seem to think of as 'normal' – yet often it takes illegal means to attain, for example via the use of anabolic steroids.

Learning point 2

- When you think of a physically fit man, what image pops up in your mind?
- What is the extent of your knowledge of techniques used by elite trainers to create screen-ready bodies for actors' filming days?
- At what point do you think a 'regular' desire for a muscular, masculine body becomes destructive?

Treatment

There are medications that can be discussed with a doctor that can help alleviate symptoms associated with eating difficulties. Cognitive Behavioural Therapies (CBT) and a specific variant, Dialectical Behaviour Therapy (DBT), can be helpful and are often the front-line treatment for individual men. For boys, family-based therapies are often offered and the family unit will need to be a part of the assessment, treatment process and recovery. Different clinicians have written about the need to allow a man's gender into the therapy room so as not to negate modern pressures on men to be 'a man'. The difficulties of living up to constraining stereotypes and expectations of manhood should be part of the therapeutic recovery process when tackling eating difficulties.

With disordered eating, some group therapies are useful, but this can come with its own problems, as many groups are 'women-only' spaces, given that most people who experience eating difficulties are female. As it stands, we do not have clear evidence as to whether all-male groups might be an answer to this, although this may be an avenue worth exploring as it can mitigate the isolation and loneliness that many men feel as they try to get help. It is important to try things that are offered – sometimes we surprise ourselves when we discover that what we are trying is effective. Talking is not compulsory but knowing that there are other men going through this with us can be an enormous help.

Conclusion

As a man with eating difficulties, I know first-hand what it can feel like to struggle with partial recovery or for eating problems to dominate one's life at different points. In this chapter I have shared some of the things we already know about boys and men with eating issues by exploring some commonly held misconceptions. For example, men are more likely to experience eating difficulties related to overeating instead of undereating. Another example was the idea that when men go to get help and support, they are often given an atypical diagnosis (described above). While men can struggle with similar eating difficulties to women, this chapter has highlighted a potential new area of concern which we are currently calling MODE, or muscularity-oriented disordered eating, where a preoccupation with muscle, eating for muscle and sustaining muscle at all costs can impair boys' and men's lives if left unchecked.

References

Baghurst T, Griffiths S & Murray S (2018) Boys and girls prefer hyper-muscular male action figures over normally-muscular action figures: evidence that children have internalized the muscular male body ideal. *North American Journal of Psychology* **20** (1) 159-69.

Cohn L & Lemberg R (Eds.) (2014) *Current Findings on Males with Eating Disorders*. Hove: Routledge.

Contois E (2020) *Diners, Dudes, and Diets: How gender and power collide in food media and culture.* Chapel Hill: University of North Carolina Press.

Delderfield R (2018) *Male Eating Disorders: Experiences of food, body and self.* London: Palgrave MacMillan.

Pope H, Phillips KA & Olivardia R (2000) *The Adonis Complex: The secret crisis of male body obsession.* New York: Simon and Schuster.

MaleVoicED (2021) ARFID [online]. London: *Male Voices with Eating Disorders*. Available at: www.malevoiced.com/arfid (accessed January 2021).

Martschukat J (2021) *The Age of Fitness*. Cambridge: Polity Press.

Morgan JF (2008) *The Invisible Man: A self-help guide for men with eating disorders, compulsive exercise and bigorexia*. London: Routledge.

Murray SB, Nagata JM, Griffiths S, Calzo JP, Brown TA, Mitchison D & Mond JM (2017) The enigma of male eating disorders: A critical review and synthesis. *Clinical Psychology Review* **57** 1-11.

Murray SB, Accurso EC, Griffiths S & Nagata JM (2018) Boys, biceps, and bradycardia: The hidden dangers of muscularity-oriented disordered eating. *Journal of Adolescent Health* **62** (3) 352-355.

Zayas LV, Wang SB, Coniglio K, Becker K, Murray HB, Klosterman E & Thomas JJ (2018) Gender differences in eating disorder psychopathology across DSM-5 severity categories of anorexia nervosa and bulimia nervosa. *International Journal of Eating Disorders* **51** (9) 1098-1102.

7. What's sexuality got to do with it? Considering eating difficulties in the LGBTQ+ community

By James Downs and Lawrence Smith

Summary

Professionals have long noted that eating difficulties are overrepresented in the LGBTQ+ community, but a lack of understanding about the relationship between sexuality, gender and eating problems often leads to LGBTQ+ individuals not receiving the most effective support in their treatment and recoveries (Williams *et al*, 2018). At worst, they may be left feeling their experiences are invalid or misunderstood.

This chapter will take a broad approach to exploring how the interrelationship of food, eating, body image and sex is relevant for people experiencing eating difficulties, irrespective of their sexual orientation and/or gender identity. Referencing research and personal experiences of the two authors – both gay men with lived experience of eating difficulties – this chapter aims to widen perspectives and highlight the ways in which those who identify as LGBTQ+ may be better understood and supported in treatment.

Introduction

It has been well-evidenced that LGBTQ+ adults and adolescents are at greater risk of developing eating difficulties than their cisgender and heterosexual counterparts (Parker & Harringer, 2020). Research has also highlighted unique concerns experienced by LGBTQ+ people in relation to food, eating and body image (Nagata *et al*, 2020) as well as the barriers to accessing specialist support that can exist for this group.

These factors combine to tell a story of inequity and oppression; where LGBTQ+ people are more likely to experience eating difficulties, less likely to have their experiences understood, and have less opportunity to access the help they need.

This makes the road to recovery a longer and lonelier one for many LGBTQ+ individuals. Yet this doesn't have to be the case. By recognising and dismantling risk factors and barriers to being understood and cared for, experiences of eating difficulties and receiving support can be improved, and people no longer need to struggle in silence.

Learning point 1

Before you read further, take a moment to pause and reflect on your understanding and experiences of LGBTQ+ communities and individuals.

- Is this a subject you feel confident talking about, or would you like to learn more about LGBTQ+ experiences?
- Are you currently aware of any particular risk factors, unique characteristics of eating difficulties, or barriers to accessing support for LGBTQ+ people experiencing eating problems?

It's OK not to have answers to these questions, but it is perhaps worth noticing your starting point when reading this chapter and approaching this subject. We each have our experiences and assumptions about different groups of people and their lives. Developing our knowledge and understanding – and indeed our openness to different perspectives which may challenge what we currently know – is an important aspect of learning about and including diverse experiences in our thinking.

Risk factors

When we ask the question, "what makes somebody more likely to develop a health difficulty or illness?", very often we look to characteristics of the individual in question as the causal factor(s), i.e. genetics, personality traits, or other inherent factors situated in the individual. The research into LGBTQ+ experiences, however, suggests that risk factors for eating difficulties are as much rooted in social factors as they are in individual characteristics. The ways in which LGBTQ+ people are viewed and treated by others is important in shaping how at-risk or protected they are from developing difficulties with food, eating and body image.

Parker and Harringer's (2020) review of studies into eating difficulties amongst LGBTQ+ populations describes how research has been able to identify and describe risk factors which are more 'distal' (pertaining to wider social behaviour and cultural attitudes), or more 'proximal' (closer to the individual and their characteristics). For example, stigma and discrimination at a societal level is associated with increased risk of disordered eating behaviours. At a more personal level, factors that are not specific to LGBTQ+ identity, but which may be of equal or heightened prevalence amongst LGBTQ+ people, include co-occurring mental health difficulties such as problems with mood or anxiety, demographic factors such as age, social isolation and a lack of belonging, body image dissatisfaction, and social media use (amongst others).

Factors associated with eating difficulties that relate specifically to LGBTQ+ identities include, but are not confined, to:

- internalised negative beliefs about self-worth on the basis of sexual orientation and/or gender identity
- experiences of discrimination as well as fear of experiencing discrimination – e.g. from friends, family and in the workplace
- experiencing bullying on the basis of sexual orientation and/or gender identity or non-conforming expressions of gender
- discordance between biological sex and gender identity
- increased pressure to conform to body image standards upheld by sections of the LGBTQ+ community.

Current research suggests that such risk factors are not uniform across different LGBTQ+ groups. For instance, Watson *et al* (2016) found that higher levels of anti-bisexual discrimination amongst women was related to increased incidence of disordered eating behaviours, and coping via psychological internalization and detachment as well drug and alcohol use were important mediating factors. For sexual minority men, the use of dating apps has been shown to be a relationship risk factor associated with eating difficulties, which may relate to increased pressure to meet certain aesthetic standards (Miller & Behm-Morawitz, 2020).

These are just some examples of the factors at play in the development and maintenance of eating difficulties among LGBTQ+ people. More research is needed to identify the protective factors that make for healthy relationships with food, eating, exercise and body image across identities also.

Lawrence on the pressures associated with body image and dating in the -LGBTQ+ community:

> *"I want to be desired. Yes for my personality and ethics, but also for my (currently non-existent) coke-can-crushing abs. Gay men are told on a daily basis that our physique is integral to our sense of self, which feels even more heightened in the gay community. Someone likes your post on Instagram? They're gay? You're chatting on private message? Surely this can only lead to conversations – and pertinently, images – of a sexual nature. So you want to present the best version of yourself, the most attractive version. But if you don't have the ideal body of the men we see on our timeline? That's points knocked off your score immediately."*

We would suggest that situating the struggles associated with sexuality and gender identity and eating difficulties within LGBTQ+ individuals themselves is shortsighted. Instead, locating resilience not in the individual but across place, community, individual and policy creates a model of interrelated systems which can predict health as well as vulnerability (Friedli, 2009). Looking at the social and cultural factors which drive the increased risk of eating difficulties may help us realise that dismantling risk and developing protective factors is a social rather than individual task. This, for example, includes changing the attitudes which lead to risk factors such as minority-based bullying and discrimination in the first place. When considering eating difficulties amongst LGBTQ+ people, the development of an inclusive culture and support for social justice for minorities is not irrelevant – it's necessary.

Learning point 2

Before you read further, take a moment to think about your understanding of the issues faced by individuals who identify as LGBTQ+ in relation to eating difficulties. Perhaps there is someone you know who has these experiences, someone you are supporting, or yourself.

- Can you identify any factors relating to the LGBTQ+ community that might be involved in the experiences of the person you are supporting, or your own?
- What can you do in your personal life and/or workplace to help dismantle the discrimination and pressures faced by people in the LGBTQ+ community?

Experiences of eating difficulties, treatment and finding support

While it is important to understand LGBTQ+ experiences in general, and for more research to be done into these populations, remembering that each individual has different lived experiences is vitally important. Assumptions about who may encounter eating difficulties and why – including assumptions about the experiences of LGBTQ+ individuals – are often a significant barrier in feeling understood and receiving the help and support needed.

James on refraining from making assumptions:

"Professionals have often seized upon the fact that I am gay to explain why I have the difficulties I have. The idea that acceptable narratives to explain what I was going through were limited to either childhood abuse or sexual orientation issues left me feeling confused and isolated. I was 'invalid' – ironically a term we used to use to describe the sick.

My total rejection of my body wasn't about rejecting my sexual orientation. Whilst I didn't have an issue with my sexual orientation, I did have an issue with my sexuality in general. It wasn't about being attracted to men, it was about having a sexuality at all.

*My problems with eating, exercise and body image were about **being in my body** and finding it hard to come to terms with all of the drives, desires, sensations and emotions that come with being human. Growing up, I had never learnt to regulate any of these – to channel my mental, physical or emotional energy. Sexuality was just a part of this picture."*

This example goes to show how, in addition to experiencing unique factors contributing towards eating difficulties, LGBTQ+ people may also face challenges in accessing treatment and support. When they do access support they may not be met with culturally competent professionals who are able to treat them in an inclusive way. Where friends and family are also unsupportive, this can be an especially isolating experience. Research has demonstrated that transgender people in eating disorders treatment settings have often found clinicians' misunderstandings of gender can make treatment more likely to be ineffective or even harmful for them (Duffy *et al*, 2016). Undertaking training in cultural and clinical competency in transgender health, facilitating access to gender-affirming interventions and using correct pronouns (by asking how individuals identify rather than assuming), have been shown to improve transgender people's experiences of treatment (Bowman, 2018).

Lawrence on feeling excluded in treatment:

"In a field that was overwhelmingly female focused, my gender was more of a hurdle to overcome than my sexuality. I was already feeling confused by my mental health and sexuality, so being recommended books by therapists wherein the author would only refer to people with eating difficulties with female pronouns further complicated my relationship with my gender and sexuality. I hope other people who are in the position I was in have access to the full range of services. Were I to engage with services now, I would make

my sexuality take on the importance it has in my everyday life – is it my predominant character trait? Is it central to my identity? In some ways, yes; in other ways, it's not. It all goes into the melting pot of what makes me 'me'."

Experiences of eating difficulties themselves may be shaped by experiences of gender, sexuality and cultural factors within LGBTQ+ groups and subgroups. For instance, changes in sexual function and body image that can occur alongside other bodily changes such as weight loss may be experienced differently, especially where sexual behaviour and desirability is entangled with perceptions of self worth (Fussner & Smith, 2015). Among sexual minority men, the use of steroids and a drive towards muscularity have been indicated as both predictors and components of eating difficulties (e.g. Griffiths *et al*, 2017).

These are just a few experiences which may be more prominent within LGBTQ+ groups. The essential point to remember is that eating difficulties are experienced by diverse groups of people in diverse ways. It is important not to assume what may or may not be involved in any one individual's experience of eating difficulties, and to have space for everything to be on the table without judgement. This can be invaluable.

James on the limitations of treatment:

"Rarely has there been space to talk about sex or sexuality in my treatment, unless it was to be hijacked by a professional using my sexual orientation to write-off my eating difficulties as being caused by a problem I would 'grow out of'. As a result, I wasn't able to talk about the abusive relationships I was in, my inability to control my untamed libido, or how I would use sex for affirmation and proof that I was worth something – even if it was just as an object. There wasn't space to talk about the risks I would take because I felt worthless, or about how buying food for binge eating made me financially desperate enough to accept money for sexual favours.

All of these factors were important in maintaining my eating disorder, and the complex relationship between body image, sex, eating and exercise were all things that I needed to talk about.

Treatment is still not confident about being inclusive of these kinds of difficulties. I recently delivered training for a specialist eating disorders service where staff said they didn't talk about sex because it rarely came up. Maybe they aren't asking the right questions."

Those supporting LGBTQ+ individuals with eating difficulties, therefore, would ideally provide an accepting and affirming environment, informed by an awareness of the types of issues discussed in this chapter, but never overlooking or excluding individual experiences. While more work needs to be done towards researching which approaches best help LGBTQ+ people with eating difficulties, encouraging findings have emerged from interventions which have attended to some of the specific challenges these groups might face (for instance around body image, discrimination and stigma) while still being affirming of diverse identity statuses (e.g. Brown & Keel, 2015). Meyer's (2015) mapping of the resilience factors of sexual and gender minority communities points to the role of peer support, positive role models and policy-level interventions which can support individual health.

Lawrence on finding social support:

> *"When I was suffering, I felt completely alone – not just in my day-to-day life, but in society at large. When I searched for help, I couldn't see anyone who looked like me. Knowing now that there are charities, groups, research programmes and social media accounts dedicated solely to minority groups with eating difficulties, I feel so hopeful for people who are now in the position that I once was.*
>
> *When carried out in a healthy and positive way, connections between people with lived experience of eating difficulties can be such a powerful tool – to be recognised by someone who has had a similar path as you can provide some true mutual resilience."*

Learning point 3

Having read this chapter, take a moment to reflect on what you may have learnt about experiences of eating difficulties amongst the LGBTQ+ community.

- Is there anything that surprised you in this chapter?
- Are there any networks you can access, either locally or remotely, which could provide positive peer support and connection?
- Are there any ways in which you might change how you support someone with eating difficulties, or how you understand your own experiences? What might you do, or see, differently?

Summary

Eating difficulties are often complex, multifaceted and situated within context. This chapter has discussed how people from LGBTQ+ backgrounds may have lives situated within the context of additional pressures and risk factors which may make them more likely to develop eating difficulties and less likely to be able to access support that is inclusive and relevant to their needs. Improving the experiences of LGBTQ+ people experiencing eating difficulties starts with listening to and understanding these difficulties, without casting judgement or making assumptions. Each of us being willing to do what we can to make our spaces, treatments and individual behaviour more affirming and inclusive can make a difference.

Useful resources

Stonewall: Leading LGBTQ+ advocacy charity including links to advice, resources and other LGBTQ+ organisations: www.stonewall.org.uk

Switchboard: LGBT+ helpline - 0300 330 0630, open 10am–10pm every day. Email support: chris@switchboard.lgbt. Online chat is also available through their homepage: https://switchboard.lgbt

MindLine Trans+: a nationwide confidential emotional, mental health support helpline for people who identify as transgender, agender, gender fluid and non-binary: 0300 330 5468. https://bristolmind.org.uk/help-and-counselling/mindline-transplus/

Gendered Intelligence: Network for Therapists and Counsellors aims to support therapists and counsellors to enable a positive experience in a therapy setting for trans people (and their families): http://genderedintelligence.co.uk/

LGBTQIA Health Education Centre report on body image, obesity and eating disorders (2017), including useful questions to ask and a guide to terminology: www.lgbtqiahealtheducation.org/wp-content/uploads/2018/04/EatingDisordersBodyImageBrief.pdf

References

Bell K, Rieger E & Hirsch JK (2019) Eating disorder symptoms and proneness in gay men, lesbian women, and transgender and gender non-conforming adults: comparative levels and a proposed mediational model. *Frontiers in Psychology* **9** (2692). https://doi.org/10.3389/fpsyg.2018.02692

Bowman MK (2018) The lived experience of transgender individuals with eating disorders. College of Science and Health Theses and Dissertations. p255.

Duffy ME, Henkel KE & Earnshaw VA (2016) Transgender clients' experiences of eating disorder treatment. *J LGBT Issues Couns.* 10 (3) 136–49. https://doi.org/10.1080/15538605.2016.1177806.

Brown TA & Keel PK (2015) A randomized controlled trial of a peer co-led dissonance-based eating disorder prevention program for gay men. *Behav Res Ther* **74** 1–10. https://doi.org/10.1016/j.brat.2015.08.008.

Friedli L & World Health Organization (2009) *Mental health, resilience and inequalities* [online]. Available at: www.euro.who.int/__data/assets/pdf_file/0012/100821/E92227.pdf (accessed August 2021).

Fussner LM & Smith AR (2015) It's not me, it's you: perceptions of partner body image preferences associated with eating disorder symptoms in gay and heterosexual men. *J Homosex* **62** (10) 1329–44. https://doi.org/10.1080/00918369.2015.1060053.

Gordon AR, Austin S, Pantalone B, Baker DW, Eiduson RAM & Rodgers R (2019) Appearance ideals and eating disorders risk among LGBTQ college students: the being ourselves living in diverse bodies (BOLD) study. *J Adolesc Health* **64** (2) S43–4. https://doi.org/10.1016/j.jadohealth.2018.10.096.

Griffiths S, Murray SB, Dunn M & Blashill AJ (2017) Anabolic steroid use among gay and bisexual men living in Australia and New Zealand: associations with demographics, body dissatisfaction, eating disorder psychopathology, and quality of life. *Drug Alcohol Depend* **181** 170–6. https://doi.org/10.1016/j.drugalcdep.2017.10.003.

Meyer IH (2015) Resilience in the study of minority stress and health of sexual and gender minorities. *Psychol Sex Orientat Gend Divers* **2** (3) 209–13. https://doi.org/10.1037/sgd0000132.

Miller B & Behm-Morawitz E (2020) Investigating the cultivation of masculinity and body self-attitudes for users of mobile dating apps for men who have sex with men. *Psychology Men Masculinities* **21** (2) 266–77. https://doi.org/10.1037/men0000221.

Nagata JM, Ganson KT & Austin SB (2020) Emerging trends in eating disorders among sexual and gender minorities. *Current Opinion in Psychiatry* **33** (6) 562-567.

Parker LL & Harriger JA (2020) Eating disorders and disordered eating behaviors in the LGBT population: a review of the literature. *Journal of Eating Disorders* **8** (1) 1-20.

Watson LB, Velez BL, Brownfield J & Flores MJ (2016) Minority stress and bisexual women's disordered eating: The role of deleterious coping. *Counsel Psychol* **44** (8) 1158–86. https://doi.org/10.1177/0011000016669233.

Williams EP, Russell-Mayhew S & Ireland A (2018) Disclosing an eating disorder: A situational analysis of online accounts. *The Qualitative Report* **23** (4) 914-931.

8. Social media and living with eating difficulties

By Wendy Solomons, Nick Hawkes, Nuha Chowdhury

Illustrations by Annie Clarke

Summary
Many of us live significant parts of our lives online. In fact, almost everything we do in 'real life' has an online counterpart. But social media and social networking sites (SNS) have some unique qualities: they are specifically designed to hold our attention; there is a frequent focus on self-presentation and performance (with the potential for personally felt shame or even public shaming when 'standards' are not met); they cast long shadows (contributions made long ago can be retrieved, ruminated on and criticised); hidden algorithms can construct interpersonal 'echo chambers' and personal 'rabbit holes'; and they are increasingly hard to avoid. This chapter looks at the significance of different social media for people with eating difficulties, exploring their relationship with body satisfaction, identity, health and wellbeing, how they tap into vulnerabilities and perpetuate difficulties, as well as how they can support recovery.

Social media as part of contemporary life
Social media – digital forms of communication and information sharing via apps or website on computers, tablets, mobile phones and other devices – provide opportunities for entertainment, discovering new information and ideas, and engaging with existing and new communities of people. Different platforms may focus primarily on text, audio or video-based communications. Much has been written about the impact of social media on our wellbeing, accompanied by alarming headlines and public concern. Yet robust research suggests that findings are less clear-cut, the relationships more nuanced (eg, Huang, 2017; Coyne *et al*, 2020). Trolling and cyberbullying can be terrible, for example, but online communities can also provide a haven for those who are bullied and excluded in other parts of their lives. To ask whether social media is 'good' or 'bad' for us may be the wrong question – we might as well ask whether it is good or bad to go outside. It depends where we are going, when, to do what, and with whom, and how we are feeling to begin with.

How are social media relevant to eating difficulties?

It is hardly surprising that the difficulties we face – including problems around eating, body dissatisfaction or our relationships to these – can unfold in the virtual world as much as in any other area of our lives. Eating difficulties, including those which can be diagnosed as 'disorders', take many forms, but they often centre around preoccupations with eating, weight, shape and appearance, and our ability to control these. This can be tied in with distress about other areas of our lives – relationships, for example, or traumatic things that have happened or are still happening, or worries about our future. There are often wider concerns about our identities and value in life (*"Am I successful / attractive / lovable / good enough?"*) and how we compare to others (*"Are they 'better' than me?"*). Then comes the idea that perhaps our lives and relationships could be different if only our eating and bodies were as we (or maybe other people) might want them to be.

Attempts to control our eating or body appearance can seem like a solution, and may even bring some initial benefits, serving to distract from other problems or pain, making us feel a bit better about ourselves, or bringing some change in how other people treat us. In societies that put so much emphasis on appearance and 'success' (in all its different forms), this is a common experience as we compare ourselves to those around us. Sometimes such concerns are manageable, fleeting or balanced by other aspects of life. Sometimes, though, there is a kind of 'tipping point': thoughts, emotions and behaviour (positive or negative) around control of eating and bodies (including compulsive exercise or purging) become preoccupations. They can take up an increasing proportion of time and energy each day, and become 'overvalued': that is, our judgement of ourselves (whether we are 'good enough') becomes overly dependent on our eating or our bodies; and the dominating value given to these aspects of life forms the psychological core of most 'eating disorders' (Fairburn, 1997).

There can be initial or sporadic 'hits' of positive experiences, feelings of achievement or social validation. These can often reinforce vicious cycles, increasingly convincing us that meeting such targets is the only way to feel good. The focus of attention narrows further, like an obsession accompanied by compulsive repetitive behaviours. Other areas of life – relationships, interests that might have provided a balance – can become pushed aside. This is the 'rabbit hole' of an eating difficulty or 'disorder' (ED).

Figure 8.1

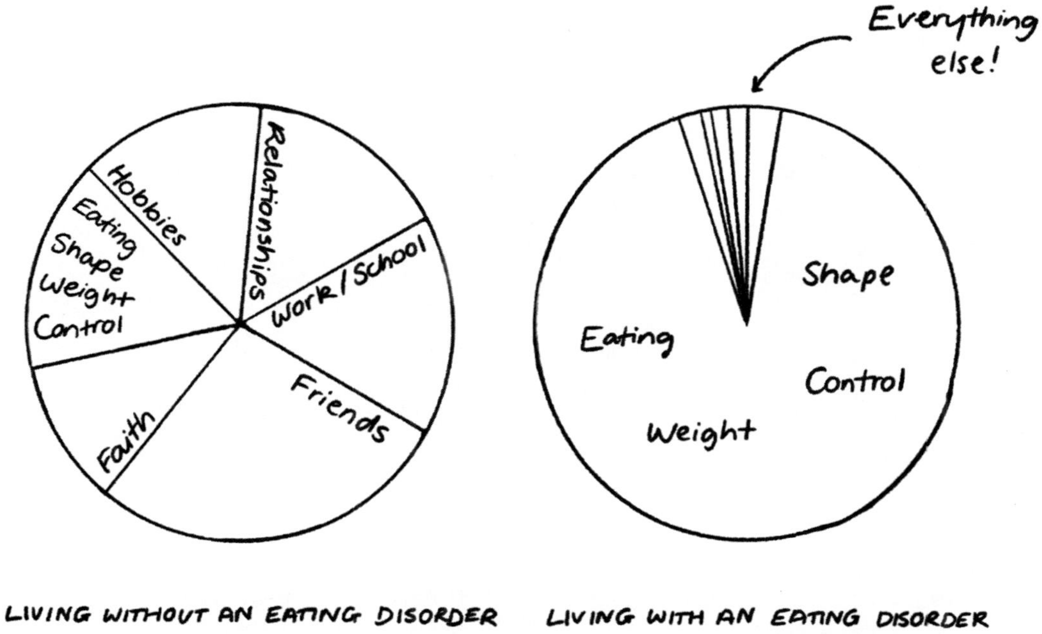

Learning point 1

Take a look at Figure 8.1, above, and reflect on some of your own experiences. Ask yourself:

- How would this look for me? What occupies my thoughts, feelings and actions?
- And what about my time online – what occupies my attention and activity on social media?

The narrowing preoccupations with weight, shape, appearance and control that accompany eating difficulties are not only mirrored in social media use, but can be actively accelerated and maintained by the nature and technological aspects of SNS that capture and hold attention and reinforce particular types of behaviour over others. Figure 8.2 builds on the work of Fairburn (2008) in highlighting some vicious cycles associated with the overvaluation of eating, shape, weight and control (ESWC) that can be involved in the development and maintenance of eating difficulties – each illustrated here with examples of how social media can become part of these processes.

Figure 8.2

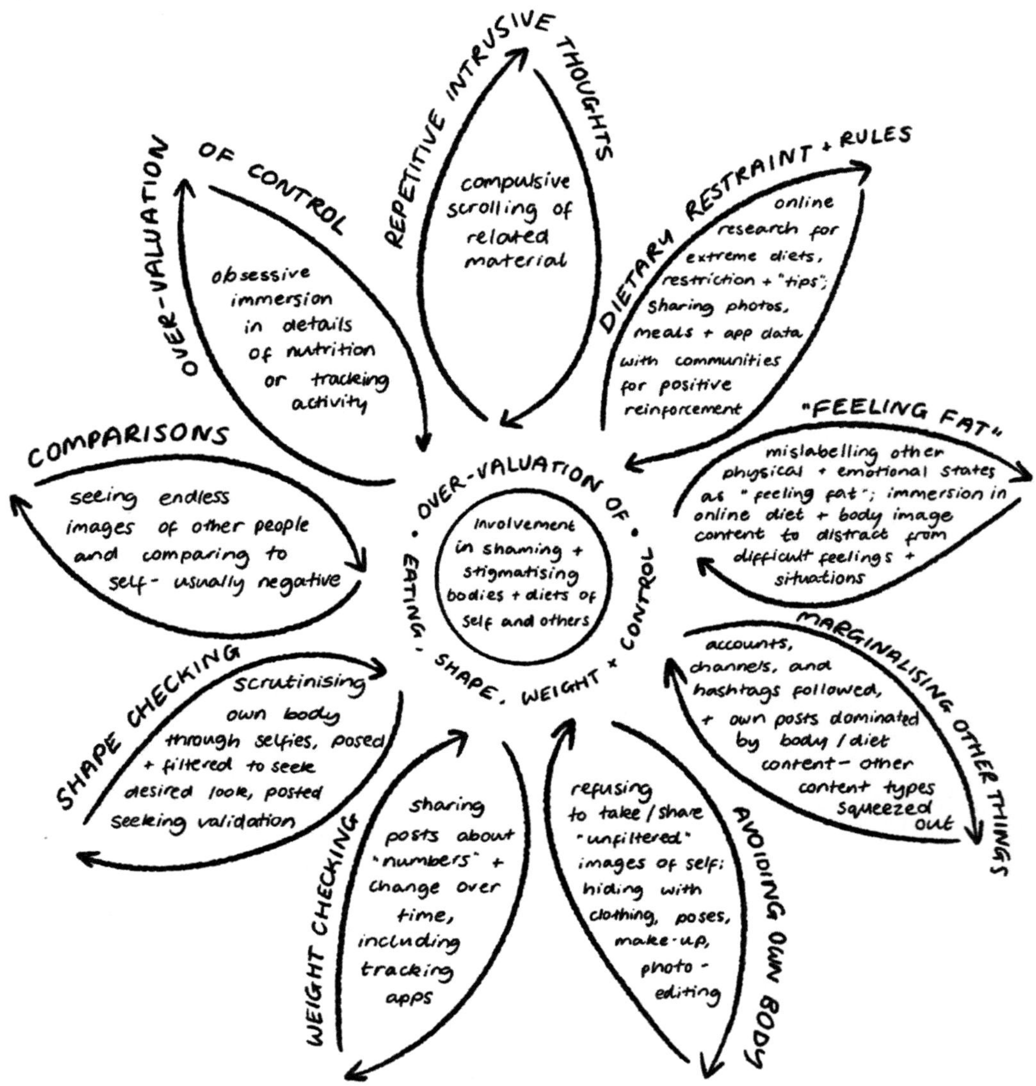

Social media and comparisons: into the rabbit hole

While social comparisons are normal, the nature of social media takes things to a whole new level, leading to unrealistic comparisons where we are almost certain to 'fall short'. Historically, people lived in relatively small communities. Where once we could compare ourselves to family members, work or classmates, now we can compare ourselves against millions of stories and images (of homes, of families, of work, of holidays, of leisure – and, yes, of meals and bodies). And although the internet can allow us to see a huge diversity of living situations, a great deal of social media, especially what is promoted and prioritised on SNSs, focuses on the lives of the relatively privileged, and those who conform to dominant societal ideals of beauty or success. These can appear to be pictures of how our own lives 'should' be. It's easy to forget that they are carefully selected, edited and manipulated, as well as potentially endless, representing unrealistic comparisons that are impossible for most of us. Even though we may 'know' this, this degree of unfair comparison can be damaging to mental health (Meier & Gray, 2013). 'Passive' use of social media (e.g. scrolling and consuming), tends to be worse for mental wellbeing than active involvement and communication (Verduyn *et al*, 2021).

Economics and technologies of social media: deepening the rabbit hole?

It's easy to forget that social media platforms are developed as businesses, designed to harvest people's attention in order to sell this to advertisers. The nature of these platforms (e.g. hashtags, links, liked/followed/recommended accounts, 'influencers' and algorithms) means that, once we have shown interest in particular types of online content, we will increasingly be presented with similar material, and brought into contact with communities who hold similar – or perhaps more extreme – interests. This may initially be welcome, especially for those who feel isolated by their experiences. However, it can also take us further into personal rabbit holes, creating 'echo chambers' that fail to challenge or to balance particular preoccupations (eg, Tan *et al*, 2016). When posting a picture of a 'weight loss journey' to a particular diet-focused community results in many 'likes' – not balanced by the views of others outside this community – these reinforce the dependence of self-esteem on weight control, looking a certain way, or being part of this particular group.

The value that societies place on weight and appearance is inevitably represented in online content, and in turn advertised products like fitness apps and diets plans. Kim Kardashian's 'diet lollipop' was one notorious example. It is hard to avoid this type of content, but for those experiencing eating difficulties, social media's algorithms can quickly parallel and accelerate internal preoccupation, deepening the rabbit hole effect. Societal 'diet culture' and associated weight stigma (including negative comments or 'trolling' of those who do not conform) is widespread online. It is detrimental to many, but also implicated in the development and maintenance of eating difficulties (Puhl & Suh, 2015).

There is a continuum: some content (e.g. 'healthy eating', exercise and fitness programmes) is normalized, even endorsed by government bodies; some is less clear (eg, 'clean' or fad diet promotion, or more extreme focus on 'lean', muscular bodies); and some moves more obviously into to realm of pro-ED (eg, pro-ana) material. The borders are not always clear. Apps that increase pre-occupation with diet- or weight-related detail and 'numbers' are particularly hazardous (Levinson *et al*, 2017). Yet these may offer SNS components that foster a sense of community identity that is particularly attractive to those who are already feeling socially isolated or low in self-esteem, but which can make them harder to leave.

Finding ways out of the rabbit hole

The path out of eating difficulties can be hard. It is likely to require support from others – either trusted friends and family, or professionals – so a first step is to seek this support. Making changes to social media use is only one part of the wider picture. Social media use – like the thoughts and actions linked to eating distress – tend to become automatic habits. It takes conscious decisions and actions to change that. Much of the process involves first increasing awareness of what you are doing and the impact it has, before actively experimenting with different ways of using social media.

Learning point 2

Take a moment to reflect on your own use of social media, and ask yourself:

- How much time each day do I spend on social media? On what sites/apps?
- Check in with yourself: how am I feeling? Do this before, during and after using particular sites, across different days. This could general mood, stress level, self-criticism – and concerns about body/eating/weight in particular.
- Are there any patterns here?

It can help to make a note of this… it might be helpful to use old-fashioned pen and paper!

Alternatively, 'Recovery Record' and 'Rise Up' are examples of apps that can be used to self-monitor behaviours that maintain eating difficulties – specific social media use could be tracked as a 'target' behaviour.

Broadly, there are two approaches to adapting social media use to support wellbeing:

- Identifying and reducing or interrupting behaviours that lock in eating difficulties, and related mental health difficulties.
- Finding ways in which social media can help to nurture other elements of life, identity and positive wellbeing.

Where you've noticed some negative impacts of particular social media use, some practical ways of interrupting this include:

Using general advice on managing social media – for instance experimenting with:

- switching off devices for short periods (and use a separate alarm clock, so you can turn your phone off at night)
- using a timer to help you keep track of time online (some apps include time limiters or feedback on use)
- turning off notifications for apps, and moving the apps off the home screens into a separate folder – so you can choose to go there if you want, but they don't get to demand your attention

Remember to check-in *during* SNS use too: it might be great for a short time, but endless scrolling tends to become progressively less helpful.

Then think about how you are 'fed' different content.

- check settings, and how each app uses your data.
- take the time to 'manage your preferences', and then delete, mute, block or unfollow particular accounts, users or key words.
- it may be necessary to delete entire apps (at least temporarily), or even to delete your own account and build a new one from scratch, to interrupt the influence of your data history on the algorithms that determine what content is pushed at you.

In parallel with these 'limiting' techniques, think about how your social media usage might positively support other aspects of your identity and interests, outside of eating difficulties.

Learning point 3

Reflect on your values and what you want from life. Ask yourself:

- What matters to you, outside of eating – or appearance-related concerns?
- What values are important to you? What sort of a person do you want to be – and what qualities to you have that you'd like to nurture?
- What interests or activities – enjoyed in the past, or that you see others doing, or that you might like for the future – 'fit' with these?
- What aspects of social media reflect this? Are there different sites or people to follow, who might help you develop these areas, and these aspects of your identity?

If you have your own personal experience of eating difficulties, consider discussing these questions with other people. Eating difficulties can make you forget these other, important areas of yourself. It can also feel hard to 'let go' of people, groups and identities that you have been engaged with, even if you know that they are harming you. This process may need to be taken gradually, supported by other people.

Begin to fill your 'feed' and devices with apps or content that meet these interests and values. Of course, finding new areas of social media to explore isn't the whole story – and ideally this will also lead to developing activity and relationships 'in real life' too. Here are some examples from people who are experts by their own experiences of eating difficulties, and who have developed other interests and identities as part of their recovery – online and beyond.

Figure 8.3

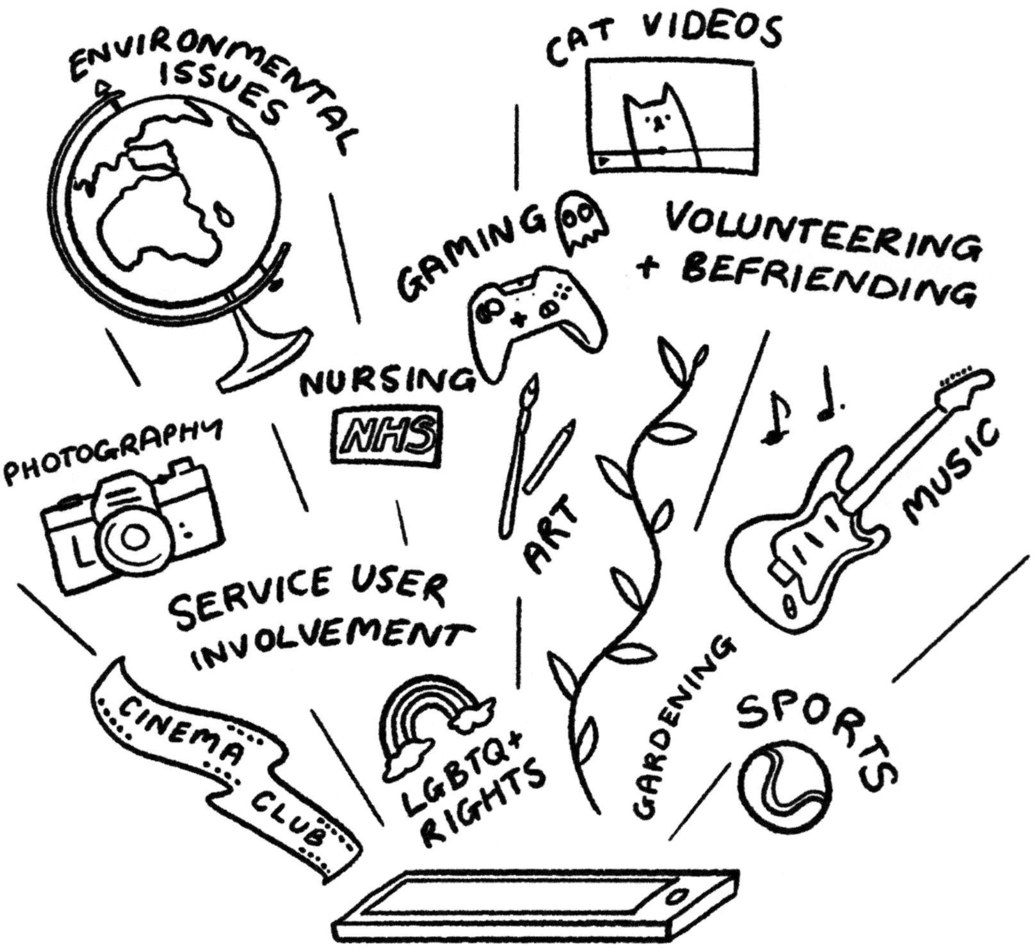

At some point you may need to decide whether you want to be involved with content that is related to eating difficulties, but in a positive or more healthy way. Some people benefit from groups that actively promote a different approach to weight and appearance (eg, 'pro-recovery', body positivity or HAES (health at every size). Some feel supported by a non-judgmental community who have had some similar experiences but want to take a different path now. For others, this type of focus just maintains the preoccupation with eating and appearance, so doesn't help and can even be 'triggering' – or can lead to feeling pressure to support others at the expense of one's own wellbeing. Paths to 'recovery' are complicated, so material posted on multi-user sites will reflect this and it's not always possible to predict what you'll find here. Everyone is different, issues are not always clear-cut, and you may need different things at different times on your own path.

Learning from my experience: social media and life beyond eating difficulties

I knew social media was having a negative impact on my wellbeing so I tried unfollowing some people and accounts relating to eating disorders. I figured I could use social media to find inspiration for baking and cooking which was something I used to enjoy, but soon fell down the same rabbit hole. Baking recipes led to 'healthy eating' content, which quickly sucked me in towards diet culture… In the end, I had to delete my whole profile and start again. I decided to steer clear of any content to do with food as it seemed inevitable that I would always be led back to diet culture in some way.

It's taken a while to find a way to remain on social media without it having some sort of negative effect. Diet culture seems to be everywhere and almost impossible to avoid. Now I tend to follow animal-related content, and particularly enjoy watching videos of cats doing stupid things. I know it seems silly, but it never fails to put a smile on my face – and my friends and I share them, so it's an easy way to keep in touch. I know some people find apps like Headspace helpful for relaxation, too.

Social media now helps me explore the others parts of me that aren't related to my eating disorder. I've discovered new hobbies, and inspiration for exciting things me and my friends can try together.

Conclusion

The paths into and out of eating difficulties are varied. Social media are unlikely to be the main 'culprits', or solutions, but they do pose particular challenges for those experiencing a range of eating difficulties. With some thought and support, however, there are ways to limit their worst impacts, and even use them to support paths to wellbeing.

The world of social media changes quickly, though. Some of the recommendations made here may become out-of-date within just a few years. Organizations like BEAT, and resources from FREED (below), are a good place to keep in touch with developments affecting those experiencing eating difficulties, including the fast-moving challenges of life online.

With thanks to Wen Jin for input in the early stages of this work

Resources

BEAT – UK eating disorder charity – includes information, resources and peer support, including social media: www.beateatingdisorders.org.uk/
www.beateatingdisorders.org.uk/your-stories/eating-disorders-and-social-media

Freedom from ED (South London and Maudsley NHS Foundation Trust)
Social Media and Apps – Friends or Foes? A guide to help address your concerns about body image, eating disorders and mental health. https://freedfromed.co.uk/img/guides/Social_Media_And_Apps-FREED.pdf

References

Brownell KD (1991) Dieting and the search for the perfect body: Where physiology and culture collide *Behavior Therapy* **22** (1) 1-12.

Coyne SM, Rogers AA, Zurcher JD, Stockdale L & Booth M (2020) Does time spent using social media impact mental health?: An eight year longitudinal study. *Computers in Human Behavior* **104** 106-160.

Eikey EV & Madhu C, Reddy MC (2017). "It's Definitely Been a Journey": A Qualitative Study on How Women with Eating Disorders Use Weight Loss Apps. Proceedings of the 2017 CHI Conference on Human Factors in Computing Systems. Association for Computing Machinery, New York, NY, USA, 642–654.

Fairburn CG (2008) *Cognitive behavior therapy and eating disorders*. Guilford Press.

Huang C (2017) Time Spent on Social Network Sites and Psychological Well-Being: A Meta-Analysis. *Cyberpsychology, Behavior, and Social Networking* **20** (6) 346-354.

Levinson CA, Fewell L & Brosof LC (2017) My Fitness Pal calorie tracker usage in the eating disorders, *Eating Behaviors* **27** 14-16.

Meier EP & Gray J (2013) Facebook Photo Activity Associated with Body Image Disturbance in Adolescent Girls. *Cyberpsychology, Behavior, and Social Networking* **17** (4) 199-206.

Puhl R & Suh Y (2015) Stigma and eating and weight disorders. *Current Psychiatry Reports* **17** 552-561.

Tan T, Kuek A, Goh SE, Lee EL & Kwok V (2016) Internet and smartphone application usage in eating disorders: A descriptive study in Singapore. *Asian Journal of Psychiatry* **19** 50-55.

Verduyn P, Gugushvili N & Kross E (2021) The impact of social network sites on mental health: distinguishing active from passive use. *World Psychiatry: Official journal of the World Psychiatric Association (WPA)* **20** (1) 133–134.

9. Mirror, mirror, on your wall: The impact of fashion on eating difficulties

By Ameerah Khadaroo and Jekaterina Rogaten

Ella is a young woman who likes hanging around with her friends, dressing up to the occasion and spending quite a lot of time on her phone. As time goes by and without her necessarily making an active choice, she gradually finds herself engaging in restricted eating and quite strict dieting. Why do women like Ella feel that they need to change their eating patterns?

Fashion and beauty advertisements are all around us. You see fashion advertisements on your daily commute to work, on billboards, in shop windows during your leisurely walks, in multiple magazines scattered around coffee tables, on TV around every 20 minutes and, of course, on your social media feed. These advertisements repeatedly present how you should look, and for women the message is quite clear: one needs to be relatively tall, slim, young and Caucasian. Men are also increasingly becoming fashion conscious, although beauty standards for males are more diverse. In general, they experience less pressure to fit stereotypical images and standards of physical appearance. In this chapter, we will look at how fashion impacts on our relationship with food, primarily focusing on how the acceptance of socially constructed beauty standards affects eating behaviour.

'I'm on this new diet, it's very effective. Well, I don't eat anything and when I feel like I'm about to faint I eat a cube of cheese.' (Emily, from The Devil Wears Prada)

The fashion industry has for years been criticised for giving minimum consideration to the health and wellbeing of fashion models: for example, some models are "eating just three apples a day to suppress hunger" (Dauxerre, 2017). Drawing on her lived experience as a professional former French model, Victoire Maçon Dauxerre, who also wrote a book about her life as a disappearing model, drew attention to fashion models being at high risk of suffering from eating difficulties just so they can fit the clothes they are asked to advertise. She described her experience battling anorexia and bulimia. Since leaving her modelling career she has become an ambassador, promoting change within the industry to reduce the likelihood of models like herself going through the experiences she went through.

Victoire's experience is not an exception, but rather the norm. Many young fashion models embark on a modelling career that gradually pressurises them to lose weight drastically (subsequently spiralling into eating difficulties), so that they can fit into size zero clothing. A survey of 3,000 models conducted by researchers from a Danish beauty industry group revealed that 94% of the sample was severely underweight (Rosenbaum, 2016). Unfortunately, the health compromise involved is often dismissed, with the focus being on becoming a successful and beautiful model whose 'perfect physique' is admired by all. This is strongly motivated by unrealistic demands from the industry such as looking skinny and flawless, which can influence the model's lived experience of reaching their professional goals – no matter what it takes.

A recent qualitative research study examining the experiences of fashion models further highlighted the extremes that models resort to in order survive in this harsh industry, such as self-imposed starvation (Super & Khadaroo, 2019). Other scholars have also repeatedly identified eating difficulties as a serious health issue among fashion models (see Zancu & Enea, 2017, for a review).

Although there are increasingly more efforts made to promote the wellbeing of fashion models, including displaying more acceptance for diverse body shapes and sizes (e.g. Boohoo and Adidas), it is just not enough and many young female models are still being trapped in cognitive distortions of their body image. For example, some women might catastrophize with the thought of failing to meet the thin ideal, and this subsequently fuels feelings of anxiety, depression and self-blame in cases where a strict restriction on one's diet is not adhered to. This can even lead them to develop thoughts that others think they are "too fat". In fact, this pressure to comply with unrealistic beauty standards does not just impact on models. Women have similar experiences in other fashion career paths. For example, Josi Maria, a 24-year-old German social influencer recently lost her life battle against anorexia (Saunt, 2020).

'This... stuff? Oh. Okay. I see. You think this has nothing to do with you...' (Miranda Priestly from The Devil Wears Prada)

Although you may think that the pressure from the fashion industry only affects models and influencers who are being paid to reflect beauty ideals, this is far from the truth. A systematic review of existing evidence on eating difficulties among fashion models concluded that the prevalence of eating difficulties is no higher in fashion models than non-models (see Zancu & Enea, 2017 for a review). So, how does fashion gain such control over our relationship with food?

Whether you are interested in fashion or not, fashion advertising affects your attitudes and behaviour. What is perceived as beautiful and fashionable is largely a matter of what society labels as being so. From a sociocultural perspective, beauty is largely defined by the means through which people obtain messages from society that shape the conceptualization of beauty ideals (Poloskov & Tracey, 2013).

The desire to look good and fashionable is strongly influenced by the creation of schematic beauty ideals (e.g. beauty associated with being super slim, looking young or being Caucasian), that are relatively uniform and universally shared ideas of how specific groups of individuals should look (Zones, 2000, p87). This brings us closer to understanding how fashion affects the creation of beauty schema and our relationship with our bodies. Furthermore, a large body of research spanning the past 70 years that looks at conscious and unconscious information processing and how it affects our judgements, concludes that people like things they are familiar with, even if they are not consciously aware or remember seeing those things (Bornstein, 1989). Thus, what we perceive as beautiful and what we like is largely influenced by our environment. Indeed, we are constantly surrounded by messages of a 'one size fits all' beauty standard.

Learning point 1

- Many people underestimate the number of adverts they see daily. Remember, we are only consciously aware of a small number of these and even if we are not consciously aware of most of them, they still affect us.
- What body shape/size do you perceive as beautiful for a woman?

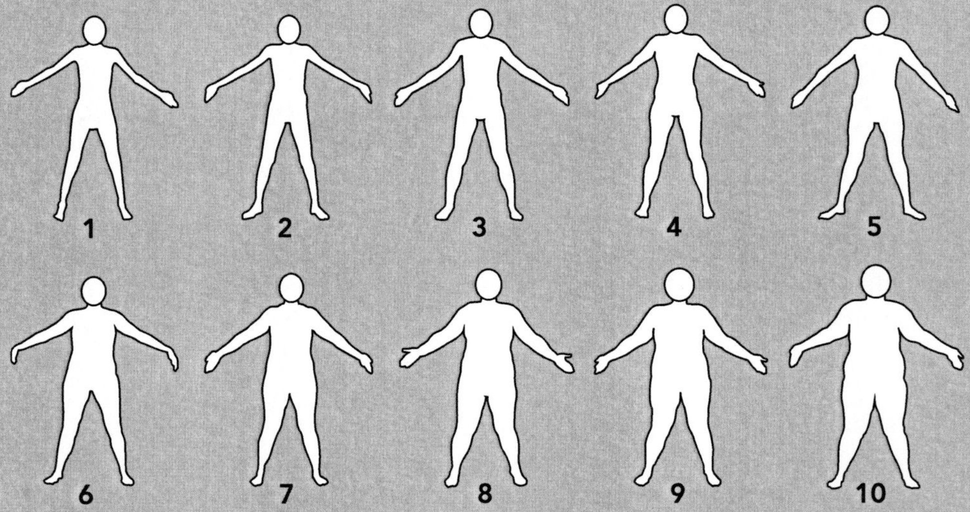

Figure 9.1 (Source: Swami *et al*, 2008, p1755)

For the next day, pay attention to all the advertisements you come across. Fill in this table for every female model you see:

Model's ethnicity	Model's age (estimated guess)	Model's body size (as shown in the pictures above 1-10)

Compare how your beauty standard relates to the models you see in the advertisements. What number have you picked as an ideal body image?

The images in Figure 9.1 above presented two models in each of the established five BMI categories: emaciated (<15 kg/m2), underweight (15–18.5 kg/m2), normal (18.5–24.9 kg/m2), overweight (25.0–29.9 kg/m2), and obese (>30 kg/m2). The images representing normal BMI are 5 and 6 (Swami *et al*, 2008).

"I'm just one stomach flu away from my goal weight" (Emily from The Devil Wears Prada)

Eating is an aesthetic and moral practice (Holla, 2020). In line with Maslow's hierarchy of needs theory, we are generally motivated to fulfil our basic needs (e.g., physiological needs) before moving up the hierarchy to meet higher needs such as esteem and self-actualization. When discussing the impact of fashion on eating difficulties, although the starting point remains the physiological needs, the need for food is deliberately and drastically altered to reach higher needs. For instance, achieving self-actualization and higher self-esteem by developing a fashionable self that reflects the internalization of stereotypical beauty standards and the thin ideal makes the body an object through which a fashionable self and identity is created.

In an endeavour to self-actualize and in the absence of objective and diverse beauty standards, it is common to find people comparing themselves to others to know where they stand (Festinger, 1954). Women's increasing awareness of beauty standards and ideals often cause them to compare their self-perceived appearance with ideal standards of beauty, and this has been shown to predict lower self-esteem with the internalization of the thin ideal as a moderating factor (Balcetis *et al*, 2013). Furthermore, in line with objectification theory which explains a tendency to view the self, in particular one's body or specific aspects of the body as an *object*, females experience considerably more sociocultural pressures that influence how they evaluate themselves with a focus on their body, and this is strongly linked to their sense of self-worth (Arroyo *et al*, 2014). Closely self-monitoring one's appearance to meet beauty ideals and reach the ideal physical self suggests that social needs are satisfied, eliciting a positive feeling of a sense of belonging.

The beauty standards imposed by society and the media can have a substantial influence on the formation of the ideal self. For women, beauty standards have become an important tool that shapes their own self-identity with increasing emphasis on appearance self-monitoring (Britt, 2015). The discrepancy between ideal physical self and perceived actual physical self can give rise to psychological tension and potential negative emotions, leading to the experience of severe body image concerns such as body dysmorphic disorder or mood disorders that can cause many women and men to feel dissatisfied with their body. Often, they are just not happy with how they look and they struggle to meet societal expectations around fashion and beauty. This can create a feeling of self-doubt – 'Am I good enough?' combined with negative emotions resulting from body dissatisfaction that can trigger disordered eating behaviours such as anorexia or bulimia in the pursuit of unattainable beauty standards.

Past research showed that exposure to thin ideal images, including images based on social comparisons, promoted negative mood and body dissatisfaction in women (Tiggemann *et al*, 2009). Sadly, fashion media is also plagued with digitally enhanced images and cosmetic surgery, which further feed into the creation of an ideal self that is far from being realistic or achievable. Internalising a desire to meet unattainable beauty standards in many instances requires a drastic modification in eating habits.

When examining how fashion can impact the way we form beauty standards and evaluate our own bodies in relation to these standards, it leaves us to wonder if people are sufficiently aware of this fake appearance-based reality created by the media. For example, the so-called perfect tanned bikini body with no trace of any blemishes, cellulites, stretch marks or wrinkles. And if so, are they well equipped to react appropriately and healthily to this issue?

Learning point 2

Before you continue reading, think about your own beauty standards.

- How similar is your ideal physical self to the average model body size, shape and general appearance of the skin?
- When looking at social media pictures, can you accurately spot if any image was digitally altered or taken using a filter?

'Everybody wants to be us' (Miranda Priestly from The Devil Wears Prada)

Social comparisons based on appearance are common among young people, especially during the process of identity formation. They regularly compare how they look, their body size and shape, with their peers and people who they classify as role models, such as fashion influencers, fashion models and celebrities. Recent research has shown that Instagram use with beauty-related images negatively impacted self-rated attractiveness, which also correlated with anxiety, low self-esteem, depressive symptoms and body dissatisfaction (Sherlock & Wagstaff, 2019). This social comparison is further strengthened when some form of reward or incentive is associated with people who invest highly in fashion and appearance (for example, media attention, fame, success, status, popularity). However, the major pitfall here is the experience of a decline in self-acceptance, which can be followed by an obsession to go to extremes to look like role models.

Therefore, the younger generation's exposure to fashion media and how fashion-related information is processed and internalised (with an impact on health and wellbeing) should be very closely monitored and challenged. There needs to be greater recognition of the role played by celebrities as powerful fashion role models and adequate measures are put in place to regulate the impact of fashion media on people both within and outside the fashion industry. This is an even more pressing issue when faced with the Covid-19 pandemic. Current research shows that people used more social media during lockdowns as a coping mechanism (Gao *et al*, 2020). This period was also highlighted as being particularly challenging for children and young people with an eating difficulty, given the experience of social isolation, limited physical exercises and disruption to their everyday life. Notably, a recent study showed that stress and anxiety brought about by the pandemic were associated with negative body image in the context of physical and social distancing (Swami *et al*, 2021). In fact, these findings are supported by other research revealing that, during lockdown, adolescents and young women used social network sites considerably more, which positively correlated with body dissatisfaction, increased drive for thinness and a higher risk of suffering from eating difficulties (Vall-Roqué *et al*, 2021).

Learning point 3

- Have a look at these two images (one original and one altered) and list how many features in each image have been changed/enhanced using digital filters.

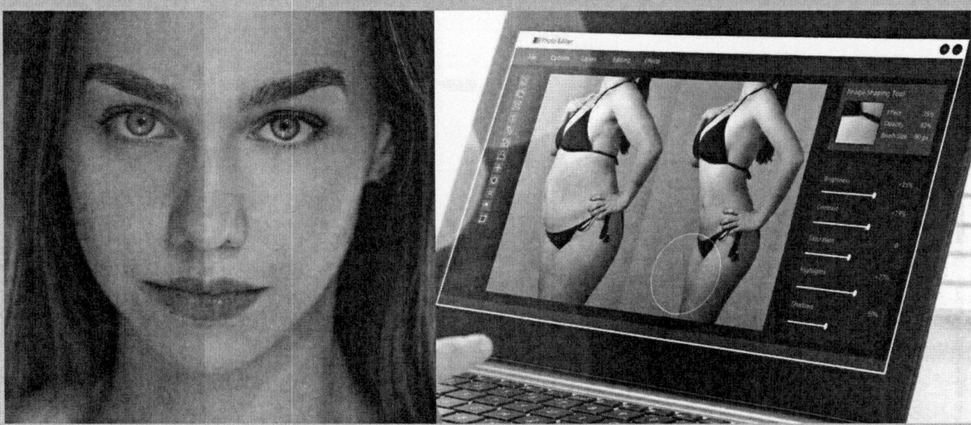

Figure 9.2

- How often do you use digital filters when taking pictures of yourself and how does this affect your relationship with your body and food?

Examples of manipulation are shown in the images presented in Figure 9.2 above (Kleemans *et al*, 2018, p. 98): Instagram photos emphasising face (removing eye bags), skin (removing wrinkles), or body (on the right: reshaping legs and waist to appear slimmer).

New research looking at the link between image-centred social media platforms and identity formation among young people concluded that new online appearance-focused interaction platforms, especially when selfie filters are involved, play a key role in increasing interpersonal uncertainty that can trigger body dysmorphic disorder and other forms of body image distortions (Tremblay *et al*, 2021).

"Alright everyone, gird your loins!" Nigel from 'The Devil Wears Prada'

The new 'fashionable' workout era is here. Over the last decade some attention has been drawn to a shift from a traditional approach to beauty and fashion (e.g. red lips, pretty dresses, dainty look etc.) to a more health and fitness representation of beauty, with a sharp rise in health and fitness magazines as a dominant source of weight-loss and body-shaping messages (Conlin & Bissell, 2014). However, research evidence shows that there was no difference in the depiction of the thin ideal in models in beauty and fashion magazines (e.g. *Cosmopolitan*, *Glamour*, and *Marie Claire*) or those in health and fitness magazines (e.g. *Shape*, *Fitness*, and *Women's Health*). Although fashion and beauty from a health and fitness perspective is expected to revolve around healthy and 'normal' body weight, research such as that by Conlin and Bissell points towards a representation of a thin and glamourous ideal that is *still* more appearance based (i.e. a perfect toned physique) than health focused (i.e. healthy body images). This is alarming, as despite the growing trend for a fit and healthy body, the association between a perfect body and restrictive eating still prevails, which signals that the risk of suffering from eating difficulties in the pursuit of the ideal physical self is still present in disguise. Therefore, this raises an important question: when will the fashion and beauty industry and media step in and work towards the conceptualization and representation of the perfect body as one which is simply about a healthy BMI that works for everyone?

Learning point 4

- Think about whether your beauty standards have changed over time with more focus on 'looking fit'.
- Reflect upon the extent to which this has influenced your eating behaviours.

Conclusion

While one may believe that only people directly involved in the fashion world such as models and influencers are at risk for eating difficulties when facing the pressures and expectations of the industry, it is equally important to note that everyone is, to a certain extent, affected by it. However, there is hope, with some brands starting to diversify their advertisements and include people of various body shapes and sizes. Paired with the new trend of fitness, healthy eating and wellbeing, there is also the hope that the fashion industry can use its widespread influence for the better and reduce, or even reverse, the negative impact it currently has on our relationships with our bodies and our food.

References

Arroyo A, Segrin C & Harwood J (2014) Appearance-Related Communication Mediates the Link Between Self-Objectification and Health and Well-Being Outcomes, *Human Communication Research* **40** (4) pp,463-482.

Balcetis E, Cole S, Chelberg MB & Alicke M (2013) Searching out the ideal: Awareness of ideal body standards predicts lower global self-esteem in women. *Self and Identity* **12** (1) pp99-113.

Bornstein RF (1989) Exposure and affect: Overview and meta-analysis of research 1968–1987. *Psychological Bulletin* **106** (2) pp265-289.

Britt RK (2015) Effects of self-presentation and social media use in attainment of beauty ideals. *Studies in Media and Communication* **3** (1) pp79-88.

Conlin L & Bissell K (2014) Beauty ideals in the checkout aisle: Health-related messages in women's fashion and fitness magazines. *Journal of Magazine and New Media Research* **15** (2) pp1-19.

Dauxerre V (2017) *Size Zero: My Life as a Disappearing Model*, William Collins.

Festinger L (1954) A theory of social comparison processes. *Human Relations* **7** (2) pp117-140.

Gao J, Zheng P, Jia Y, Chen H, Mao Y, Chen S & Dai J (2020) Mental health problems and social media exposure during COVID-19 outbreak. *Plos One* **15** (4) e0231924.

Holla SM (2020) Food in fashion modelling: Eating as an aesthetic and moral practice. *Ethnography* **21** (1) pp26-47.

Kleemans M, Daalmans S, Carbaat I & Anschütz D (2018) Picture perfect: The direct effect of manipulated Instagram photos on body image in adolescent girls. *Media Psychology*, **21**(1), pp.93-110.

Poloskov E & Tracey TJ (2013) Internalization of US female beauty standards as a mediator of the relationship between Mexican American women's acculturation and body dissatisfaction. *Body Image* **10** (4) pp501-508.

Rosenbaum S (2016) Models keep getting skinnier and skinnier. *The New York Post*. Available online at: https://nypost.com/2016/06/09/models-keep-getting-skinnier-and-skinnier/#:~:text=A%20Danish%20beauty%2Dindustry%20group,of%20them%20are%20woefully%20underweight.

Saunt R (2020) German influencer who documented her anorexia battle on social media dies aged 24 after going without food for two days before flying to Gran Canaria on holiday. *DailyMail*. Available online at: www.dailymail.co.uk/femail/article-9074807/Influencer-documented-anorexia-battle-social-media-dies-aged-24.html (accessed August 2021).

Sherlock M & Wagstaff DL (2019) Exploring the relationship between frequency of Instagram use exposure to idealized images and psychological well-being in women, *Psychology of Popular Media Culture* **8** (4) pp482–490.

Super EF & Khadaroo A (2019) *The well-being of fashion models: A qualitative study* (Unpublished master's thesis). University of the Arts: London.

Swami V, Horne G & Furnham A (2021) COVID-19-related stress and anxiety are associated with negative body image in adults from the United Kingdom. *Personality and Individual Differences*, **170**, 110426.

Swami V, Salem N, Furnham A & Tovée MJ (2008) Initial examination of the validity and reliability of the female photographic figure rating scale for body image assessment. *Personality and Individual Differences*, **44**(8), pp.1752-1761.

Tiggemann M, Polivy J & Hargreaves D (2009) The processing of thin ideals in fashion magazines: A source of social comparison or fantasy? *Journal of Social and Clinical Psychology* **28** (1) pp73-93.

Tremblay SC, Tremblay SE & Poirier P (2021) From filters to fillers: An active inference approach to body image distortion in the selfie era. *AI and Society*, **36**(1), pp.33-48.

Vall-Roqué H, Andrés A & Saldaña C (2021) The impact of COVID-19 lockdown on social network sites use, body image disturbances and self-esteem among adolescent and young women. *Progress in Neuro-Psychopharmacology and Biological Psychiatry*, **110**, 110293.

Zancu SA & Enea V (2017) Eating disorders among fashion models: A systematic review of the literature. *Eating and Weight Disorders-Studies on Anorexia Bulimia and Obesity* **22** (3) pp395-405.

Zones JS (2000) Beauty myths and realities and their impacts on women's health. *Gender through the prism of difference* pp87-103.

10. Eating difficulties: Holy self-hatred and the summit of perfection

By Tracey Wade, PhD; Ivana Osenk, BPsychHons; and Madelaine de Valle, BPsychHons

Blackbird Initiative, Órama Institute, Flinders University, Adelaide, South Australia, Australia

Summary

The title of this chapter comes from a quote from Saint Catherine of Siena (1347-1380). She was a high achiever but died from causes likely related to anorexia nervosa in her early 30s. She said: "Make a supreme effort to root out self-love from your heart and to plant in its place this holy self-hatred. This is the royal road by which we turn our backs on mediocrity, and which leads us without fail to the summit of perfection." This chapter explores the relationship between perfectionism and eating difficulties. First, we define perfectionism. Second, we consider its impact on mental health and productivity. Third, we discuss evidence that perfectionism can be decreased. Fourth, we look at what else improves when perfectionism is decreased. Finally, we summArise what we think are the active elements of perfectionism interventions (that is, the bits that really work). A take-home message is that it is possible to decrease perfectionism and its harmful consequences while still pursuing high standards.

Perfectionism defined

Despite being a popular target for research in psychology, perfectionism has been difficult to define. Various theories have been suggested, but these have differed based on the views of each researcher, and to summArise all the definitions of perfectionism is beyond the scope of this chapter. However, researchers generally agree that perfectionism involves setting yourself overly high, and often unrealistic, standards for what you want to achieve, along with making huge efforts to reach these standards, self-criticising when you don't reach them, and dismissing your achievements even when you actually do meet your standards

(Shafran *et al*, 2002). If you're thinking that perfectionists don't win either way – either they don't reach their standards and feel bad, or they discount their achievements when they do – then we agree.

A common question that people have is about the difference between pursuing *perfectionistic* standards and pursuing *high* standards. In other words, what does 'turning down the dial' on perfectionistic standards look like, and what effect does it have? The main differences between pursuing perfectionistic standards versus high standards are about the *difficulty* of the goals that you set yourself, the *intensity* with which you work towards your goals (that is, how much effort you put in to achieve them), and the *savoring* of your accomplishments (that is, whether you stop to enjoy the sense of achievement when you reach your goals). Perfectionism involves trying to achieve flawlessness in a relentless, excessive manner, basing your self-worth entirely on your achievements, and disregarding your successes (for example, "I have to achieve 100% on this test otherwise I am a failure"). Pursuing excellence, on the other hand, allows for *attainable* standards, where you put in a 'good enough' effort to reach your goals and celebrate your successes. We highlight the differences between these two approaches in more detail in Table 10.1.

Table 10.1: Differences between aiming for perfectionistic standards versus high standards

Perfectionistic Standards	High Standards
Setting high goals and working hard towards them but 'almost perfect' is seen as failure: all or nothing thinking	Setting high goals, working hard towards them to be the best you can be, knowing that any outcome helps you to improve
Spotting tiny imperfections in your work and yourself: selective attention for imperfections, ignoring accomplishments	Taking pride in your accomplishments and tending to support others
Tending to be *pushed* toward your goals by a fear of *not* reaching them	Tending to be *pulled* toward your goals by a desire to achieve them
Setting goals that are out of reach or extremely difficult to achieve	Setting goals that are high but not out of reach, enjoying going a little further once your goals are reached
Being so concerned about achieving goals and avoiding failure that you don't enjoy the process of growing/striving	Enjoying the process of chasing a goal as much or more than the actual reaching of the goal itself
Beating yourself up a lot and feeling bad about yourself when you don't meet your standards	Bouncing back fairly easily from disappointment, 'getting back on the bike' more quickly
Feeling much more afraid to fail than most other people	Not enjoying failure but seeing it as a way to get better

Perfectionistic Standards	High Standards
Taking constructive criticism as an attack, reacting defensively to it Being self-critical, believing that beating yourself up will help you to get better results Worrying so much about doing something imperfectly that you freeze and can't do anything at all	Seeing criticism as valuable information to help you improve your future performance Being more likely to use self-compassion Being more likely to approach your valued goals

Research supports the idea that there are important differences between pursuing perfectionistic rather than high standards. Striving for perfection is related to increased depression and anxiety, compared to striving for high standards, which is unrelated to mental health difficulties (Blasberg *et al*, 2016). In addition, while perfectionistic strivings are related to better academic achievement, only the healthy pursuit of high standards seems to protect against harmful outcomes of successful learning (Osenk *et al*, 2020). We discuss this a little more in the next section.

Learning point 1

Before reading further, you may like to consider the following questions:

- Why are perfectionism and eating difficulties so closely linked?
- Is there anything you would add to our definition of perfectionism?
- How would you explain the differences between perfectionistic standards and high standards to a person living with an eating difficulty?

Perfectionism, mental health and productivity

People with perfectionism are more likely to develop eating difficulties, and perfectionism also makes it more challenging to recover from eating difficulties. People with perfectionism are more likely to experience other mental health challenges, too, like anxiety related to social situations, panic attacks, obsessions and depression. Especially worryingly, people with more perfectionism also have more thoughts of suicide and suicidal behaviours than people with less perfectionism (Egan *et al*, 2011; Limburg *et al*, 2017).

People with perfectionism base a lot of their self-esteem on how well they meet very high standards in areas of life that are important to them. Unfortunately, because the standards they set themselves are so demanding, they often 'fall short of the mark', which leads them to self-criticise. Like perfectionism, self-criticism is also linked to poorer mental health, including eating difficulties, depression, anxiety and suicidality. On top of all that, self-criticism is associated with problems in relationships with others (Warren *et al*, 2016). As you can see, perfectionism and self-criticism are bad news!

You may be thinking, "Okay, perfectionism and self-criticism may be bad for my mental health, but I need these things to keep me motivated and productive". This is a common belief, but research suggests that it is not true. People who expect perfection of themselves or tend to self-criticise have worse productivity and more stress and burnout at work. As students, they face more barriers to academic success, including procrastination (putting things off), anxiety about tests, and study-related stress and burnout (Osenk *et al*, 2020). Similarly, self-criticism is linked to poorer progress towards goals, which seems to be due to self-critical people ruminating (repeatedly going over negative things in their head) and procrastinating. In short, perfectionism and self-criticism are not your friends when it comes to getting things done, as you will see in the short case study illustration below.

Case study

Sally experienced perfectionism in various domains in her life, including her standards for eating and appearance, study, work and social interactions. She felt she could never perform to her desired standard. This perfectionism had resulted in an eating difficulty (Bulimia Nervosa), constant procrastination in her study assignments and avoidance of tutorials in case she could not answer questions, sticking to old routines in her rehabilitation work rather than using new protocols "in case they failed", and avoiding social interactions when she was feeling depressed. Things spiralled down over her first few years at university, where she reached the point of not handing in assignments and avoiding most social interactions. She had become quite depressed and did not reach out to lecturers or counselling service staff, or ask for extensions, as this would all be a sign of failure. Ultimately, the university wrote to her an informed her that she would be suspended for five years given she had not submitted assignments or talked to anyone about the reasons for this. To them, she seemed just another disengaged student. They said if she could write and explain by a certain date, they would reconsider. Sally felt that she could not adequately explain her situation in a letter and so the due date went by and Sally was suspended.

Self-compassion

It is one thing for us to be able to say what *doesn't* work, but it's more useful to know what *does* work. That is where self-compassion comes in. Self-compassion means being kind and understanding with yourself during difficult times, when you make a mistake, or when you don't achieve what you set out to do. People who are more self-compassionate tend to have better mental health in the same areas in which people with perfectionism or self-criticism are more likely to struggle, including eating difficulties. Also, they are more likely to achieve their goals or cope well when they don't reach their goals, and they are less likely to procrastinate or worry about studying (Warren *et al*, 2016). Self-compassion is the force that gets you up after you fall off the bike, dresses all the wounds, and then tells you to get back on and have another try. So, if you have perfectionism or self-criticism, all is not lost! Developing self-compassion is one way to tackle this. There is more information on Compassion Focused Therapy for Eating Disorders (CFT-E2) in Chapter 28.

Learning point 2

Before you continue, consider the following:

- Have you experienced any mental health challenges that could be related to perfectionism?
- Are you someone who tends to self-criticise or use self-compassion when things go wrong?
- Can you think of any ways you could include some more self-compassion in your life to help you be more resilient and productive?

Evidence that perfectionism can be decreased

To date there are three meta-analyses that have looked at the effectiveness of perfectionism interventions, and these interventions are all based on cognitive behaviour therapy (CBT). This therapy is delivered in different ways depending on which area of mental health is being targeted, but all CBT interventions are based on the understanding that beliefs (interpretations of an event, or the meaning you take from an experience) lead to emotions, which lead to behaviours. Helping people develop more flexible beliefs allows them to choose from a wider range of reactions to an event, some of which will be more helpful than others.

The earliest meta-analysis on perfectionism interventions included eight studies (Lloyd *et al*, 2015). It looked at differences in participants' perfectionism from the beginning to the end of an intervention. There was a large reduction in perfectionism. This was followed by another meta-analysis, which included ten studies (Suh *et al*, 2019). They focused on comparing intervention groups to control groups. People who received the intervention ended up with significantly lower perfectionism than the control group, both in terms of perfectionistic strivings and perfectionistic concerns, and the difference between the groups was medium-sized. So far, so good – CBT for perfectionism significantly reduces perfectionism.

Evidence that decreasing perfectionism improves general mental health

The two meta-analyses discussed above also showed that perfectionism interventions reduce depression and anxiety, even though these aren't what the interventions focus on. The first noted that there was a moderate reduction in anxiety and depression (Lloyd *et al*, 2015). The second examined face-to-face and online interventions, where eight were conducted on people with perfectionism, one targeted people with an eating difficulty, and one targeted people with perfectionism and obsessive-compulsive disorder (a type of anxiety disorder). They too found significant, medium-sized decreases in depression and anxiety. They also found face-to-face and online interventions to be equally effective (Suh *et al*, 2019).

The third study included nine studies of perfectionism interventions that also examined the impact of the intervention on disordered eating or body image concerns. They concluded that perfectionism interventions caused a large decrease in disordered eating and body image concerns – even bigger than the decreases that we mentioned above for depression and anxiety (Robinson & Wade, 2021).

The evidence we have suggests that, while doing as few as three out of a set of eight treatment modules is enough to decrease perfectionism, it takes more than that to reduce anxiety, depression and disordered eating (Wade *et al*, 2019). It may be that decreasing perfectionism is the pathway to improving mental wellbeing, and reducing your perfectionism needs to happen before you can apply new skills to make changes outside of perfectionism.

Active elements of interventions

We have summArised the 'active elements' (the parts that seem to be most important) of perfectionism interventions in Table 10.2. They may not apply to everyone who is struggling with perfectionism. For example, not everyone experiences procrastination and avoidance, which happen when you can't bear the idea of not getting something right the first time. One thing we do know, and that young people who struggle with perfectionism tell us, is that this is really difficult work to do on your own. Getting support is critical, because the perfectionism will try to tell you that you are not doing well enough, not making enough changes, and not trying your hardest. Having someone on your side, whether it be a therapist, an online therapy, a friend, or a family member, can really help you maintain perspective on the bigger picture and keep going when you feel discouraged.

Learning point 3

Before you continue, consider the following:

- Which of the active elements listed in Table 10.2 seems most useful to you?
- Is there one you would like to try out?
- Can you find an inspirational quote about the necessity and usefulness of failure?

Table 10.2: Active elements of interventions that decrease perfectionism

Theme	Examples
Pros and cons of perfectionism	Identify the pay-offs of perfectionism and be radically honest about the costs. Where do you want to be in one year's time?
Expanding self-evaluation	We're all different for a reason, each with our own unique gifts to offer, not just in the area of achievement. Spend more time nurturing these other areas, which celebrate the journey, not the outcome.
Self-criticism to self-compassion	Recognise that self-compassion is more productive than self-criticism – try it and see!
Self-monitoring	Changing a habit takes practice. Become aware of how perfectionism impacts across your life, and how vicious cycles are created that maintain perfectionism.
Thinking styles	All-or-nothing and black and white thinking maintain perfectionism, so set guidelines and not rules.
Behavioural experiments	The only way to learn if changing your behaviour works for you, is to try it and see. Make some specific predictions about what might happen if you do things differently, then try doing it, and evaluate the outcome afterwards.
Procrastination and time management	Set deadlines that let you move on, so you don't get stuck trying to perfect one project at the expense of another. The mantra needs to be 'just do it' – get started with small steps, which move you towards the bigger goal.
Adjusting goals and expectations	Consider loosening the standards that suggest only one outcome is acceptable.
Recognising the benefits of mistakes	Failure is key to moving forward; trial and error are essential for learning and achievement.

Self-assessment and resources

You will find a self-assessment tool in Table 10.3 to help you consider whether you experience perfectionism. If you answer 'most of the time' to most of the questions, then working on your perfectionism is highly likely to be helpful for your mental health, including your eating. In the reference list you will find a self-help book that can help you start this journey (Shafran *et al*, 2018). You can also find helpful free worksheets on the Centre for Clinical Interventions website: www.cci.health.wa.gov.au/Resources/Looking-After-Yourself/Perfectionism (accessed November 2021).

Table 10.3: The Clinical Perfectionism Questionnaire

Modifications have been made to questions 2 and 8, please consult the original questionnaire for reproduction purposes: Fairburn, C.G., Cooper, Z., & Shafran, R. (2003). Clinical Perfectionism Questionnaire. Unpublished scale, University of Oxford, Oxford, UK.

1	Over the past month, have you pushed yourself really hard to meet your goals?
2	Over the past month, have you tended to focus on what you *have not* achieved, rather than on what you have achieved?
3	Over the past month, have you been told that your standards are too high?
4	Over the past month, have you felt a failure as a person because you have not succeeded in meeting your goals?
5	Over the past month, have you been afraid that you might not reach your standards?
6	Over the past month, have you raised your standards because you thought they were too easy?
7	Over the past month, have you judged yourself on the basis of your ability to achieve high standards?
8	Over the past month, have you done more than you needed to just to get by?
9	Over the past month, have you *repeatedly* checked how well you are doing at meeting your standards (for example, by comparing your performance with that of others)?
10	Over the past month, do you think that other people would have thought of you as a 'perfectionist'?
11	Over the past month, have you kept trying to meet your standards, even if this has meant that you have missed out on things?
12	Over the past month, have you avoided any tests of your performance (at meeting your goals) in case you failed?

Glossary

Control groups: Control groups are usually people on the waitlist for an intervention who complete assessments. This allows the researchers to measure changes over time in people who *do* versus *do not* undergo an intervention.

Meta-analysis: The best way to figure out if treatments can decrease perfectionism is to use 'meta-analyses'. For a meta-analysis, researchers tip all individual studies about an intervention into one bucket and use an overall average result to more accurately estimate the effects of an intervention than a single study (because there can be lots of variation in single studies).

References

Egan SJ, Wade TD & Shafran R (2011) Perfectionism as a transdiagnostic process: A clinical review. *Clinical Psychology Review* **31** 203–212.

Limburg K, Watson HJ, Hagger MS & Egan SJ (2017) The relationship between perfectionism and psychopathology: A meta-analysis. *Journal of Clinical Psychology* **73** (10) 1301–1326.

Lloyd S, Schmidt U, Khondoker M & Tchanturia K (2015) Can Psychological Interventions Reduce Perfectionism? A Systematic Review and Meta-analysis. *Behavioural and Cognitive Psychotherapy* **43** 705-731.

Osenk I, Williamson P & Wade TD (2020) Does perfectionism or pursuit of excellence contribute to successful learning? A meta-analytic review. *Psychological Assessment* **32** 972–983.

Robinson K & Wade TD (2021) Perfectionism Interventions Targeting Disordered Eating: A systematic review and meta-analysis. *International Journal of Eating Disorders.*

Shafran R, Cooper Z & Fairburn C. (2002). Clinical perfectionism: a cognitive–behavioural analysis. *Behavior Research and Therapy* **40** 773-791.

Shafran R, Egan S & Wade TD (2018) *Overcoming Perfectionism. Second Edition*. London: Little, Brown Book Group.

Suh H, Sohn H, Kim T & Dong-Gwi L (2019) A review and meta-analysis of perfectionism interventions: Comparing face-to-face with online modalities. *Journal of Counseling Psychology* **66** 473-486.

Wade TD, Kay E, de Valle MK, Egan SJ, Andersson G, Carlbring P & Shafran R (2019) Internet-based cognitive behaviour therapy for perfectionism: More is better but no need to be prescriptive. *Clinical Psychologist* **23** 196-205.

Warren R, Smeets E & Neff K (2016) Self-criticism and self-compassion: Risk and resilience: Being compassionate to oneself is associated with emotional resilience and psychological well-being. *Current Psychiatry* **15** 18–33.

11. Understanding eating difficulties among Muslim populations

By Justin Thomas and Alaa Galadari

Chapter summary

In the biblical book of Ecclesiastes, we read: '...nothing new under the sun'. It's a phrase commonly used in Arabic, too: *La jadeed tahta shams*. Despite our tendency to view eating difficulties as something new, symptoms of a modern malaise, they aren't. When we look back across the centuries, we can identify problems that are in many regards similar to conditions that contemporary psychiatry would call eating disorders. However, one apparent difference is that these historical cases are very frequently connected with religious belief and practice – religiosity. This chapter will explore how Islam and being a Muslim might influence eating difficulties, and it offers practical points that might inform those involved in the care treatment and prevention of eating difficulties among Muslim individuals and communities.

Introduction

Anorexia mirablis is Latin for 'miraculously inspired loss of appetite'. Often referred to as 'holy anorexia', this condition is attributed to several prominent holy women in medieval Christendom. Perhaps the most well know of these female ascetics is Catherine of Sienna. Writing about Catherine in her book, *Holy Anorexia*, Bell (1985) describes Catherine as adopting an extreme form of dietary restraint, bordering on self-starvation. Catherine is also said to have engaged in self-induced vomiting (Bell, 1985). Such behaviours arguably contributed to Catherine's death at the relatively young age of 33 (the supposed age Jesus was crucified). Another female ascetic was Beatrice of Nazareth. She claimed that even the smell of food would make her throat close up, while the aroma of meat would make her vomit. Such behaviours have been explained as self-mortification, overcoming the 'sinful' flesh to purify the spirit. In her analysis of these holy women, Brumberg writes:

> '*...in the earlier era (13th to 16th centuries) control of appetite was linked to piety and belief;...the modern anorectic strives for perfection in terms of society's ideal of physical rather than spiritual beauty.'* (Brumberg, 1988, p53)

Do our religious beliefs or practices have implications for our eating difficulties?

To this day, however, the world's major religions continue to influence billions of people's dietary practices. For example, Islam, Judaism and several Christian denominations all prescribe forms of fasting. The idea that some contemporary eating difficulties might still be intertwined with religiosity is an interesting proposition, a hypothesis that has been explored by a small number of research studies (Thomas *et al*, 2018; Sipila *et al*, 2017; Pittock, 2014; Huline-Dickens, 2000; Joughin *et a*., 1992). This research has generally looked at populations where Judeo-Christian religious traditions are dominant, noting the elevated rate of religiosity among individuals diagnosed with an eating disorder.

In one of our studies, the first to explore the question among young Muslim women, we found a significant positive correlation between Islamic religiosity and eating disorders symptoms. In other words, higher levels of religiosity were associated with higher levels of eating disorders symptoms among young Muslim women in the United Arab Emirates (UAE) (Thomas *et al*, 2018). In general, religiosity has been reported as being higher among Muslims compared to other (Christian, Hindu, Jewish) groups (Loewenthal *et al*, 2001) and the UAE constitution enshrines Islam as the official religion of the state. Such findings point to the idea that religion and religious traditions may still play some role in influencing the onset, course or maintenance of eating difficulties. This relationship may be particularly notable in communities where religiosity remains a dominant social force.

Don't assume religiosity, but leave the door open for its discussion

The first point to make is that levels of religious commitment among Muslims are highly variable. Assuming a person's religiosity, based on a name and a nominal faith affiliation, can be a big mistake. So while we don't make assumptions, it can also be helpful to at least indicate that religion is something that is 'OK' to discuss. Religion is not off the table.

The Muslim world

As in medieval Christendom, the Muslim world offers up several examples of eating difficulties from before the modern era. The earliest written account is from 9th century Syria (Hajal, 1982). It is the case study of a teenage Prince, al-al – Mu'tazzbillah, who is described as refusing food without any apparent physiological cause. His physician, Bukhtishu Ibn Jibrail, uses a kind of behaviour therapy (token-economy), to coax the prince back into accepting nourishment.

Much of the discussion about eating disorders in the modern Muslim world centres on Western acculturation (adopting Western social norms) and globalization. Since the 1990s, the psychiatric research literature began to report cases of anorexia nervosa among populations, where this condition had hitherto gone unreported or undiagnosed. Majority-Muslim countries such as Egypt, the United Arab Emirates, Oman, Kuwait and Saudi Arabia all began reporting cases of diagnosed eating disorders, or elevated levels of eating disorders symptoms around this time (Abou-Saleh *et al*, 1996; Al-Subaie, 2000; Eapen *et al*, 2006; Nasser, 1986; Nasser, 1992).

One interpretation of the rise in eating difficulties among Muslim populations was the idea of increased exposure to Western body image ideals, which, during the latter half of the 20th century had placed growing emphasis on thinness. In the *Anatomy of an Epidemic*, Gordon describes this fixation on thinness as the thin body cult (Gordon, 2000). What is a cult, if not a fledgling religion?

For many Muslim nations, globalization and the spread of Western media has also coincided with rapid, intranational social change and rising levels of obesity. For example, the Arab Gulf states (Kuwait, Saudi, UAE etc.) have experienced the boom of oil revenues, which has radically transformed the landscape, the economy, access to education and gender-roles. Such rapid social changes are widely viewed as fertile ground for the emergence of eating difficulties (Gordon, 2000; Gordon, 2001), especially in contexts where the thin body cult is actively promoted.

One concrete example that the thin body cult taking root in Muslim lands is the popularity of a doll called Fulla. Launched in 2003 by a Dubai-based company, Fulla is the Muslim competitor to Barbie. At approximately the same height as Barbie, Fulla is thinner (waist 9.8 vs 10.5 mm.), and even more tubular (hips 11.4 vs 13.5), see figure 11.1. The manufacturers of Fulla claim the doll was developed to reflect Muslim values, which she expresses through her accessories, for example her hijab, prayer carpet and prayer beads. However, despite the explicit Islamic trimmings, Fulla is a poster girl for the thin body cult. With more than 1.5 million units sold, Fulla is one of the best-selling fashion dolls in the Muslim world (Harrod, 2012).

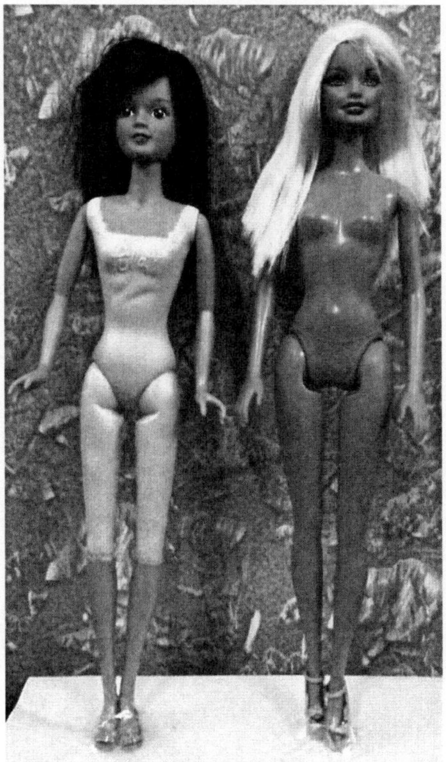

Figure 11.1: Fulla and Barbie
Source: Photograph by Justin Thomas (2013)

Research among Muslim populations has shown a clear link between body image dissatisfaction and eating difficulties (Thomas *et al*, 2010). In contrast, there are non-Western populations (India and China) where body image concerns are absent, and eating difficulties appear to be expressed in more psychosomatic terms, with reference to vague physical discomfort associated with eating (Khandewal *et al*, 1995; Lee *et al*, 1993; Lee, 1991). In addition to the clear link between body image concerns and eating difficulties reported among Muslims, there are also numerous studies suggesting that Western acculturation, in general, is also predictive of eating difficulties. Hill and Bhatti, for example, studied adolescent girls attending a school in Lahore, Pakistan. They found that the girls most exposed to Western culture also had the highest levels of abnormal eating attitudes and body dissatisfaction (Hill & Bhatti, 1995). Similar studies and findings are also reported among Muslim populations in Egypt (Nasser, 1986; Nasser, 1992) and Saudi Arabia (Al-Subaie, 2000).

Learning point 1

To what extent might media-promoted body images impact our eating difficulties?

To what extent might uncertainty and rapid social change influence our eating difficulties?

Dismissing the thin body cult

We might use the media, big business and psychoeducation to undermine the idea that female worth is bound up with physical appearance. There are some excellent examples of this in Western nations. However, I can find no examples in the Muslim world. This should change. In some Muslim nations, imported magazines alter their content to respect religious and cultural norms. Eating disorders advocacy groups might call for the same pressure to be applied to unhelpful body image tropes. Ultimately the challenge is to undermine the very notion of an 'ideal' body image.

Muslims in the West

Muslims living in Western nations tend to be minority communities, and much of the research exploring eating difficulties among ethnic minorities is applicable here. In addition to links between appearance ideals and eating difficulties, research among minorities tends to link eating difficulties and acculturative stress (the mental and emotional challenges of adapting to a new culture). Even among second and third-generation immigrants there can still be an acculturative tension between traditional cultural identity and Western outlooks: do I wear my hijab, or do I go with the LA Lakers baseball cap? One study undertaken amongst schoolgirls of Asian origin in the UK found that eating difficulties were associated with traditional (in-group), rather than Western, (out-group) cultural orientations.

This study suggests that the stress caused by cultural adjustment may sometimes be a more significant influence on eating difficulties than even Western body image ideals (Hill & Bhatti, 1995).

We also know that children from minority communities experience more adverse childhood events (this is true for the US). It could also be that such events, particularly peer-victimization experiences (bullying), contribute to the development of eating difficulties among Muslim communities in the West. We know that, in general, school-age bullying is predictive of eating difficulties (Copeland *et al*, 2015).

An additional challenge for Muslim minorities is access to assessment and treatment that is culturally sensitive, appropriate and responsive. A better approach involves taking into consideration its 'meaning' for the patient and members of his/her society. Human suffering should not be removed from its cultural context; it should be understood within it.

Cultural competence and religio-culturally attuned interventions

That Islamic religiosity can be associated with eating disorders symptoms among some Muslim women (Thomas *et al*, 2018) suggests that pastoral care and spiritually attuned/integrated forms of psychotherapy may prove helpful for some. This would be particularly true for Muslims with relatively high levels of religiosity: those who spontaneously express their experiences in religious themes and perhaps even explicitly request faith-affiliated interventions.

Practitioners involved in delivering psychotherapeutic interventions with Muslim clients might draw upon Islamic/cultural bridging concepts to make therapy more appropriate and religiously and culturally relevant (detailing these is beyond this chapter's scope). There has been some work done towards developing spiritually attuned cognitive behaviour therapy for depression (Thomas & Furber, 2015). This work might prove a useful starting point. However, specific religious and cultural knowledge aside, adopting and developing cultural competence is essential.

A more culturally capable approach would involve clinicians taking into consideration their own preconceptions about the patient's culture. This approach would recognize how different the patient may or may not be from other members of society. This also involves identifying differences in the patient's conceptualization of eating difficulties and other mental illnesses. It entails understanding the patient's definitions of self in relation to the family and the community as a whole (Bhui & Morgan, 2007).

An example of a culturally capable approach is the adaptation of The Body Project for women in Saudi Arabia. This preventative approach aims to reduce body dissatisfaction and eating difficulties as well as reducing the development of eating disorders. Their manual includes activities to be practiced both in sessions and at home. An example of cultural adaptations to the approach involved behavioural exercises. Visiting the pool in a swimsuit was changed to dressing in fitted clothes, and posting a video of their home workout to YouTube was replaced with posting a self-affirmation text on social media (AlShebali *et al*, 2021).

Despite limitations to the preliminary study, such as the number of participants and the lack of a control group, it confirmed the feasibility of culturally adapting this preventative program and showed preliminary effectiveness. In recent decades, there have been great strides to encourage psychotherapists and counsellors to develop culturally competent practices. This is undoubtedly an area where further progress should be made.

Learning point 2

How might our experiences of bullying impact our eating difficulties?
How aware are we of other cultures and aspects of that culture that might influence eating difficulties?

Preventing peer-victimization, promoting compassion

In some nations, Muslims, especially Muslim women, can be highly visible minorities. Ensuring zero-tolerance for hate speech and all forms of victimization across our societies and institutions is essential. Beyond zero-tolerance, however, schools and workplaces should actively work hard to encourage cultures of tolerance, compassion and kindness. Reducing victimization experiences will reduce eating difficulties and mental health problems in general.

Ramadanorexia: fasting and the onset of eating difficulties

Wherever Muslims live, they are likely to have had some aspects of their lives shaped by Islam's source materials: the Quran and the hadith (sayings and doings of the prophet). This body of work extends to eating and dietary practice, from prohibitions against particular foodstuffs and over-consumption to exhortations about eating with the right hand. A familiarity with Islam's rich literature on eating and dietary practice might certainly help a therapist working with Muslim clients. For example, in response to a man who pledged to keep a continuous fast, the prophet said: "…I fast, and I break my fast…" (Sahih al-Bukhari: Hadith 5063). This hadith is often taken as a discouragement of extreme asceticism within Islam.

Fasting, however, is part of Islam, especially during the Holy Month of Ramadan. This is a time when Muslims are called to fast between sunrise and sunset. Ramadan can potentially be a difficult time for Muslims with a vulnerability to eating difficulties. This is an issue well-articulated by Sameera al Romaithi in her book, *You Are What You Eat* (Al-Romaithi, ND).

Case study: the intersection of Ramadan and eating difficulties

Samira is an Emirati, born and raised in the United Arab Emirates. In 2004 she was diagnosed as suffering from anorexia nervosa. Samira chose to share her experiences, hoping to help others with similar difficulties. In her book, Samira describes how her meals became highly ritualised, with minimal variation on a very low-calorie theme. She also discusses being heavily invested in the shopping and food preparation process while simultaneously and cunningly avoiding food consumption. However, diverging from the classic portrayal of anorexia, Samira traces the onset of her eating difficulties to the holy month of Ramadan.

> *'I abused the good intentions behind the holy month and will forever be ashamed. It was an anorexic's dream come true. I could go all day without eating a thing, have my dose of exercise by horseback riding, and then at Iftar (the breaking of the fast) eat only the little set of 'safe' foods I had prescribed for myself: a green apple, a 90-calorie cereal bar and a glass of orange juice.'*
> (Al-Romaithi, ND)

Samira recovered, and when we last spoke to her she was doing great. She is still keen to help prevent the onset of eating difficulties in her community. We hope this chapter and the following practice/learning points make a small contribution to this aim.

Public health messaging and timing

Religious fasting may be misappropriated and end up making eating difficulties worse. Within the Islamic tradition, even outside of Ramadan, religious fasting is frequently advocated as a means of expiating (wiping out) past sins and misdeeds. With Muslim clients who demonstrate high levels of religious commitment, an exploration of such ideas may be helpful. Exploring Islam's call for moderation and the condemnation of excess (excessive fasting) might also prove a useful focus for prevention-orientated health messaging and awareness raising. Just before the start of Ramadan would be an excellent time to launch eating disorders awareness campaigns and events within Muslim communities.

Conclusion

In conclusion, understanding the complex relationship between mental health conditions and culture could change the way we deal and interact with these conditions. This chapter explored how being Muslim affects eating difficulties and provided some points on how to manage and prevent eating difficulties in a culturally capable way. It discussed how one should not assume religiosity, but should leave the door open for its discussion. It highlighted the role of media and comprehensive psycho-education to undermine the idea that female worth is bound up with physical appearance. It emphasized the role of reducing victimization experiences in order to reduce eating difficulties and mental health problems in general. And finally, how cultural competence and religio-culturally attuned interventions could make all the difference. Becoming aware of one's own cultural values and biases, valuing others' worldviews and developing culturally appropriate interpersonal skills, can all feed into culturally competent practice. An approach that is more culturally congruent would result in better engagement between the patient and the practitioner.

References

Abou-Saleh MT, Younis Y & Karim L (1996) 'Anorexia Nervosa in an Arab Culture'. *International Journal of Eating Disorders*, **23**, pp207-12.

Al-Romaithi S (ND) *You are what you eat* [online]. Abu Dhabi: The Death Diet. Available at: www.thedeathdiet.com/usr/downloads/The_Death_Diet.pdf [accessed August 2021].

AlShebali M, Becker C, Kellett S, AlHadi A & Waller G (2021) Adapting the body project to a non-Western culture: a dissonance-based eating disorders prevention program for Saudi women. *Eating And Weight Disorders - Studies On Anorexia, Bulimia And Obesity.* doi: 10.1007/s40519-021-01104-9

Al-Subaie AS (2000) 'Some Correlates of Dieting Behaviour in Saudi Schoolgirls'. *International Journal of Eating Disorders* **28** pp242-46.

Bell RM (1985) *Holy Anorexia*. London: University of Chicago Press.

Bhui K & Morgan N (2007) Effective psychotherapy in a racially and culturally diverse society. Advances in Psychiatric Treatment. *Cambridge University Press* **13** (3) pp187–193. doi: 10.1192/apt.bp.106.002295.

Brumberg JJ (1988) *Fasting Girls: The emergence of anorexia nervosa as a modern disease*. Cambridge: Harvard University Press.

Copeland WE, Bulik CM, Zucker N, Wolke D, Lereya ST & Costello EJ (2015) 'Does childhood bullying predict eating disorder symptoms? A prospective, longitudinal analysis'. *The International Journal of Eating Disorders* **48** (8), pp1141-1149.

Eapen V, Mabrouk AA & Bin-Othman S (2006) Disordered eating attitudes and symptomatology among adolescent girls in the United Arab Emirates. *Eating Behaviors* (**7**) pp53-60.

Gordon RA (2000) *Eating Disorders: Anatomy of a social epidemic*. 2nd edn. Oxford: Blackwell.

Gordon RA (2001) Eating disorders East and West: A culture-bound syndrome unbound. In: Nasser M, Katzman MA & Gordon RA (eds.) *Eating Disorders and Cultures in Transition*. New York: Brunner-Routledge.

Hajal F (1982) Psychological Treatment of Anorexia: A case from the Ninth Century. *Journal of the History of Medicine and Allied Sciences*. XXXVII(3) pp325-328.

Harrod H (2012) 'Little girls, big business', *The Telegraph*, 12/June/2012. Available at: www.telegraph.co.uk/culture/9314640/Little-girls-big-business.html

Hill AJ & Bhatti R (1995) Body shape perception and dieting in preadolescent british asian girls: Links with eating disorders. *International Journal of Eating Disorders* **17** (2) pp175-183.

Huline-Dickens S (2000) Anorexia nervosa: some connections with the religious attitude. *The British Journal Of Medical Psychology* **73** (1) pp67-76.

Joughin N, Crisp AH, Halek C & Humphrey H (1992) Religious Belief and Anorexia Nervosa. *International Journal of Eating Disorders* **12** (4) pp397-406.

Khandewal SK, Sharan P & Saxena S (1995) Eating disorders: An Indian perspective. *International Journal of Social Psychiatry* (**41**) pp132-146.

Lee S (1991) Anorexia Nervosa in Hong Kong: A Chinese perspective. *Psychological Medicine* (**21**) pp703-711.

Lee S, Ho TP & Hsu LKG (1993) Fat phobic and non-fat phobic anorexia nervosa: A comparative study of 70 Chinese patients in Hong Kong. *Psychological Medicine* (**23**) pp999-1017.

Loewenthal KM, Cinnirella M, Evdoka G & Murphy P (2001) Faith conquers all? Beliefs about the role of religious factors in coping with depression among different cultural-religious groups in the UK. *British Journal of Medical Psychology* **74** (Pt 3) pp293-303.

Nasser M (1986) Comparative study of the prevalence of abnormal eating attitudes among Arab female students at both London and Cairo universities. *Psychological Medicine* **16** pp621-25.

Nasser M (1992) *Screening for abnormal eating attitudes in a population of Egyptian secondary school girls*. Doctor of Medicine (DM), Southampton University, UK.

Pittock A (2014) How are anorexia nervosa and spirituality connected, and what implications does this have for treatment. *Royal College of Psychiatrists: Spirituality and psychiatry special interest group newsletter* (**31**) pp1-14.

Sipila P, Harrasova G, Mustelin L, Rose RJ, Kaprio J & Keski-Rahkonen A (2017) '"Holy anorexia" - relevant or relic? Religiosity and anorexia nervosa among Finnish women', *International Journal of Eating Disorders* **50** pp406-414.

Thomas J, Abdulrahman A & Khan S (2010) Eating attitudes and body image concerns among female university students in the United Arab Emirates. *Appetite* **54** pp595-598.

Thomas J & Furber M (2015) Culturally and Spiritually Attuned Psychotherapy in the UAE. In Al-Karam CY and Haque A (eds.) *Mental Health and Psychological Practice in the United Arab Emirates*. London: Palgrave Macmillan.

Thomas J, O'Hara L, Tahboub-Schulte S, Grey I & Chowdhury N (2018) Holy anorexia: Eating disorders symptomatology and religiosity among Muslim women in the United Arab Emirates. *Psychiatry Research* **260** pp495-499.

12. Ordered and disordered eating in traditional Jewish communities

By Esther Altmann

Summary

The scourge of disordered eating, dieting and body preoccupations has affected Jewish women across the denominational spectrum, much as it has affected women across cultures and countries, particularly in the Western world. Jewish women are as likely as non-Jewish women to use their bodies as a repository for psychological distress and trauma, and as a socially sanctioned way of expressing anxiety, despair, self-doubt and struggles with self-esteem. Many Jewish women of all ages have chronic eating concerns and negative feelings about their bodies. Jewish men, similarly, have also been influenced by a culture of body worship and dieting. Although this chapter will focus on the psychology and experiences of Jewish women, it is important to note that Jewish men also suffer from Disordered Eating Pathology (DEP), similar to men in the general population.

Jewish identity and disordered eating

Jewish identity represents a broad spectrum, from Jews who are atheists to those who are ultra-orthodox and adhere strictly to the dictates of Jewish law and traditions. In addition to great variability along the dimension of faith and practice, there is also variability in socioeconomic status, educational levels, ethnicity, race and national identities. As with the population in general, all these factors mediate the expression and experiences of DEP.

Since Judaism represents a complex blend of culture, beliefs and traditions, the psychotherapist who is inquiring and knowledgeable about specific religious practices and identities will be most able to provide empathic, productive treatment. (For more information about Jewish denominations, see Schlosser, 2006.)

The role of the body in Judaism

In contrast to the centrality of the perfected, glorified body in the contemporary psyche, Judaism discourages the idealization of the body. In rabbinic texts, bodies are discussed with great respect and viewed as transient instruments through which the fundamental religious goals of worship, study and *chesed* (acts of loving kindness) are realised. The Torah (Hebrew Bible) is explicit in stating that the human body is created *Bi'tzelem Elokim*, in the image of God, with each person containing a spark of the divine. In addition to caring for the body, Jewish law mandates that an ill person is obligated to seek medical care. In fact, maintaining one's health is so important that the Talmud prohibits Torah scholars from living in a city that does not have a physician. Access to good medical care is deemed an important consideration in choosing where to live (Goldwasser, 2010). Furthermore, caring for and visiting the sick, *bikur cholim*, is a central act of *chesed* in Judaism. And most importantly, eating difficulties fall into the Talmudic category of *Sakanat Nefesh*, a danger or threat to life. Judaism mandates that no effort should be spared when a life is at risk. Thus, traditional Judaism views the body as sacrosanct and mandates its proper care.

Food and eating in the Talmud

The Talmud, the central text of Jewish law and theology written between 200-500 CE, is replete with rabbinic discourse about a variety of foods to eat or avoid in order to support health and wellbeing. Although many of these ancient Talmudic recommendations are not supported by our modern understanding of nutrition, it is clear that preparation and consumption of food for rituals and for daily needs were often on the rabbinic mind.

Interestingly, in the tractate of the Talmud that discusses *Yom Kippur*, the Day of Atonement, the rabbis distinguish between eating a minimum amount of food 'to be satisfied' versus consuming an amount of food that 'merely settles the mind' (Babylonian Talmud, Yoma, 79). This ancient rabbinic argument resonates with our current diet culture in which the goal is often to eat just the minimum required to maintain body functioning rather than to savor a meal and feel fully satisfied at its completion. It is the feeling of satisfaction after dining that the rabbis consider the prerequisite for saying the Grace after Meals, the benediction recited after consuming a meal that includes bread.

Jewish practices and disordered eating

In contemporary Jewish life, food is integral to life-cycle celebrations and the observation of the Sabbath and festivals. Food is also a means of providing comfort in times of loss and mourning. Many families also uphold unique food traditions that originate from the diverse countries Jews have inhabited over the millennia.

These food traditions, transmitted across generations, are also a source of Jewish identity and culture.

Unfortunately, these traditions have not been powerful enough to combat the tyranny of the 'thinness ideal' from seeping into the psyches of Jewish women. This has even been the case in ultra-orthodox communities, which generally try to shield themselves from broader cultural influences deemed contrary to Jewish precepts. In addition to the pervasive visual saturation of an unattainable body ideal, mental health professionals have wondered whether there may be a link between DEP, Jewish rituals and the sociocultural and historical context of religious Jewish life. Several factors have been suggested connecting Jewish practices to DEP.

First, it has been suggested that young orthodox Jewish women develop DEP because they feel pressure to marry young and have large families, with children often born in quick succession. The notion of a 'superwoman ideal' in which young women feel that they have to excel on all fronts – personal, professional and familial – is also deeply ingrained within traditional Jewish communities. Thus, an eating difficulty may be a way for a young woman to signal she does not feel psychologically ready to take on the responsibilities of a wife and mother, or that the dual demands of academic success and marriage at a young age is simply overwhelming.

However, these pressures can be alleviated and the risks of DEP can be reduced in several ways. Parents can mitigate overwhelming expectations by paying close attention to their child's emotional development and unique psychological needs regarding readiness for marriage and professional success. Psychotherapists can play a crucial role in buffering societal and parental pressure to marry young, thereby helping young women modulate their internalised perfectionistic tendencies to strive for excellence in all areas.

Second, it has been suggested that Jewish rituals and festivals, so intertwined with food and lavish meals, may interact with disordered eating. Delighting in Sabbath and festival meals is indeed a deeply embedded tradition and a time when families come together. Large Sabbath meals are not only a weekly occurrence, but each Sabbath includes two elaborate meals – a Friday night dinner and a Saturday afternoon lunch. For individuals struggling with DEP, these sumptuous meals may cause distress and anxiety. Some individuals restrict their caloric intake before or after the Sabbath and holidays in order to indulge in the delicious, abundant food during these festive meals. This behaviour may intensify problematic eating patterns by precipitating bingeing, purging or food restriction to compensate for actual overeating or merely the perception of indulgence. Families may need to be aware of symptomatic behaviours and be flexible in their approach as to how these struggles are navigated.

Third, in stark contrast to elaborate festive meals, the Holocaust's haunting images of skeletal victims hover over the pathology of self-induced starvation and may represent a collective communal legacy of trauma. One theory is that an unconscious, collective identification with grandparents who survived the Holocaust, or with relatives who perished, may underlie eating difficulties in the Jewish community. In some families, food, either consciously or unconsciously, represents safety from annihilation and may therefore be fraught with meaning and its importance over-emphasized.

Fourth, it is also the case that, within *halacha* (Jewish law), food is highly regulated: blessings are recited before and after meals, hands are washed ritually before bread is eaten, and *kashrut* laws define permissible and non-permissible foods in ways that, on the surface, may appear psychologically similar to DEP tendencies to eliminate food groups such as carbohydrates and fats. Although compelling, this comparison may be misleading. There is little clinical, material or empirical evidence to confirm a psychological connection between patients with eating difficulties and those who observe the laws of *kashrut*. Moreover, these laws have been practiced for more than 2,000 years, whereas the prevalence of eating difficulties is largely a contemporary phenomenon. Finally, Judaism is not the only religion or culture in which food is regulated and plays a central role.

Learning point 1

What role, if any, might these factors play in Jewish body dissatisfaction and disordered eating?

Clearly, there are genetic, intrapsychic and familial factors that culminate in DEP and eating difficulties. In contemporary culture at large, not everyone develops an eating disorder even though all women are bombarded by media messages promoting an unattainable thinness ideal. Similarly, in the Orthodox world, research confirms that the vast majority of girls and women do not develop DEP – though they may experience the pressures of the superwoman ideal, matchmaking, young marriage, early motherhood, keeping kosher, lavish festive meals, and the Holocaust's legacy of deprivation and trauma (Altmann, 2009). Although it is important for therapists to attune themselves to these cultural norms and stressors when working with Orthodox patients, they should not presume that these factors are central to the development or maintenance of a particular individual's eating difficulty. Moreover, although most ultra-Orthodox women live with their families until marriage, and premarital sexual relations or casual dating is prohibited, treatment providers should not assume that because a patient is Orthodox or ultra-Orthodox, they do not want to, or do not need to, explore their feelings about religious conflicts, sexuality, gender, sexual orientation, or substance abuse, for example; concerns that may be counter to the values espoused by their families or religious education.

In addition, clinicians treating DEP among religious Jews need to be aware that there are two major fast days on the calendar, *Yom Kippur* and *Tisha B'av*, in which one fasts from sundown to sunset of the next day (25 hours) and four minor fast days in which one fasts from sunrise to sunset of the same day. For those in recovery from eating difficulties, fasting may precipitate a regression or may be deemed unsafe by a therapist or physician. Patients may be reluctant to adhere to the recommendation not to fast as the desire to do so may interact with their eating pathology. Teasing apart their religious commitment from their eating pathology can be nuanced and challenging. Under these circumstances, it might be appropriate to consult with a rabbinic authority. The vast majority of rabbis are sensitive to medical recommendations and will prioritise health over religious observance.

Case study

Note: The name and personal details of the following case have been altered to protect privacy.

The case of Rebecca, an 18-year-old woman from an ultra-orthodox family, exemplifies several of the themes highlighted in this chapter. Rebecca had been suffering with anorexia for a year when she and her parents consulted me. Her parents' mandate was that she get better quickly, very quickly, so that she could attend a women's seminary abroad for post-high school study as planned. In Rebecca's community, this year of post-high school study is typically the step before seeking a suitable marriage partner. My firm recommendation that Rebecca required extended treatment and was not healthy enough to go away was not well received by her parents. Fortunately, they consulted a respected rabbi who reinforced the recommendation that treatment was essential and should supersede learning in seminary.

Over the course of therapy, Rebecca discussed her feelings about being the eldest of seven children and her parentified role in the family. She worried about her younger siblings, several of whom had psychological difficulties. Rebecca was not only a devoted sister and daughter, she was also an exemplary student and was always the first to take on additional responsibilities. Rebecca's parents worked long hours to support the family, had their own struggles with weight and dieting, and had limited capacity for empathy. Both parents were raised by Holocaust survivors who struggled to keep their traumatic histories of loss and violence at bay while they led 'ordinary' lives as new immigrants in the US.

Within the safety of the therapeutic relationship, Rebecca, a highly intelligent and capable young woman, revealed that contrary to communal expectations, she did not want to have a large family. Rebecca was able to let go of her disordered eating and body preoccupations once she felt seen and understood. Therapy supported her developing autonomy as an independent adult able to make sound decisions that took her psychological wellbeing into account. She began dating, married at 19, and had her first child when she was 21 years old. She continued to pursue her education and chose a profession that she found intellectually stimulating and fulfilling. Rebecca's husband, who was also raised in an ultra-orthodox family, supported her interest in furthering her career. After having a second child at age 24, she went on to graduate school and became a successful attorney. With psychotherapeutic support and a loving husband, Rebecca was able to attend to her evolving emotional needs, keep parental and communal pressures at bay to have many children, and pursue her ambitious career goals. Most remarkably, she was also able to create a loving family and maintain a meaningful and rich religious life on her own terms.

Prevention

Perhaps a more important question is not whether Jewish traditions contribute to the problem of DEP but rather how the incorporation of Jewish practices can help prevent the problem from arising. Some interesting research has emerged that supports the idea that religious experience can function as a potential buffer against body dissatisfaction and DEP. A series of studies by Weinberger-Litman and Latzer (2007; 2008; 2015) revealed that young orthodox women who had an internalised religious orientation, defined as more spiritual and inner focused, had a more positive body image and fewer disordered eating behaviours in comparison to women who had an externalized religious orientation, defined as more focused on communal affiliation and ritual. This research suggests that personal religious beliefs may mitigate negative feelings about the body or eating difficulties. It is also consistent with a well-documented finding that religious coping can be a helpful strategy in dealing with physical and psychological stressors and challenges.

The unique food traditions of the many holidays on the Jewish calendar may also be employed as antidotes to the destructive cultural overlay of body dissatisfaction and dieting. For example, on the Sabbath, two *challahs*, braided loaves of bread, are placed on the table to remind us of the double portion of *manna* that the Israelites received from heaven when they were wandering in the desert. This symbol of replenishment invites us to be grateful for our bounty. Similarly, on *Rosh Hashanah* (the Jewish New Year), we eat apples and honey to symbolise the hope that the year will bring sweetness into our lives and eat round *challah* to remind us of the cycles of life and renewal. Moreover, the *Passover Seder*, commemorating the liberation from enslavement, opens with the declaration, "Let all who are hungry, come and eat" (Lefkovitz, 2008).

The rabbis, in their ancient wisdom, were perhaps early practitioners of mindful eating when they mandated that each unique food group required its own blessing. For example, there are unique blessings before eating bread, fruit, vegetables, dairy products, wine and even cake and candy. The Torah also mandates reciting the Grace after Meals after consuming a major meal. These blessings and prayers encourage us to pause, reflect, and savor our food. They are small acts of gratitude and faith that nourish both body and soul and direct us to reclaim the holy sparks that lie within.

References

Altmann E (2009) Food for Thought: Eating disorders and the Jewish community. *JOFA Journal*. *VIII*(2).

Goldwasser D (2010) *Starving Souls*. Jersey City, NJ: KTAV Publishing House.

Latzer Y, Tzischinsky O & Gefen S (2007) Level of religiosity and disordered eating pathology among modern-orthodox Jewish adolescent girls in Israel. *International Journal of Adolescent Medicine and Health* **19** 511-521.

Latzer Y et al (2015) Negative religious coping predicts disordered eating pathology among orthodox Jewish adolescent girls. *Journal of Religion and Health* **54** 1760-1771.

Lefkovitz L (2008) *Judaism, body image, and food*. In: E Dorf & L Newman (Eds.) Jewish choices, Jewish voices, Volume I. Philadelphia: The Jewish Publication Society.

Weinberger-Litman et al (2008) The influence of religious orientation and spiritual well-being on body dissatisfaction and disordered eating in a sample of Jewish women. *International Journal of Child and Adolescent Health*. Vol. I. 373-387.

Schlosser L (2006) Affirmative Psychotherapy for American Jews. *Psychotherapy: Theory, Research, Practice. Training*. **43** (4) 424-435.

13. "Sleep, the main course in life's feast": the role of sleep in eating difficulties

By Annie Zimmerman and Andrew Green

Summary
Of the three pillars of good health, nutrition and exercise are compromised in eating difficulties. The third – sleep – is therefore even more important, yet professionals pay little attention to it in the context of eating difficulties. Sleep is important for physical and emotional health and for memory and learning, and poor sleep can cause many problems. Problems with sleep are common among people with eating difficulties, particularly those involving malnutrition, such as anorexia. People with eating difficulties often report sleep disturbances which negatively impact quality of life and both physical and mental health. Sleep deprivation can often hinder recovery by increasing cravings for highly palatable foods high in sugar and/or fat, such as ice cream, pizza or fried foods, which often leads to binge eating – especially during the night – thereby exacerbating the fatigue-binge cycle. It is therefore important to understand the relationships between sleep and eating difficulties, basic sleep science and how to help.

Sleep and eating difficulties
While the role of sleep is often overlooked in the context of eating difficulties, there is a two-way relationship with problems often occurring together. Insomnia is related to an increased risk of eating disorders and sleep difficulties are linked to poorer treatment outcomes for eating disorders (Cooper *et al*, 2020). People with eating difficulties, particularly those involving malnutrition such as anorexia, often report sleep disruption, which can negatively impact quality of life and both physical and mental health (Delvenne *et al*, 1992). This should be taken seriously: people with sleep and eating difficulties experience more severe disordered eating, and the interaction may increase mortality rates.

Learning point 1

Reflect on what and when you eat. Have you noticed any associations with how well you sleep? Do certain foods alter how well you sleep, for example going to bed with a full stomach, or eating sugary foods before bed?

One explanation for the association is likely to be malnutrition, which damages almost every system, including neurological and hormonal functioning. Orexin, a neuropeptide released from the hypothalamus, regulates both wakefulness and appetite. Levels of orexin increase during hunger to promote wakefulness and motivate the search for food. Additionally, malnutrition can affect the secretion of melatonin, which helps in the control of circadian rhythms and therefore the regulation of the sleep-wake cycle. Hence, malnutrition in anorexia may create sleep disturbances by dysregulating these sleep-related hormones. However, patients with eating difficulties related to binge eating (such as binge eating disorder and bulimia nervosa) are shown to experience more sleep disturbances than non-bingeing disorders (such as anorexia nervosa). This suggests that the issues surrounding sleep extend beyond poor nutrition.

There are also important links to mental health. Both sleep and eating can be negatively impacted by poor mental health. The toll of having an eating difficulty on one's emotional wellbeing and mental health is likely to influence everyday quality of life, including sleep. Eating difficulties can often stem from the need to control, in which obsessional thoughts and compulsions about eating and body image can be used to cope with uncomfortable and unbearable feelings (Brockmeyer *et al*, 2014). There is a well-established link between eating difficulties and obsessive-compulsive disorder[1]. People with eating difficulties often have high stress levels and an overactive automatic nervous system, which is critical in regulating sleep. The high stress and anxiety suffered by people with eating difficulties can make it challenging to initiate and maintain sleep. For example, obsessional thinking may keep individuals up at night and prevent them from quietening their minds and calming their nervous systems enough to fall asleep. Strategies to help patients fall and stay asleep are outlined below.

Sleep deprivation, and the associated fatigue, directly impact eating behaviour, which may in turn harm recovery. Fatigue can reduce control of eating impulses or increase obsessional thoughts about diet and healthy eating as a way to alleviate the tiredness. Alternatively, fatigue can increase cravings for highly palatable foods such as sugar, and lead to binge eating – especially during the night where cognitive control is lessened – thus exacerbating the fatigue-binge cycle. Indeed,

1 For more information see www.verywellmind.com/obsessive-compulsive-disorder-and-eating-disorders-1138191 (accessed November 2021).

women sleeping poorly are 5.5 times more likely to be diagnosed with binge eating disorder than women sleeping well (Trace *et al*, 2012). Clearly, sleep and eating difficulties influence each other and need to be considered together.

Sleep science

In order to help others to improve sleep, some knowledge of sleep science is helpful: understanding how we get to sleep and understanding the structure of sleep. See Walker (2017) for a comprehensive and accessible introduction.

Learning point 2

Before reading on, make a list of all the ways that you might try not to sleep if for some reason you needed to remain awake until 3:00am.

Three things influence when we sleep:

- The homeostatic drive.
- The circadian drive.
- Arousal levels.

A homeostatic process maintains stability in a system – regulating body temperature, for example. In the case of sleep, the longer that you have been awake, the greater is the drive to sleep. This is why daytime sleep can delay night-time sleep.

The circadian drive is governed by the body clock. If it were not reset daily by daylight it would run on a cycle of just over 24 hours (hence *circadian*, meaning about a day). Light controls the production of melatonin (the 'darkness hormone') which regulates sleep: morning daylight stops production. Similarly, unfiltered blue wavelength light from screens (computers, tablets, phones) mimics daylight and can delay sleep.

A complication with the circadian drive is that some people are naturally 'night owls', as opposed to 'larks'. Young people's sleep is typically delayed, whereas older people tend to be larks: this would be advantageous in preindustrial communities, because the period of night-time vulnerability is reduced, but it is unhelpful when fitting with regular school or work hours. Furthermore, a small minority have a continuing delay to sleep (known as delayed sleep phase disorder) where maintaining conventional routines is very difficult. It is important to be aware of this because it can manifest as insomnia.

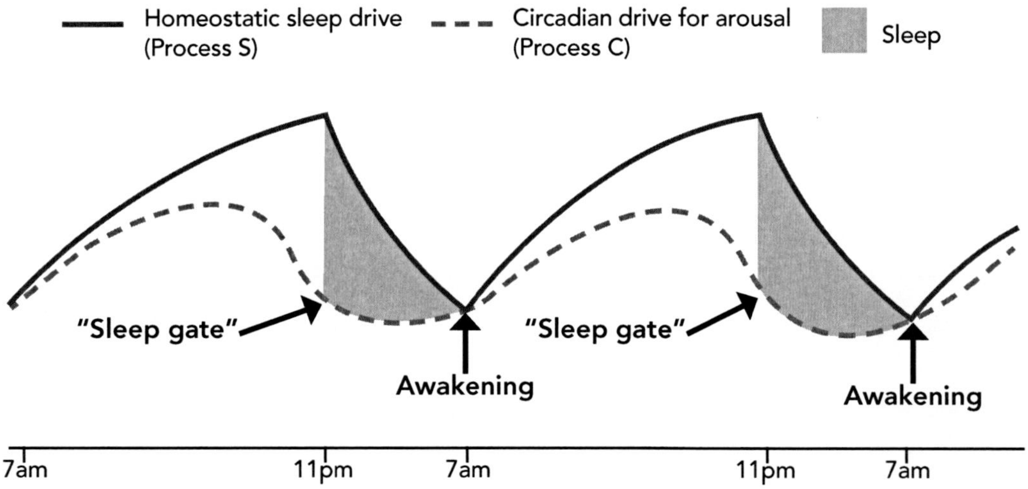

Figure 13.1

Balancing the circadian and homeostatic drives maintains a sleep pattern (Figure 13.1). However, it would make no sense if we slept according to a schedule without taking account of circumstances. Dealing with threats from predators might be a more immediate need than sleep, and evolution had to allow for flexibility: we cannot ignore imminent danger and fall asleep. It is important therefore to minimise arousal in order to fall asleep, but the problem is that our body chemistry does not distinguish between the fear on hearing an intruder, excitement because tomorrow is Christmas, anger over a neighbour's noise, or anxiety over a job interview. There is no 'sleep switch' as such, but it is a helpful analogy. Figure 13.2 shows the factors that are involved.

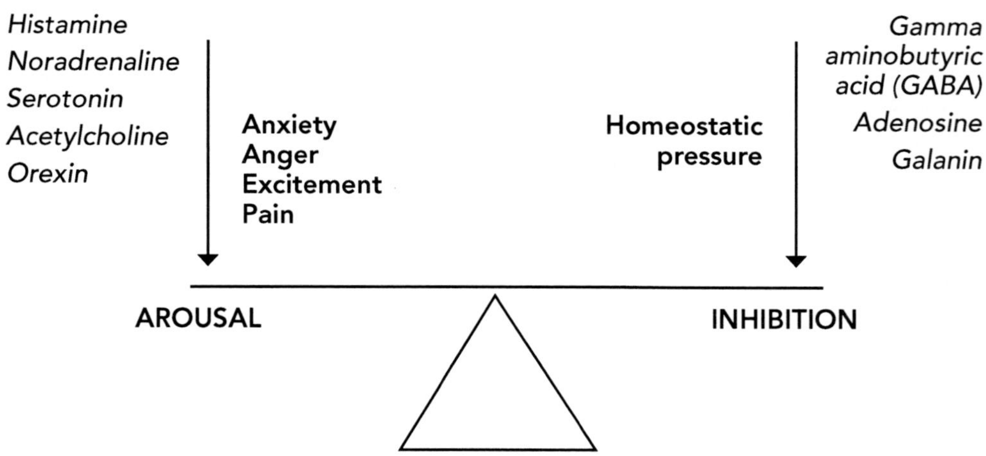

Figure 13.2: The "sleep switch"

Learning point 3

Review your answers to the question in Learning point 2: to which of the three influences does each apply? For example, having an afternoon sleep delays the homeostatic drive and going for a late run will maintain levels of arousal. Doing the opposite of these things will enhance sleep.

It is important to know that sleep is not a single state: we go through stages of sleep. Stage 1 (often experienced when fighting to stay awake in meetings) is a transitional stage. Stage 2 is light sleep, in which we spend half of the night, and from which we are easily woken. Stage 3 (stages 3 and 4 in earlier classifications) is deep sleep, in which the body is relaxed and still; being woken from it causes brief disorientation. Rapid eye movement (REM) sleep is actually a different state of being from wakefulness and non-REM sleep. The brain is as active as in waking, but the body is unable to move; it is when we tend to dream. The temporary paralysis of the voluntary muscles prevents us from acting out our dreams.

As seen in Figure 13.3, we go through four or five cycles of sleep of 90–120 minutes each. Notable points are that the deep sleep mostly occurs early in the night and that sleep becomes lighter towards morning. A stylized representation does not show the number of wakenings in the night, but an adult normally wakes between cycles and, as the night progresses, within cycles. However, if nothing catches their attention (noises outside, full bladder, snoring partner) they will return to sleep unaware of having been awake. This seems to be protective because hours of unbroken sleep would make us vulnerable, but it is reassuring to know that waking is entirely normal (although being roused from *deep* sleep is disruptive, and remaining awake for any length of time reduces total sleep time). Light sleep, deep sleep and REM sleep all are important for memory and learning. However, deep sleep is prioritised and is thought to be more restorative. It is deep sleep (as opposed to a short nap) that regulates the homeostatic drive and should be avoided in the daytime if a full night's sleep is the goal.

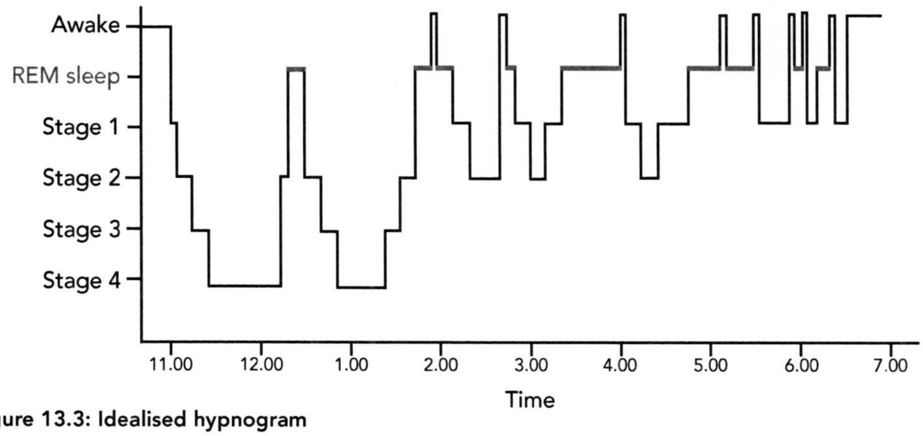

Figure 13.3: Idealised hypnogram

Maintaining a good sleep pattern

Anyone with a suspected sleep difficulty should be referred to an appropriate clinic, but much can be done to improve sleep: see, for example, Espie (2006) or Meadows (2014). Medication for insomnia is not a long-term solution and cognitive behaviour therapy for insomnia (CBT-I) is more effective. Although any individual could sign up to an online CBT-I programme, CBT-I should not be undertaken by people without a suitable qualification, experience and supervision. However, some commonsense measures can be advised by anyone.

Using the bedroom only for sleep (and sex) is suggested, because it helps to create an association and works for people with their own home. It is less easy for people in student accommodation, in the family home or in shared accommodation where some ingenuity may be required to create a 'sleeping area'.

Going to bed when sleepy maximises the chance of sleeping quickly and reduces the chance of spending time in bed worrying, or getting frustrated over not sleeping, and thereby reinforcing a negative association with the bed(room). It is important to distinguish tiredness (experienced in the body) from sleepiness (often felt in the eyes or associated with yawning).

Avoiding daytime sleep will maintain the pressure to sleep at night, but that does not override safety concerns, in the case of driving, for example. Deep sleep would delay night-time sleep, but a short nap (20–30 minutes) is encouraged if feeling sleepy before or while driving. Sitting in a chair to nap and setting an alarm should suffice to avoid deep sleep.

Rising at the same time every day is perhaps the single most useful thing for maintaining a regular sleep pattern. The key is to avoid extremes, but this does not mean that anyone rising early one day a week should get up at that time every day – and variation is also necessary in the case of shift work. If there is weekend lie-in, it is better on a Saturday morning in order not to delay sleep on Sunday night (assuming a Monday to Friday work pattern).

Calming the mind before sleep is essential. It can be useful to take time to reflect on the day and to make notes about things that need to be done. If reflecting on a difficult encounter with someone, it might help to draft a letter or email to express feelings (although usually it is best not to send it without a further period of reflection!). Another possibility is a reflective journal: putting thoughts into words is a good way to stop them rotating endlessly in the mind. Specific worries, including worries about sleep itself, can be challenged as in cognitive behaviour therapy. All these methods can help to stop the thoughts that increase arousal, but nature abhors a vacuum, and something must replace them. Imagery (for example, imagining oneself in a peaceful place) is commonly recommended, and mindfulness meditation is another possibility.

Nutrition, eating behaviour and sleep

Diet quality and patterns affect both daytime alertness and night-time sleep. Current thinking recommends that high carbohydrate intake shortens sleep, high protein intake improves sleep quality, and high fat intake reduces total sleep time. That being said, messages are contradictory, as some show that low carbohydrate intake can worsen sleep quality.

A sleep-promoting diet is balanced and varied, rich in fruits and vegetables and whole grains and lean proteins, and lower in high-sugar and heavily processed foods (Binks *et al*, 2020). The priority for those with eating difficulties should be to avoid malnutrition, which has critical effects on neuro-endocrine functioning, as detailed above.

Late night eating, or eating a substantial meal within two hours of going to bed, can negatively impact the quality of sleep. Short time periods between dinner and sleep can affect circadian rhythms and the secretion of key hormones, such as leptin, melatonin and ghrelin (Nakajima, 2018). Additionally, sleeping on a full stomach can cause gastroesophageal reflux or reduced thermogenesis, both of which can reduce sleep quality. Thus, longer time periods between sleep and dinner are advised.

Sleep-specific eating disorders

For some, eating disorders manifest specifically during sleep. Sleep-related eating disorder and night eating syndrome are examples of illnesses in which eating difficulties manifest during sleep. While both involve frequent episodes of out-of-control eating episodes during the night, individuals with night eating syndrome are usually aware and have a memory of these nocturnal eating episodes, whereas those with Sleep-Related Eating Disorder have little or no memory. Night eating syndrome is linked to binge eating and is more common in people with a higher body weight. It has been thought to be a response to a restrictive diet, in which the body compensates for the daytime restriction at night. During unconsciousness, or when individuals are close to sleep, the cognitive control required to restrict is lessened, and individuals find themselves unable to control their eating. Furthermore, eating during the night disrupts sleep and often leads to fatigue, and associated consequences.

Nikita's experience

Nikita (40) was having a combination of CBT and psychodynamic therapy for binge eating disorder and night eating syndrome. She expressed great shame that her eating at night was out of control. She reported chronic dieting involving highly restrictive behaviours during the day and would wake in the middle of the night to binge-eat highly palatable foods. She described this as a dissociated state in which she was conscious (on waking she would recall the eating) but without control over her behaviour. She became so desperate that she would lock herself in her room at night. Her night eating was directly worse during periods of stress, reaching as many as five or six episodes in one night and, consequently, she was exhausted by day.

The first step of treatment was to help her to be less restrictive in her diet, so that her body did not need to compensate by eating during the night. Through an Intuitive Eating program (Tribole & Resch, 2012), she was able to improve her relationship with food and work towards consuming a balanced, less-restrictive diet during the day. Over time, the night eating reduced as her daily calorie intake was met. As binge eating in the daytime reduced, so did the frequency of night eating, potentially helped by regulated insulin levels or hunger hormones.

The next stage was to improve her sleep hygiene. This involved limiting screen time an hour before bed, encouraging winding down activities such as reading and meditation, and ensuring that she only used her bed for sleep (rather than watching television in bed, as done previously).

Once sleep and diet were improved, the next step was to address the underlying emotional issues that were underpinning the emotional eating and night eating. This involved helping her to process childhood trauma and accept and regulate her feelings, rather than using food to self-soothe. Through a combination of Intuitive Eating, CBT and psychodynamic therapy, Nikita learnt strategies to cope with her feelings and improve her self-worth and relationship with food. Over time, the night eating and binge eating stopped, and she was able to benefit from undisrupted sleep.

Conclusion

Sleep disruption is an important clinical feature in eating difficulties which can have detrimental effects on recovery, yet professionals often pay little attention to it. There are types of eating difficulties that are directly linked to sleep, such as night eating disorder and sleep-related eating difficulties. Individuals with eating difficulties often struggle with high anxiety, obsessional thinking and stress, which can impact sleep. Similarly, poor sleep can increase anxiety, stress and fatiue which may worsen eating difficulties. An integrated approach is recommended to treat these complex, interrelated problems. Practitioners should incorporate strategies to improve sleep into the management of eating difficulties.

References

Binks H, Vincent G, Gupta C, Irwin C & Khalesi S (2020) Effects of diet on sleep: a narrative review. *Nutrients* **12** (4) 936.

Brockmeyer T, Skunde M, Wu M, Bresslein E, Rudofsky G, Herzog W & Friederich HC (2014) Difficulties in emotion regulation across the spectrum of eating disorders. *Comprehensive psychiatry* **55** (3) 565-571.

Cooper AR, Loeb KL & McGlinchey EL (2020) Sleep and eating disorders: current research and future directions. *Current opinion in psychology* **34** 89-94.

Delvenne V, Kerkhofs M, Appelboom-Fondu J, Lucas F & Mendlewicz J (1992) Sleep polygraphic variables in anorexia nervosa and depression: a comparative study in adolescents. *J Affect Disord* **25** (3) 167–72.

Espie CA (2006) *Overcoming insomnia and sleep problems*. London: Constable and Robinson Ltd.

Meadows G (2014) *The Sleep Book.* London: Orion Books Ltd.

Nakajima K (2018) Unhealthy eating habits around sleep and sleep duration: To eat or fast? *World Journal of Diabetes* **9** (11) 190.

Trace SE, Thornton LM, Runfola CD, Lichtenstein P, Pedersen NL & Bulik CM (2012) Sleep problems are associated with binge eating in women. *Int J Eat Disord* **45** (5) 695–703.

Tribole E & Resch E (2012) *Intuitive eating*. Macmillan.

Walker M (2017) *Why we Sleep*. London: Penguin.

14. Eating difficulties and the law

By Rachel Jenkins and Judy Laing

Summary

This chapter provides an overview of the law governing the treatment of eating difficulties in England and Wales. It focuses on the law on consent and the Children Act 1989, Mental Capacity Act 2005 and Mental Health Act 2007. Together, these statutes regulate the provision of medical treatment for children and adults. The chapter outlines the processes that permit compulsory admission and treatment of eating difficulties. Notably, it includes the controversial treatment of naso-gastric feeding for critically underweight patients and the use of restraint in mental healthcare, which some readers may find distressing to read. Emphasis will be placed on the legal safeguards and rights of persons who are experiencing eating difficulties.

Introduction

This chapter considers the laws that exist to provide care and treatment – compulsorily in some cases – for people with eating difficulties in England and Wales. It focuses on overlapping legal frameworks to make decisions about treatment in the Children Act 1989 (CA) for children and young people; the law of consent and the Mental Capacity Act 2005 (MCA) for persons over the age of 16; and the Mental Health Act 1983 (as amended in 2007) (MHA) for compulsory treatment for a 'mental disorder' for people of any age in a psychiatric unit/hospital. Each framework has different legal criteria and processes and may involve different professionals who make decisions about diagnosis and treatment. It is important to recognize that these laws permit treatment in many cases on the basis of medical recommendations, which may differ from and override a person's own wishes about their treatment. This means that the law can work in a paternalistic way to make decisions for others, based on the opinions and decisions of professionals who provide care and treatment for persons with eating difficulties.

Case study: a local authority v E

In 2012, a case involved a 32-year-old woman with severe anorexia nervosa who had been admitted for treatment under the MHA on 10 different occasions in six years. She had attempted to make two advance decisions to refuse life-saving treatment during that time, but had been found to lack capacity (i.e. the ability) to do so at the time. Her case came before the court again under the MCA, where the judge decided that E was not able to make a treatment decision herself and it was in her best interests to be fed, by force, if necessary.

Treatment for children and young people under the Children Act 1989

The law relating to young people's competency (up to the age of 18) and consent to treatment under the CA is complex and reflects a paternalistic desire to protect children from both external harm and their own actions. Multiple frameworks regulate the treatment of children: the CA applies to those under the age of 18; the MCA is relevant to those aged 16 and over; and the *Gillick* case applies to those under the age of 16. While the general threshold for child competency (i.e. the ability to consent to treatment) reflects the law in the *Gillick* case, this becomes more complex when a decision to refuse treatment is concerned. So-called 'Gillick competence' to consent is achieved when a child under the age of 16 sufficiently understands the information about the proposed treatment, including its purpose, nature, likely effects and prognosis. However, due to the potentially dire consequences of refusing treatment, it has been suggested that a greater degree of understanding must be demonstrated by young people to withhold their consent (Pearce, 1994).

This means that those with parental authority or the court are in some cases able to override a child's treatment refusal. In the case of children under 16, one or both parents can consent to treatment on their child's behalf, and compulsory treatment may be considered if the child actively resists their parents' decision. However, if both the child and parent(s) refuse proposed life-saving treatment, safeguarding procedures under the CA may be necessary to ensure the child's welfare.

The best interests test in the Children Act 1989

The CA is focused on safeguarding children. Part I states that children's welfare should be the paramount concern, with questions often framed in terms of what is in a child's 'best interests'. Welfare checklist criteria in the CA include consideration of a child's ascertainable wishes and feelings; their physical, emotional and educational needs; and any harm they have suffered or are at risk of suffering. This is particularly relevant when children are at significant risk of harm by refusing treatment for their eating difficulties. In these instances, the CA sets out proportionate steps to limit the effects of such harm. The main methods of safeguarding include Specific Issue Orders under section 8, Care Orders under section 37, and the Inherent Jurisdiction of the Court under section 100 of the CA (MARSIPAN, 2014: CR189).

A Specific Issue Order

Where medical intervention is deemed necessary by professionals, a Specific Issue Order may be invoked. A 'section 8 order' provides 'directions for the purpose of determining a specific question which has Arisen, or which may Arise, in connection with any aspect of parental responsibility for a child'. This can be used to pass a nasogastric tube if a child is critically underweight and at risk of severe malnourishment.

A Care Order

A Care Order is another means through which treatment can be given to children facing significant risk of harm. Following an investigation into a child's circumstances, it can be applied if the child's welfare is endangered due to care given or withheld. Local authorities may apply for Care Orders where children are not receiving appropriate or food-related treatment for their eating disorder within the family setting.

The inherent jurisdiction of the court

The final notable safeguarding procedure is the Inherent Jurisdiction of the Court. Where wider-ranging and longer-term issues exist, section 100 can be used to authorize treatment against a child's will. The main aim of this jurisdiction is to fill any gaps in statutory schemes and ensure protection and treatments for extremely vulnerable children, who are likely to suffer significant harm in the absence of such intervention. It permits detention and medical care in the absence of child or parental consent where necessary.

Whilst the CA applies to those under the age of 18, the MCA also applies to those aged 16-18. As explained below, the MCA and its Code of Practice is used by professionals to assess mental capacity to consent to treatment (including any treatment for eating difficulties) and to make decisions on behalf of those aged 16 and over who lack the capacity to consent.

Consent and treatment decisions under the Mental Capacity Act 2005

The MCA grants adults with capacity the 'absolute right to refuse... treatment' (reflecting what Lord Donaldson said in the case of *Re T* in 1992 at para. 688H). The law starts with a presumption that a person has capacity to consent (section 1(2)) but this can be displaced if there is any evidence that the s/he lacks capacity. The MCA sets out a two-stage test for capacity, which is based on the particular decision that has to be made at that point in time.

- **The functional test in section 3 MCA**

  The first is described as a functional test (section 3), which says that a person lacks capacity and is 'unable to make a decision' if they cannot do any of the below:

  1. Understand the information relevant to the decision.
  2. Retain that information.
  3. Use or weigh that information as part of the process of making the decision.
  4. Communicate their decision (whether by talking, using sign language or by any other means).

- **The diagnostic test in section 2, MCA**

  This is followed by a diagnostic test (section 2) where capacity may be rebutted if a 'permanent or temporary impairment/disturbance in the functioning of the mind or brain is evident'. A prior diagnosis of an eating disorder may be relevant to this test, as it can indicate the existence of a mental disturbance and may be difficult to rebut. The MCA says that professionals/decision makers must take all practicable steps to enable a person to make their own decision (section 1(3)) and must not treat a patient as unable to make a decision simply if their determination is seen as unwise (section 1(4)). We can see how this works in a case called *Kings College v C & V* in 2015, in which a patient's belief that life would never 'regain (its) sparkle' was determinative, despite this meaning a refusal of life-saving treatment.

- **The MCA principles**

  The ability to make 'unwise' decisions is the third of five MCA key principles, including:

  - the presumption of capacity (Principle 1)
  - supporting individual decision-making (Principle 2)
  - best interests (Principle 4)
  - the least restrictive alternative (Principle 5).

The 4th and 5th principles apply only when a 'causative nexus' (Herring & Wall, 2015) is established between the functional and diagnostic tests, meaning that a patient lacks capacity and a decision can be made in their 'best interests'.

- **The best interests test in section 4, MCA**

  The MCA does not state definitively what is in a person's best interests, however section 4 sets out certain non-exhaustive criteria that may be considered before reaching a decision. One of the factors means involving the patient as far as possible and, as set out in section 4(6), considering past and present wishes, in addition to any feelings, beliefs or values that may influence their decision (Department for Constitutional Affairs, 2007: Chapter 5). This would include taking into account any religious, moral or cultural beliefs. Another factor is to consider the views of any carers/family members in making a best interest decision.

- **Case law examples**

  In the context of eating difficulties, the application of the MCA has been framed in the light of cases such as *Aintree University NHS Foundation Trust v James*, which means that welfare must be considered in the widest possible sense. To a large extent, this reflects the provisions of the CA, which also aims to maximise a patient's welfare through best interest decision-making. Similar principles are reflected in MCA cases, which aims to foster empowerment, even in circumstances of incapacity. For example, when deciding best interests in the case of *Ms X* who lacked capacity for treatment for anorexia, the judge stressed that the patient "retains an interest in life, and has plans for her future". So, through taking a balancing approach to determining her best interests, the patient's future interest in life outweighed her current desire to refuse treatment as a result of her anorexia.

  For those assessed as lacking capacity, in addition to decisions being made in a person's best interests, the least restrictive alternative must be considered before any treatment/care-plan can be implemented (section 1(6)). Following this, if the proposed treatment involves restraint, it must be reasonably believed that it is proportionate and necessary to prevent harm, as set out in section 6. Under certain circumstances, this may also be subject to the MCA's Deprivation of Liberty Safeguards (DoLS).

- **Deprivation of Liberty Safeguards**

  Where treatment meets the threshold for a deprivation of liberty, it must be authorised under the DoLS scheme following a Court of Protection order or under section 4B if a court decision is pending. The professional in a care home or hospital responsible for the person's treatment initiates this procedure and, if authorised, the deprivation of liberty authorisation lasts for 12 months.

This complex system will be replaced in future with a new Liberty Protection Safeguard (LPS) process. As introduced in the Mental Capacity (Amendment) Act 2019, LPS provisions have been designed to put the rights and wishes of those people at the centre of process. While they have similar goals to DoLS (which will run alongside LPS for the first year after its implementation), LPSs aim to provide a more streamlined service and broaden the scope to compulsorily treat persons in a medical emergency, without gaining prior authorisation. The target date for LPS implementation is now 1 April 2022[1].

Summary

With many people suffering from eating difficulties being found to lack capacity for food related treatment, these legislative routes to care are highly significant to individuals and their families. Fundamentally, the MCA is concerned with empowering individuals through a patient-centric approach (Department for Constitutional Affairs, 2007: Chapter 2), often through the best interests framework when applied to eating difficulties. However, this empowerment approach is often restricted by the current inconsistency in the management or psychological treatment of persons living with eating difficulties in the UK. This, in part, results from two overlapping legal regimes – the MCA and MHA – which can make it challenging for all concerned to know which one is most applicable.

Compulsory treatment under the Mental Health Act 1983/2007

The MHA provides a legal basis for compulsory admission and treatment to a psychiatric unit/hospital of persons with a 'mental disorder'. The MHA has no age restrictions, so can be used to treat both adults and children. In 2018-19, there were about 46,000 detentions under the Act, and almost 2,000 of them (just over 4%) were for young people aged 17 and under (NHS Digital, 2020).

The definition of mental disorder and criteria for admission

The MHA is used by mental health professionals to admit and treat a person suffering from a mental disorder in the interests of their own health or safety, or for the protection of other people. Consent is not required here as the process involves compulsion. The definition of 'mental disorder' in section 1 is very wide to include 'any disorder or disability of mind'. In practice, this includes a wide range of recognized psychiatric conditions. Guidance in the accompanying MHA Code of Practice lists clinically recognized conditions that would typically fall within this wide definition, and eating difficulties diagnosed as anorexia, bulimia or binge eating are included (DoH, 2015; 26). Additionally, the MHA requires that

1 More information is available at: www.gov.uk/government/publications/liberty-protection-safeguards-factsheets (accessed November 2021).

the disorder must result either in a risk to the individual's own health/safety, for example of suicide or self-harm (though it extends to psychological as well as physical harm); or a risk to others. The professionals involved in the process make decisions about the diagnosis and assessment of risk, as well as the availability and appropriateness of any potential in-patient treatment. The Code of Practice advises that the least restrictive alternative should always be considered, and compulsory powers should be used as a last resort only in the most severe cases, where there is a risk to the person's life.

Routes to compulsory admission

There are three different routes to hospital under different sections of the MHA – this compulsory admission process has traditionally been referred to as 'sectioning'. Under section 2, a person is admitted as an in-patient for an assessment of their mental health for a period of up to 28 days. Under section 3, admission for treatment is permitted for a period of up to six months, though this can be renewed for further periods of time depending on the nature and severity of the condition. Section 4 allows for an urgent admission for 72 hours in a crisis situation. The route used will depend on the individual circumstances, the nature of the disorder and the particular care and treatment needs.

The compulsory admission process

The process is coordinated by a professional with mental health expertise, typically a social worker known as an Approved Mental Health Professional (AMHP). The MHA states that s/he must personally interview the person in a 'suitable manner' (section 13(2)) and coordinate the assessment process, including arranging medical recommendations to support the application. One of these may be provided by a person's GP and the other must be provided by a clinician, such as a psychiatrist or psychologist, with specialist expertise in mental health. One of the main challenges can be finding a suitable hospital bed, particularly for young people, as there is an acute shortage of suitable in-patient facilities for children and adolescents (Education Policy Institute, 2020). There are also problems accessing specialist services, such eating disorder services (NHS England, 2015: 17).

Compulsory treatment

Once in hospital, under section 3, medical treatment can be given to a person for their mental disorder – but not for any unrelated physical condition. Typically, the treatment given to the majority of in-patients is medication and/or talking therapies. Guidance for treating eating difficulties from the National Institute for Health and Care Excellence (NICE) recommends that medication should not be offered as the sole treatment, and a range of different psychological treatments are suggested for persons with eating difficulties, including Cognitive Behavioural Therapy, or family focused therapy for children and young people (NICE Guidelines NG69, 2020).

The definition of 'medical treatment' in the Act is broad however, and includes invasive procedures such as naso-gastric tube feeding for in-patients with a mental disorder such as anorexia, if it is clinically indicated as being in their best interests. This happened in the case of *B v Croydon Area Health Authority* in 1995 for example, where the judge said that treating the symptoms (i.e. a refusal to eat) is just as important as treating the underlying disorder. Naso-gastric tube feeding was therefore justified as treatment for the symptoms of the patient's particular mental disorder under the MHA. NICE guidance recommends that feeding people without their consent in this way should only be carried out by multi-disciplinary teams who are competent to do so (NICE, 2020: 1.12.3), and that compulsory powers should only be used where a person's physical health is at serious risk due to their eating disorder (NICE, 2020: 1.12.1-1.12.2).

Legal rights

Being detained can be a difficult and disempowering experience (Akther *et al*, 2019). The MHA Code of Practice states that in-patients should be treated with equality, dignity and respect throughout the admission, detention and discharge process (DoH, 2015: 24). Professionals are also encouraged to involve in-patients fully in decisions about their care and treatment and give effect to their views and preferences in care, treatment and discharge plans (DoH, 2015: 23-24). In-patients have important legal rights to an Independent Mental Health Advocate during their MHA admission, to complain about their treatment under the MHA, as well as access to an independent Mental Health Tribunal to review their continued detention. In-patients should be given information about these rights as soon as they arrive in hospital and should regularly be kept informed of their rights, so they know how to exercise them (DoH, 2015: Chapter 4).

Carers and relatives are also given some important powers in the MHA to be informed and consulted about decisions to invoke the Act's powers. This comes in the form of the Nearest Relative role, which is given to a family member, ideally someone who knows the person well, to support them during the admission process. The Code of Practice recognizes that carers should be involved in MHA decisions and that a person's nearest relative should be identified as soon as possible by the AMHP during an assessment for possible admission (DoH, 2015: Chapter 5). There are government plans to reform the MHA which are briefly discussed in the section below.

Law reform proposals

The government announced a White Paper, *Reforming the Mental Health Act*, in January 2021 with proposals to reform the current legislation in England and Wales (Department of Health and Social Care, 2021). The White Paper was subject to consultation in early 2021 and new legislation is likely to be introduced in 2023/24. The proposals are numerous and wide ranging and would result in some significant changes to the admission criteria, processes and safeguards for detained in-patients. Included in the White Paper are recommendations for:

- new guiding principles in the Mental Health Act which include promoting patient choice and autonomy and treating the patient as an individual
- amending the criteria to include a higher risk threshold for compulsory detention
- strengthening independent advocacy and tightening the safeguards for compulsory treatment, especially relating to invasive procedures such as electroconvulsive therapy (ECT)
- introducing advance choice documents for treatment for mental disorder
- including more regular reviews before an independent Mental Health Tribunal
- replacing the Nearest Relative with a new Nominated Person role with more extensive powers. The person fulfilling the role would be based on the wishes of the detained patient provided s/he has mental capacity. These changes could lead to stronger legal rights and improved protection for detained patients, including persons with eating difficulties who are detained under the MHA.

Conclusion

The majority of treatment for eating difficulties is provided on a voluntary basis in England and Wales and compulsory treatment should be viewed as a last resort for severe cases, where life is at significant risk. When compulsory treatment takes place however, it can be an extremely traumatic and disempowering experience. The guiding principles to using the law for professionals focus on promoting dignity, respect and participation, but the reality for many patients can be quite different, as the evidence and research studies often tell us. It is important for everyone involved to remember that the law includes a range of important rights and support, such as rights to information and access to independent advocacy, as well as placing emphasis on the views and wishes of the person about their treatment. Every effort should be made by professionals and services involved to promote these legal rights, to facilitate support mechanisms, to build relationships, trust and actively involve persons with eating difficulties in their care, treatment and discharge decisions and plans. We know from research evidence that these factors are key to positive treatment experiences and successful recovery for persons with eating difficulties such as anorexia nervosa (Tan *et al*, 2010; 17).

References

Akther S et al (2019) Patients' experiences of assessment and detention. *Brit J Psych Open* **5**(3).

Department of Health (2015) *Mental Health Act 1983: Code of Practice* TSO, London. [online]. Available at: https://assets.publishing.service.gov.uk/government/uploads/system/uploads/attachment_data/file/435512/MHA_Code_of_Practice.PDF (accessed August 2021).

Department of Health and Social Care, *Reforming the Mental Health Act* (January 2021) [online]. Available at: www.gov.uk/government/consultations/reforming-the-mental-health-act/reforming-the-mental-health-act (accessed August 2021).

Department for Constitutional Affairs (2007) *Mental Capacity Act 2005: Code of Practice* [online]. TSO, London. Available at: https://assets.publishing.service.gov.uk/government/uploads/system/uploads/attachment_data/file/921428/Mental-capacity-act-code-of-practice.pdf (accessed August 2021).

Education Poverty Institute (January 2020) *Access to child and adolescent mental health services in 2019* [online]. Available at: https://epi.org.uk/publications-and-research/access-to-child-and-adolescent-mental-health-services-in-2019/ (accessed 6 January 2021).

Herring J & Wall J (2015) Autonomy, Capacity and Vulnerable Adults: Filling the Gaps in the Mental Capacity Act. *Legal Studies* **35** (4) 698-719.

Law Commission (2017) *Mental Capacity and Deprivation of Liberty*, Law Commission No 372 [Online]. Available at: www.lawcom.gov.uk/project/mental-capacity-and-deprivation-of-liberty/ (accessed August 2021).

MARSIPAN (2014) *Management of Really Sick Patients with Anorexia Nervosa* CR189 [0nline]. Available at www.rcpsych.ac.uk/docs/default-source/improving-care/better-mh-policy/college-reports/college-report-cr189.pdf?sfvrsn=6c2e7ada_2 (accessed August 2021).

NHS Digital (2020) *Mental Health Annual Statistics 2018-19* [online]. Available at https://digital.nhs.uk/data-and-information/publications/statistical/mental-health-act-statistics-annual-figures/2018-19-annual-figures (accessed 6 January 2021).

NHS England (2015) *Access and Waiting Time Standard for Children and Young People with an Eating Disorder* [online]. Available at: www.england.nhs.uk/wp-content/uploads/2015/07/cyp-eating-disorders-access-waiting-time-standard-comm-guid.pdf (accessed August 2021).

National Institute for Health and Care Excellence (2020) *Eating Disorders: recognition and treatment*, NICE Guideline NG69 [online]. Available at: www.nice.org.uk/guidance/ng69 (accessed August 2021).

Pearce J (1998) Consent to Treatment During Childhood The Assessment of Competence and Avoidance of Conflict. *The British Journal of Psychiatry* **165** (6) 713-716. Available at: www.cambridge.org/core/journals/the-british-journal-of-psychiatry/article/consent-to-treatment-during-childhood/89C4AFD9051EE8021369F66DD19D98B1 (accessed August 2021).

Social Care Institute for Excellence (2017) *Mental Capacity Act (MCA): MCA in Practice: Best Interests Principle* [online]. Available at www.scie.org.uk/mca/practice/best-interests (accessed 11 January 2021).

Tan JAO, Stewart A, Fitzpatrick R & Hope T (2010) Attitudes of patients with anorexia nervosa to compulsory treatment and coercion. *International Journal of Law & Psychiatry*, **33** 13-19.

Cases

A Local Authority v E [2012] EWCOP 1639, COP

Aintree University Hospitals NHS Foundation Trust v James [2013] UKSC 67

An NHS Foundation Trust v Ms X [2014] EWCOP 35

B v Croydon Area Health Authority [1995] Fam 133, CA

Kings College NHS Foundation Trust v C & V [2015] EWCOP 59

Re T (An Adult: Consent to Medical Treatment) [1992] 3 WLR 782

Statutes

Mental Health Act 1983 (as amended in 2007)

Children Act 1989

Mental Capacity Act 2005

Mental Capacity (Amendment) Act 2019

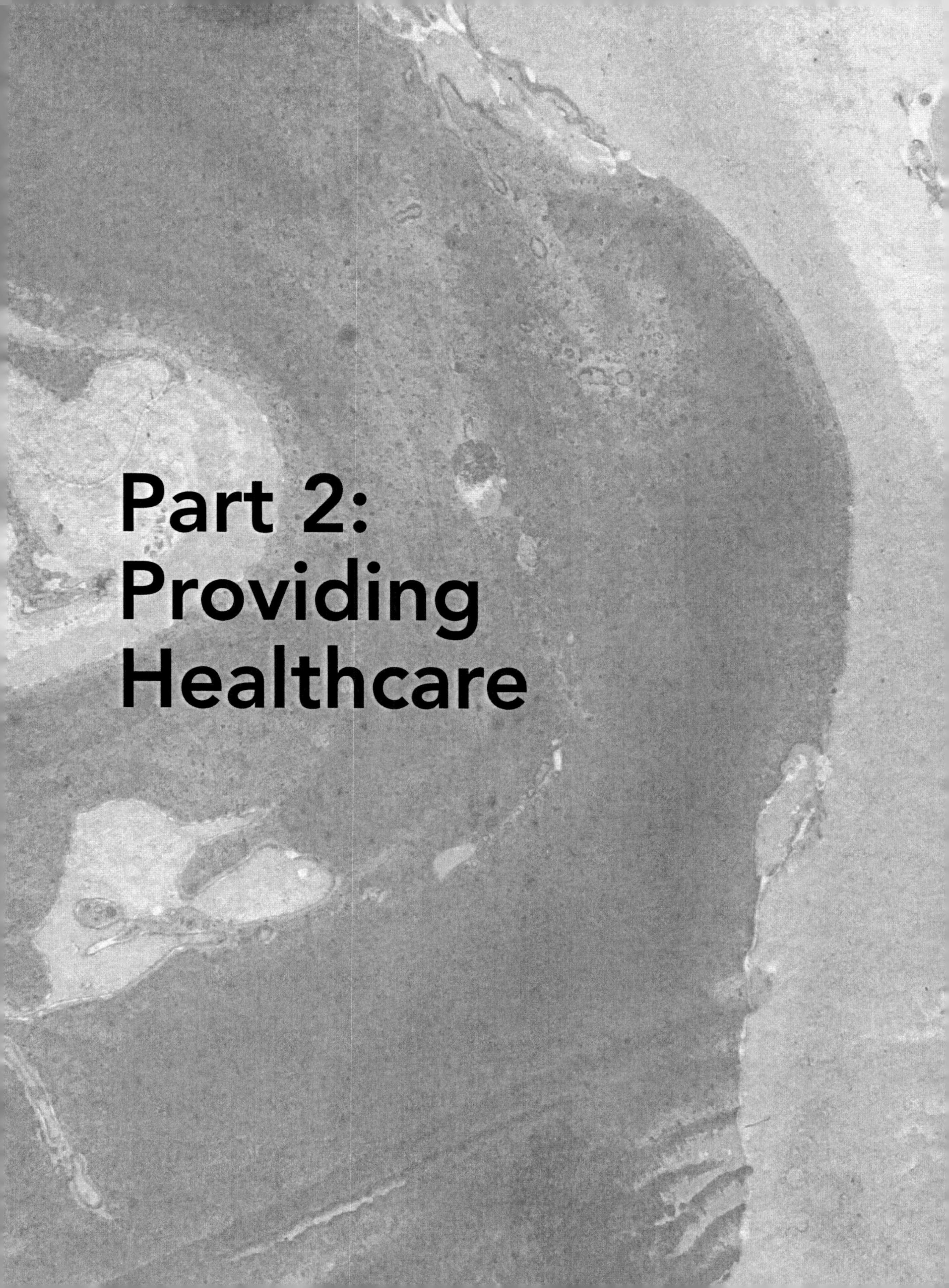

Part 2: Providing Healthcare

15. Seeking NHS treatment and support for eating difficulties

By Emily Rothwell, Jess Griffiths, Andrew Radford

Summary

In this chapter, we help guide people through the process of seeking treatment for eating difficulties. Our aim is to support those who are personally affected (whether or not they are formally diagnosed with an eating disorder, or supporting a loved one), and to provide tips to professionals supporting people affected by a range of eating difficulties. We recognize that each person's experience of being diagnosed with an eating disorder and accessing help and support is individual. We will share reflections from both our professional and personal experiences, which will help highlight some of the potential barriers to seeking help, and how to try to overcome these in order to have the best chance of recovery.

Recognising that help is needed

It is often said that the first step to recovery is recognising that there is a problem. While this may seem a straightforward idea, realising that you are experiencing difficulties with eating and being open about it isn't always simple. This can make seeking help for an eating disorder more difficult.

It is important to remember that eating disorders often serve a function. For example, it may be that thoughts and behaviours relating to food and eating provide a greater sense of control, or feelings of safety and comfort. The eating disorder might also numb difficult emotions or offer a way of communicating (Gregertsen *et al*, 2017; Serpell & Treasure, 2002). These functions will be individually different, and can make it difficult for someone to recognize the need to access help. For some, the prospect of looking for treatment can seem overwhelming. Even if someone is aware that things may not be quite right at the moment, it can be hard to equate this with needing to seek help.

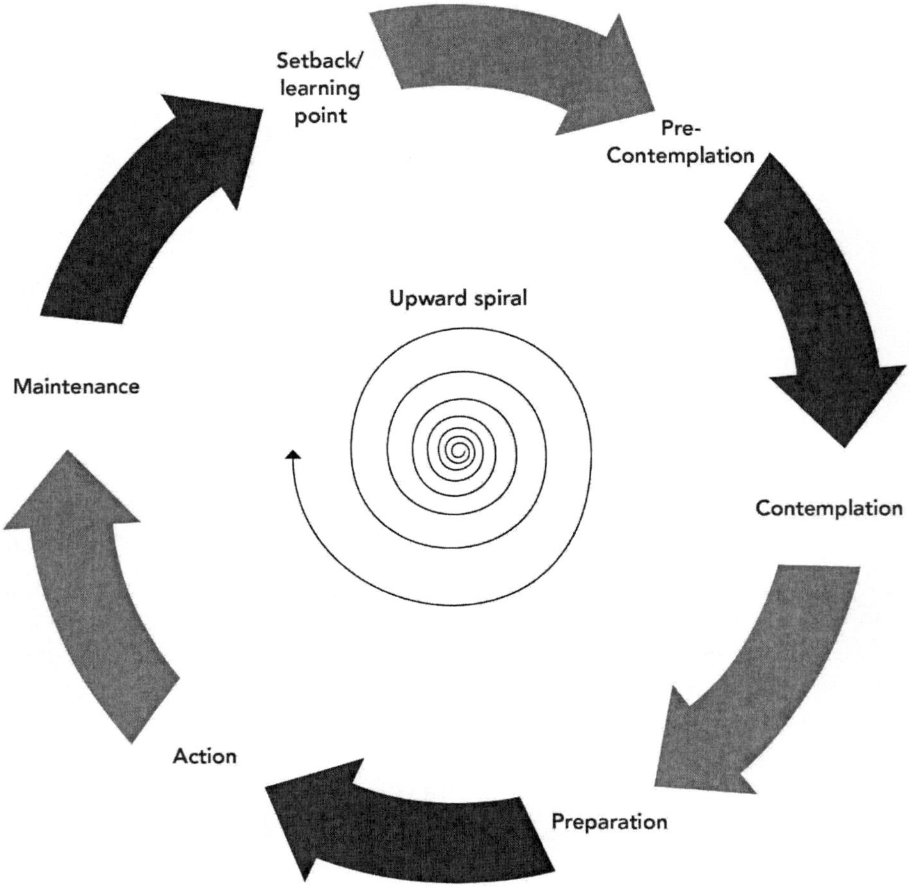

Figure 13.1. Stages of Change Cycle, adapted from work by Prochaska and DiClemente (1983). Figure taken from Beat's website

The Stages of Change cycle (Prochaska & DiClemente, 1983) highlights the different stages that a person may go through when changing their behaviour, and this can be held in mind when considering recovery from an eating disorder.

People often begin in the 'pre-contemplation' stage, where they are unable to recognize that change is needed. Over time and with support, this can move to the individual contemplating change, preparing for this and then putting the necessary changes into action. This will not resonate with everyone's experiences, but it can be a helpful cycle to hold in mind. More information on this can be found on Beat's website.[1]

1 www.beateatingdisorders.org.uk/

Here, Emily reflects on her experiences of contemplating change:

> *"Thinking back to my own experiences, when the eating disorder first started taking hold of my life, I had no idea. I remember being sat waiting for my maths class to begin and saying to my friend that people kept commenting on what I was eating but I didn't know why. I felt confused and annoyed by the comments as I couldn't see that there was a problem, and I just wanted people to leave me alone.*
>
> *When thinking about what I would say to people in this situation, it would be that you are not alone. I felt like no-one could understand what I was going through and like everyone was against me, which was scary and isolating. It can feel terrifying to reach out to others, but I would encourage you to try to, whether this is through messaging a close friend or loved one, or logging onto one of Beat's online support groups. For those supporting someone, I now see how lucky I am that others didn't leave me alone, despite how I kept pushing people away. It took being in treatment for a number of years for me to accept that I needed help, and to recognise that I wasn't in control of my behaviours, but this point did come. I share this to offer hope that things can change, even if this process is gradual and the situation feels hopeless."*

Learning point 1

Take a moment to consider the following points:

1. If you are currently experiencing eating difficulties, reading about barriers to help-seeking could raise many different emotions. Take a moment to consider if anything has resonated with you, and think about where you may be in terms of the Stages of Change cycle. Is there anyone you feel able to share this with? Beat's helpline is open every day if you wish to talk this through.
2. If you are currently supporting someone affected by eating difficulties, consider where they might be in terms of the Stages of Change cycle. Remember that this may not match where you currently are in terms of wanting things to change, as often those supporting someone are already in action mode. If there is a mismatch between these stages, it could be helpful to try to have a conversation about this. The best times for these conversations tend to be away from mealtimes so that feelings of anxiety aren't too heightened. Writing a note or sending a message can also be a helpful way of giving the person time to consider what is being said, and to think about how to respond.

Preparing to seek help

After recognising the need to seek help, the next step for a person experiencing eating difficulties is to share their concerns with someone. Often people feel worried about disclosing an eating disorder because of fear of stigma and feelings of shame (Ali *et al*, 2017; Becker *et al*, 2010), as well as social factors such as the belief that difficulties should not be discussed outside of the family (Cachelin *et al*, 2001). If you are feeling this way, we encourage you to reach out to Beat's helpline to discuss these worries.

Jess reflects on seeking help:

> *"The first person I told about my eating disorder was a close friend I'd known from school. We were both studying at separate universities at the time. I was far away from home and living in shared halls with 16 other people. My eating was chaotic and my behaviours were causing me to steal food from my housemates. I didn't feel I could open up to anyone I lived with and didn't know of any support within the university. I didn't feel I could tell my parents as I felt so ashamed of what I was doing. When I spoke to my friend, she listened without judgement and arranged for me to see a doctor at the medical centre within the university. She attended the appointment with me to ensure I communicated all that was going on at the time."*

Seeking professional support for eating problems can include accessing specialist eating disorder services. In the UK, the most common way to get this is by being referred to an eating disorder service by a GP. Unfortunately, most GPs are not trained in identifying and treating eating disorders when they were medical students. While many have taken opportunities to catch up since then, GPs have often reported lacking confidence in recognising eating disorders and many have been found to have substantial gaps in their knowledge (Waller *et al*, 2014).

There are certain steps that can therefore be taken to help someone to get the most out of their GP appointment:

1. Try to book a double GP appointment, to allow you to have enough time to talk your concerns through. It may be that there is a GP at the surgery who has a specialist interest in mental health, so it could be helpful to ask for them when booking the appointment.
2. Take Beat's First Steps GP leaflet (found on Beat's website) to the appointment. This has a section that explains to the GP why and how they

should refer you for specialist assessment and treatment without delay. GPs have told us that they have found it useful when a patient has given them this.

3. Write down any thoughts, feelings, behaviours or symptoms which you have noticed in relation to the eating difficulties, and how this is impacting on your day-to-day life.
4. Write down any questions you would like to ask the GP.
5. Consider whether attending with a friend or family member would provide you with support.

Specialist eating disorder services are increasingly allowing people to refer themselves directly without needing to go via their GP. These services may also allow family members to make a direct referral. This change is being led by children's and young people's services in England (NHS England, 2015), but is also starting to be adopted in the rest of the UK and by adult services (Beat, 2020). Check the website of your local eating disorder service to see if it allows self-referral, and how to go about this. If it's not clear, Beat's helpline advisors should be able to help.

Learning point 2

1. If you are experiencing eating difficulties and have yet to share these with anyone, take time to consider what is stopping you. Following this, try to think whether there are any benefits of other people knowing. Is there anyone who you would feel comfortable talking to or sending a message about how you are feeling and what is going on for you? One step towards this could be to look at Beat's website and access support through here.
2. If you are supporting someone experiencing eating difficulties, it is really important to have a collaborative approach. The person could feel very anxious about taking this next step to ask for help, so might need encouragement from you to face that fear. It's also important that you don't speak for them and allow them to verbalise their thoughts. Maybe ask them how you can support them through this and think through plans together? This could involve sitting with them while they make a phone call, or attending the appointment with them and waiting in the car park. Ensure to 'check in' with the person, so that you're not assuming what they need.

Tips for professionals

Often the most helpful way to understand more about eating difficulties is to speak to those who have been affected. We asked people with lived experience of eating disorders what they would like professionals to know in regard to treatment and support. They told us that it is important to remember:

- Eating disorders are not a choice, a teenage phase, or someone being 'attention seeking'.
- Anyone can be affected by an eating disorder, no matter their age, gender, race or weight – they do not discriminate.
- It is important to be aware of both the physical and psychological impact of the eating disorder – please focus on the whole person.
- Language matters – terms such as 'resistant to change' or 'treatment resistant' can be harmful and cruel.
- It can be incredibly distressing to be weighed, so please be sensitive and ask the person how you can support them with this.
- Difficulties around eating often occur alongside other problems – be mindful of what else may be going on for the person. This could include low mood, anxiety, obsessive compulsive difficulties or a diagnosis of autism.
- It is important to refer to specialist services straight away, rather than delaying to 'see how things go'.
- Signposting to Beat's services can provide helpful support and reduce how isolating things may feel.

Overcoming barriers

While many people seeking help for eating difficulties start treatment within a fairly short period, there are times when this doesn't happen. This could be for a variety of reasons – some of them are justified, but many of them are not and services are not always able to give the care they should be able to.

If you or your loved one are experiencing difficulties accessing support, it is important to keep on trying. We recognize how exhausting this can feel, so it can be helpful to reach out to friends and family for support around this. Beat's website has detailed guidance around both overturning poor decisions, and understanding when a decision is the right one.

Additional support

There are several eating disorder charities in the UK offering a wide range of services to help people move towards recovery and support families and carers. We have mentioned Beat several times in this chapter as it is the largest of these UK-based charities and offers a wide range of services, mostly online or by telephone. Many other charities cover a specific geographical area and provide counselling, peer support and other face-to-face services. Most local charities (and many professionals offering private services) are listed on Beat's HelpFinder: https://helpfinder.beateatingdisorders.org.uk/ (accessed November 2021)

While recovery from an eating disorder can often feel an abstract concept or unattainable, we know that it is possible with the right help and support, so it is important to always hold on to hope. At times it may feel too distressing or exhausting, so it is at these times we encourage you to reach out for support and to think about what recovery means for you and the reasons to keep going.

References

Ali K, Farrer L, Fassnacht DB, Gulliver A, Bauer S & Griffiths KM (2017) Perceived barriers and facilitators towards help-seeking for eating disorders: A systematic review. *International Journal of Eating Disorders* **50** (1) 9–21.

Beat (2020) *Best practice recommendations for eating disorder services accepting self-referral* [online]. Available at: https://beat.contentfiles.net/media/documents/self-referral-final.pdf (accessed September 2021).

Beat (2020) *Overcoming Bad Decisions* [online]. Available at: www.beateatingdisorders.org.uk/support-services/overturning-bad-decisions (accessed July 2021)

Becker AE, Hadley Arrindell A, Perloe A, Fay K & Striegel-Moore RH (2010) A qualitative study of perceived social barriers to care for eating disorders: Perspectives from ethnically diverse health care consumers. *International Journal of Eating Disorders* ***43*** (7) 633–647.

Cachelin FM, Rebeck R, Veisel C & Striegel-Moore RH (2001) Barriers to treatment for eating disorders among ethnically diverse women. *International Journal of Eating Disorders* **30** (3) 269–278.

Gregertsen EC, Serpell L & Mandy W (2017) The Egosyntonic Nature of Anorexia: An Impediment to Recovery in Anorexia Nervosa Treatment. *Frontiers in Psychology* **8** 2273.

NHS England (2015) *Access and Waiting Time Standard for Children and Young People with an Eating Disorder: Commissioning Guide* [online]. Available at: www.england.nhs.uk/wp-content/uploads/2015/07/cyp-eating-disorders-access-waiting-time-standard-comm-guid.pdf (accessed September 2021).

Prochaska JO & DiClemente CC (1983) Stages and processes of self-change of smoking: toward an integrative model of change. *Journal of Consulting and Clinical Psychology* **51** (3) 390.

Serpell L & Treasure J (2002) Bulimia nervosa: Friend or foe? The pros and cons of bulimia nervosa. *International Journal of Eating Disorders* **32** (2) 164–170.

Waller G, Micali N & James A (2014) General Practitioners are poor at identifying the eating disorders. *Advances in Eating Disorders: Theory, Research and Practice* **2** (2) 146–157.

16. Supporting eating difficulties in primary care: the role of the GP

By Simon Atkins

Summary

This chapter aims to serve as a helpful refresher of diagnostic features and guidelines for referral for anyone working in or with primary care providers. The advice in this chapter may also help inspire confidence in the sharing of care between GPs and specialist services, especially where the latter are either thin on the ground or have rigid referral criteria. These details may also help anyone experiencing or caring for someone with an eating difficulty to know what kind of care to expect from their GP and wider services.

Introduction

One of my favourite medical books is *Suburban Shaman* by the late Cecil Helman. He was a London-based general practitioner who drew on the practices of traditional healers in his native South Africa to reflect on 21st century medicine. "With all our science, our sophisticated X-rays, MRI scans and other sophisticated gadgetry," he wrote, "I think we can learn something from them. It's [their] more holistic view of illness, that focuses primarily on the person and not just on their diseased organ." (Helman, 2006, p.9)

It is that holistic, person-centred approach to medicine that I believe family doctors are well-placed to provide to people living with eating difficulties. And given that there is a great deal of evidence that early detection improves long term outcomes for people living with these conditions, it is GPs who often know our patients over many years, who are often are well-placed to spot any changes in people's physical or emotional states. Not only that, but by having helped them through other, unrelated difficulties in the past, we will hopefully have developed levels of trust that will make people feel more confident to open up to us about any eating difficulties they may be experiencing.

But despite being in 'pole position' to help, researchers have found that family doctors still have progress to make when it comes to making detecting eating difficulties, with some estimating that GPs are diagnosing less than 70% of people who meet the criteria of clinically diagnosable eating disorders (Waller *et al*, 2014). Availability of local services also seems to be a factor that impacts timely care, with studies suggesting that doctors are less likely to make a diagnosis in areas where specialist services are scarce and the burden on primary care would therefore be high (Wood *et al*, 2019).

Setting the scene

Latest available statistics suggest that around 1.25 million people in the UK have a diagnosable eating disorder. Of these, around 25% are male (Beat, 2020). The range of eating difficulties which may not be diagnosed or experiences as an 'eating disorder' extend well beyond this. The mean age of onset is between the ages of 16 and 17 years (Joy, 2012), with studies in primary care finding that diagnosable eating disorders are twice as common in people between the ages of 16 and 20 years as they are in children between the ages of 11 and 15, or in adults between the ages of 21 and 24 (Wood *et al*, 2019).

However, the charity Beat point out that there are reports of people as young as six and as old as 70 developing eating difficulties (Beat, 2020), so it is important not to rely on stereotypes when assessing people, as those who do not 'fit the bill' may well be misdiagnosed and so not benefit from help.

It is also important to remember that, in the same way that eating difficulties can occur at any age, they can also occur at any weight (Shetty & Nicholls, 2017). A recent parliamentary report suggested that many GPs are over-reliant on a person reaching a particularly low body mass index before making a diagnosis (PACAC, 2019), which has led to many sufferers being deemed 'not thin enough' to receive support.

Learning point 1

Before you read further, reflect on your knowledge of eating difficulties, and the kinds of experiences, presentations and people that first come to mind when you think about them.

- Is there a 'kind of person' you immediately think of when you think about eating difficulties?
- What kind of characteristics do you think a typical person with an eating difficulty might have?

It is important to remember that eating difficulties can affect anyone, of any age, sex or background, and of any shape or size. Being mindful of any stereotypes we might have can help us to put them aside when considering the needs of individuals in our care.

Identifying eating difficulties

As with all good models of medical practice, making a diagnosis will depend on taking a thorough medical history and the findings of a clinical examination. Where eating difficulties are concerned, it is worth remembering that you need to be on the lookout for things that aren't said in response to your questions, as much as those that are. Because, while people may well come to discuss their concerns with you directly, either alone or brought by a concerned friend or relative, it may appear at first as though the consultation is ostensibly about something else.

Learning point 2

Take a moment to consider your experiences of eating difficulties, whether from a personal or professional point of view.

- What kinds of things may prevent people from being open about eating difficulties?
- How might these barriers be overcome? What can you do for someone you are supporting to create a non-judgemental environment, build trust and encourage yourself or someone else to seek support?

The following sections include helpful advice for general practitioners when helping people experiencing eating difficulties. They may also assist anyone seeking help from their GP for themselves or someone they care about, giving a guide of what to expect.

Common presenting symptoms

In cases where the difficulties around eating are the main presenting complaint, the following factors might be present:

- Changes in eating behaviours, for example to new types of diet that eliminate certain foods or food groups (e.g., vegetarian/vegan, lactose free, low carbohydrate).
- Excessive and impulsive exercise.
- Significant weight changes.
- Being over-concerned about body image with particular focus on size or shape.

- Self-induced vomiting or periods of fasting.
- Use of appetite suppressants, diuretics or laxatives.
- Social withdrawal, particularly from situations that involve food.

It is worth remembering that, while on the surface eating difficulties might seem to be straightforwardly about weight and body image, they are often about other factors, with the eating and/or weight being one of the few things that sufferers might be able to control in otherwise chaotic or traumatized lives (Froreich *et al*, 2016). There is a significant body of evidence pointing to a relationship between eating difficulties and previous history of childhood abuse, neglect and bullying (Seubert & Virdi, 2018), and these issues may come to light during your assessment of the patient. Understanding these potential triggers can also help with ongoing management.

Physical symptoms

The table below gives examples of physical symptoms that may affect people with eating difficulties. It is worth remembering that these may be the first symptoms they come to an appointment about.

Body system	Symptom
General	Feeling tired all the time, hot flushes, feeling faint or giddy, cold intolerance
Cardiorespiratory	Palpitations, chest pains, shortness of breath, ankle oedema
Gastrointestinal	Heartburn, reflux, constipation, bloating, piles, rectal prolapse
Endocrine	Amenorrhoea, reduced fertility, loss of libido
Dermatological	Hair loss on the scalp, lanugo hair on the face, Russell's sign (calluses on the knuckles from self-induced vomiting), brittle nails
Psychological	Depression, anxiety, OCD, insomnia, poor concentration, self-harm

Taking a history

When people are open to talking about their issues around eating or body image, it's important to try and get a handle on how long they've been struggling and how entrenched their behaviours are.

So, questions to ask would include:

- Dietary history: which specific foods or food groups they eat and which they exclude.
- Compensatory behaviours such as vomiting, use of laxatives, insulin misuse, use of diet pills and other over-the-counter supplements or alternative medicines.
- Exercise routines including types, frequency and duration.
- Any weight loss including how much and how rapidly.
- Menstrual history, focusing on when and if periods started and whether they are ongoing.
- Past or concurrent psychiatric history of anxiety, depression, substance misuse and any past traumas.
- Family history of eating difficulties, obesity and mental health issues.

Screening tools

Alongside, but never instead of, taking a full history, it might also be helpful to use a screening tool such as the **SCOFF** questionnaire, which was first developed in 1999. It is designed to raise suspicion that a person has eating difficulties rather than to provide a definitive diagnosis by asking the following questions:

Do you make yourself **S**ick because you feel uncomfortably full?

Do you worry you have lost **C**ontrol over how much you eat?

Have you recently lost more than **O**ne stone in a 3-month period?

Do you believe yourself to be **F**at when others say you are too thin?

Would you say that **F**ood dominates your life?

Each question that is answered 'yes' scores one point and an overall score of two or more points suggests the person may have an eating disorder.

Clinical examination

This will provide a baseline assessment of the general health of the person you are seeing and provide an opportunity to check for complications and other potential causes of weight loss.

It should include:

- General observation of skin and appearance for pallor, dry skin, lanugo or chill blains.
- Height and weight measurements to check body mass index.

- Pulse and sitting and standing blood pressure (bradycardia and hypotension are red flags).
- General state of hydration.
- Musculoskeletal examination to assess for muscle wasting and strength.

Your examination may then be expanded depending on other presenting symptoms or specific concerns of your patient.

Being mindful of other mental health problems, you may also want to consider screening questionnaires for anxiety (such as GAD-7) and depression (PHQ-9). But once again, it's worth re-iterating that the care of someone with eating difficulties should be seen as a marathon rather than a sprint and once red flags for urgent referral have been ruled out, it may well be appropriate to carry out more detailed assessments over the course of several appointments.

Baseline tests

Guidelines from NICE suggest the following baseline tests in the GP surgery to both assess for complications of eating difficulties and to rule out other causes of weight loss where this is present. Some of the following investigations may be required:

- Full blood count, which may show anaemia, low white cell or platelet counts.
- Plasma viscosity which may trigger further investigation of another cause of weight loss.
- Electrolytes, which may be altered by laxatives, vomiting or dehydration.
- Liver function tests may be elevated by malnutrition and albumin may be reduced.
- Blood glucose.
- ECG (checking particularly for bradycardia).

Depending on the initial test results or the clinical presentation, other appropriate tests might include:

- Calcium, phosphate and magnesium (which can all be low due to poor nutrition).
- B12, folate and ferritin.
- Thyroid function tests.
- Coeliac screening.
- Reproductive hormone profiles looking for another cause of amenorrhea (e.g., FSH, LH, prolactin and pregnancy test).

Referral

You should always refer people of any age to the appropriate local specialist services. Watchful waiting is not appropriate, and neither is holding on until someone reaches a particular BMI, not only because early referral improves long-term prognosis but also because many people with eating difficulties will have a normal BMI.

Unfortunately, because of NHS pressures and funding issues, there may be a significant wait for someone to be seen. It is therefore important to continue to follow people up in the GP surgery while they wait. Frequency of follow-up will depend upon level of risk and should include monitoring of baseline symptoms, examination findings and investigations for rapid change or deterioration, support around the impact of the eating difficulties on education or work, and ongoing care of other conditions which may otherwise be forgotten.

Red flags for emergency admission

There are some situations where emergency hospital treatment may be needed (Robinson & Jones, 2018). These include where BMI or body weight are below a safe range for age, sex and height (some guidelines suggest this would be <75% of median) and rate of weight loss of more than 1kg per week (Academy for Eating Disorders, 2015). Additionally, emergency treatment may be needed for cardiovascular instability such as bradycardia (40 beats or less per minute), tachycardia on standing, prolonged QT interval on ECG, or hypotension (including postural).

Hypothermia, concurrent infection, overall ill health or rapid deterioration and abnormal blood tests such as electrolyte imbalance or hypo-glycaemia are all red flags indicating the need for emergency care. Red flag symptoms and signs are initially managed by emergency admission to a medical rather than mental health ward.

Ongoing support and follow-up

Once someone has been assessed by specialist services they will, hopefully, be followed up by secondary care teams who will provide appropriate treatment and support. Nevertheless, primary care has a vitally important continuing role in monitoring for medical complications. This should involve periodic catch-ups to review the person's overall health and to repeat blood tests looking for signs of deterioration caused by poor nutrition (Williams *et al*, 2008).

NICE guidelines highlight the following specific points:

- Encourage people with compensatory behaviours like vomiting to book regular dental checks.
- Put an alert on the person's prescribing records that they are more at risk of drug side effects (particularly cardiac dysrhythmias) because of malnourishment.
- Sexually active women should be counselled about the increased risk of adverse pregnancy outcomes if they are underweight and about the most appropriate choices of contraception, which they should be advised to use even if they have amenorrhoea.
- Bone health should also be discussed given the higher risk of developing osteoporosis.
- Carers and close family may benefit from signposting to local organisations offering support.

These reviews will also provide a valuable opportunity to check on the person's mental health, too. Issues may come to light that their psychiatry team are unaware of and which can helpfully be fed back. And as GPs, it will be as important as ever to offer holistic care. Just as heart patients or people living with diabetes will consult with unrelated problems, people with eating difficulties will continue to have general health queries too, which need attending to in their own right.

Learning point 3

Having read this chapter, think about the following questions in light of what you have read and your own personal or professional experiences.

- Do you feel like you have a clearer understanding of the role of primary care in supporting someone experiencing eating difficulties, and what to expect from a GP?
- How might you use this information to help someone (either yourself or someone you care for in a personal or professional capacity) to access the care and support they need?

Conclusion

The statistics quoted earlier in this chapter can make for concerning reading. Not only because they tell us about the vast number of people who are living with eating difficulties, but because they also suggest that there are many more who we don't know about and so can't try and help.

So, hopefully by being more aware of the symptoms, signs and available referral pathways, those of us working in primary care will be better placed not only to help those people who actively come looking for support, but to pick up on the subtle clues that others might give when seeking help for another medical issue. By adopting a holistic, person-centred and non-judgemental approach to care we can create an environment in which people will feel able to discuss their eating difficulties and so take the first step on the road to recovery.

References

Academy for Eating Disorders (2012) *Eating disorders: Critical points for early recognition and medical risk management in the care of individuals with eating disorders* [online]. Available at www.aedweb.org/publications/medical-care-standards (accessed August 2021).

Beat (2020) *How Many People Have an Eating Disorder in the UK?* [online]. Available at: www.beateatingdisorders.org.uk/how-many-people-eating-disorder-uk (accessed August 2021).

Froreich FV, Vartanian LR, Grisham JR & Touyz SW (2016) Dimensions of control and their relation to disordered eating behaviours and obsessive-compulsive symptoms. *Journal of Eating Disorders* **4** (1) 1-9.

Helman C (2006) Suburban shaman: tales from medicine's frontline. London: Hammersmith Press.

Joy J (2012) Eating Disorders in Primary Care. *Healthcare Counselling and Psychotherapy Journal* **12** (2).

Public Administration and Constitutional Affairs Committee (2019) *Ignoring the Alarms Follow-up: Too many avoidable deaths from eating disorders* [online]. Available at: https://publications.parliament.uk/pa/cm201719/cmselect/cmpubadm/855/85502.html

Robinson P & Jones WR (2018) MARSIPAN: management of really sick patients with anorexia nervosa. *BJPsych Advances* **24** (1) 20-32.

Seubert A & Virdi P (Eds.) (2018) Trauma-informed approaches to eating disorders. Springer Publishing Company.

Shetty V, Nicholls D (2017) Clinical Review: Eating Disorders. GP Online. Available at: www.gponline.com/clinical-review-eating-disorders/mental-health/mental-health/article/1111690 (accessed August 2021).

Waller G, Micali N & James A (2014) General Practitioners are poor at identifying the eating disorders. *Advances in Eating Disorders: Theory, Research and Practice* **2** (2) 146-157.

Williams PM, Goodie J & Motsinger CD (2008) Treating eating disorders in primary care. American Family Physician **77** (2) 187-195.

Wood S, Marchant A, Allsopp M, Wilkinson K, Bethel J, Jones H & John A (2019) Epidemiology of eating disorders in primary care in children and young people: a clinical practice research Datalink study in England. *BMJ open* **9** (8) e026691.

17. The role of the psychiatrist in caring for people with eating difficulties

By Professor Paul Robinson and James Downs

Summary

This chapter is about the role and value of a consultant psychiatrist in caring for people with eating difficulties. The chapter will cover how the consultant psychiatrist is trained, the responsibilities they hold, and their role(s) as part of a wider team caring for those with eating difficulties. These will be brought to life with examples from clinical practice as well as some personal experiences and reflections.

The aim of this chapter is to inform and encourage those reading – whether healthcare professionals, or people living with or caring for someone with an eating difficulty – to better understand the role of the psychiatrist and what to expect from them as part of the team involved in providing care. In general, the term 'eating difficulties' is used, with some references to 'eating disorders' where this is relevant to the examples given. Written together by a consultant psychiatrist and a patient, this chapter represents the rewards of collaborative relationships between those providing and those receiving care. We hope it is helpful.

Learning point 1

Before reading further, take a moment to reflect on your own experiences of psychiatry – be that professional or personal.

- What have those experiences been like?
- Do you have any strong feelings about your experiences, or any assumptions about the role or value of psychiatrists?
- Do you have a clear idea of the role of the psychiatrist in supporting someone with an eating difficulty?

What is a psychiatrist?

A psychiatrist is a doctor who has basic medical training, taking 4½ to six years, basic medical experience taking one or two years, and psychiatric training usually lasting six years. This amounts to a total of between 10½ and 14 years of training. Some are additionally trained in other areas such as medicine, paediatrics, or psychoanalysis. Some pursue a research career and achieve a higher degree such as PhD or MD. Within psychiatry are different subspecialities, each of which have their own faculties, listed in Table 17.1.

Table 17.1: The faculties of the Royal College of Psychiatrists and their possible relevance to eating difficulties

Expectations of a consultant in any specialty of medicine	
Faculty	Training relevant to eating difficulties?
Academic	Possibly
Child and adolescent	Yes
Forensic	Probably not
Intellectual disability	Possibly
Medical psychotherapy	Yes
Old age	Probably not
Rehabilitation and social	Possibly
Addictions	Possibly
Eating Disorders	Yes
General adult	Yes
Liaison	Yes
Neuropsychiatry	Probably not
Perinatal	Possibly

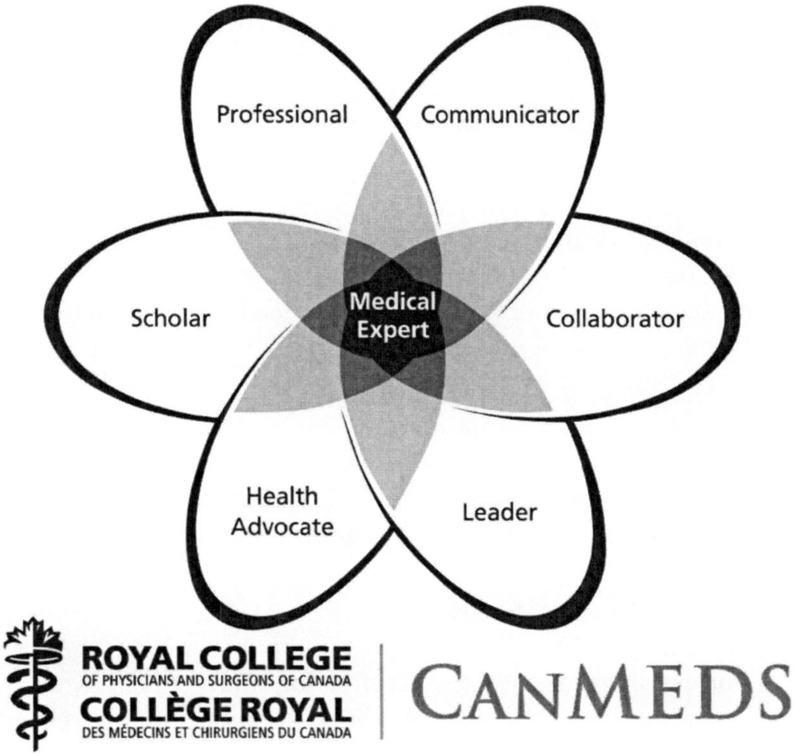

Figure 17.1: The Canmeds framework[1]

The Canmeds framework (The Royal College of Physicians and Surgeons of Canada, 2015) has been adopted by the Royal College of Psychiatrists in the UK and lists the roles that are expected of a consultant. These are:

- **Medical Expert:** This is the central role from which all others arise.
- **Professional:** That is to use a body of knowledge in pursuit of benefit for patients. Thus, the consultant psychiatrist recommends and provides the best available treatment for the people with eating difficulties who consult them.
- **Communicator:** To convey information to patients, their families and to other professionals. This means informing people with eating difficulties about the possible causes, complications and management of their problems, as well as members of the primary and secondary care teams, and, when appropriate, family members and carers.

1 Copyright © 2015 The Royal College of Physicians and Surgeons of Canda https://www.royalcollege.ca/rcsite/canmeds/canmeds-framework-e. Reproduced with permission.

- **Collaborator:** To work with other health care professionals, patients and families and the voluntary sector for the benefit of patients. In the care of people with eating difficulties this means working with primary care, specialist eating disorder services and other healthcare teams.
- **Leader:** To act as a role model and leader for doctors and other staff on teams set up to help patients. In the care of people with eating difficulties, this means giving talks to other team members and developing documents that guide best practice. For example, the consultant psychiatrist may be involved in advising inpatient medical units who admit patients for medical treatment, provide clinical leadership to teams, and be involved in developing services for the local community of people with eating difficulties.
- **Health advocate:** To make representations to local health commissioners, medical Royal Colleges and governmental bodies to improve treatment and management. For people with eating difficulties, this might mean advocating to government or through third-sector organisations such as BEAT to improve specialist services.
- **Scholar:** To keep abreast of knowledge in the consultant's field of work so as to provide the best possible up-to-date care, and to teach other staff in those methods. This can involve reading and attending conferences to stay up to date, making use of the structures of professional appraisal and revalidation to ensure that this activity is of high quality, and contributing to local, national and international teaching events to make expert training more widely available. Research projects to understand eating difficulties better and to find better treatments are covered here.

A fictional case history

The following example will help us to reflect on the different ways in which the above roles might come into play for a consultant psychiatrist working within a specialist eating disorders team:

> *John is a 17 year old with a year-long history of a restrictive eating disorder (diagnosed with anorexia nervosa). His 18th birthday is a week away and he has been referred to the adult eating disorders service by the child and adolescent eating disorders service, where he has been a patient for six months having family-based therapy. John is very attached to the child and adolescent team and feels that his eating symptoms are returning rapidly ahead of transitioning out of the service. He is seen by a nurse in the adult service and found to be depressed and losing weight quickly. The nurse asks for a consultant review for diagnosis and risk assessment.*

Helping the patient directly

How might the psychiatrist help John in the assessment of his difficulties and assist the team in providing a management plan that meets his needs?

First the psychiatrist, Dr X (who happens to be male), arranges a consultation with John. During this interview, Dr X establishes a rapport with John and finds out how he is feeling about the upcoming change in his treatment team, sympathising with the difficulty that must be causing. The aim is to establish a working alliance between John and the new team, which will be essential to its success.

Secondly, the psychiatrist must do a risk assessment, using established criteria, looking at John's BMI, his rate of weight loss and other aspects of his physical health as well as risk of self harm, which is part of his mental health assessment. This will also yield an assessment of what mental health diagnoses might affect John's well being. It seems likely that anorexia nervosa would be one of those diagnoses, and the psychiatrist will conduct a broad mental state examination and psychiatric history to see whether any other diagnoses such as depression or anxiety might also be relevant.

Having established a good working relationship with John, made a physical and psychiatric risk assessment and a psychiatric diagnostic assessment, the psychiatrist is now in a position to collect further information and develop a care plan. Further information is often obtained from a relative through having a meeting or phone call with them. The patient's consent for this is much more likely within a collaborative and trusting relationship.

Supporting the multi-disciplinary team

How might Dr X help the multi-disciplinary team to care for John?

Dr X meets regularly with the whole multi-disciplinary team. He describes his interaction with John after the nurse has conveyed John's history. His diagnostic assessment is that John is suffering from anorexia nervosa which is currently worsening in the context of the change in his treatment team. John also meets the criteria for a depressive disorder, but Dr X judges this as being related to his eating difficulties, suggesting support with this rather than medication would be the best first-line approach. John is losing weight at a rate which suggests a moderate risk of physical collapse. His vague suicidal thoughts add to the risk, which is determined to be moderate to severe.

Dr X gives a view on what treatment approaches should be used in order to improve John's physical and mental health. He suggests a combination of day care, dietetic assessment, individual therapy and family meetings with physical investigations, including blood tests, electrocardiogram and ongoing medical monitoring, including tests of muscle strength. He asks the trainee psychiatrist on the team to perform a full physical examination, suggests that the dietitian evaluates his nutritional needs, recommends continued individual therapy by the nurse and family meetings with the family therapist.

Dr X is available to give a view on what to do in the event of an urgent problem, such as a serious abnormality in John's physical tests, and at the weekly Multi Disciplinary Team (MDT) meeting he evaluates reports from each MDT member and provides advice to them in their role from a medical point of view.

The consultant psychiatrist as a fluid and flexible role

The different roles illustrated by the Canmeds model are often interdependent as well as fluid in relation to context. The 'Medical Expert' role depends on the 'Scholar' role, which keeps the doctor up to date with different research findings. In fact, all of the roles the consultant performs depend on their knowledge and understanding of diseases and their treatment.

Some roles are particularly relevant during interactions within a team setting, for example the 'Leader' role. Some roles come more to the fore when working with patients directly, such as being a 'Communicator' of information. The role of 'Collaborator' could be with patients, carers or other healthcare professionals. Some roles, such as 'Health Advocate' may be deployed with healthcare commissioners.

It can be argued that all roles are in play in all of these interactions. Perhaps the consultant who spends time in a laboratory investigating biochemical contributions to disease might use their interpersonal skills somewhat less, but only until they have to present their findings at a conference. It is, however, in the one-to-one interactions with patients that the interpersonal roles become primary.

Learning point 2

We all have many different roles and identities in our lives. Some of these compliment each other, some compete, and some can even cause us difficulties. Take some time to write down all the different roles you have in your life.

- What do you notice about these many roles? Which are in your personal life, which are professional? Are some both?
- Are there any roles you experience or view as more positive or more negative? Are some more difficult, others more natural? Which are more important to you, which are more central to your sense of who you are? Are there some you could do without?

- How does it feel to reflect on the different roles you take in your life? If you've written them down, does it matter if your page looks messy or confusing? Do you feel your roles need to be more integrated, or are they able to co-exist?

Managing organisational tensions as a consultant psychiatrist

The 'Health Advocate' role can take the consultant to encounters which are more about the organization of care than its delivery, and can even place the consultant in a vulnerable position, as the following example demonstrates:

> *A consultant psychiatrist was seeing a patient outside the hospital system, who was also being treated at the hospital. The consultant was concerned to learn that the hospital, with which he had an unpaid contract, had not brought together all the professionals involved in the patient's care to discuss her case and minimise risk. The consultant wrote a strongly worded letter to the head psychologist in the hospital unit. The manager became very angry that the unit had been criticised and cancelled the consultant's unpaid contract, ending the consultant's role in the eating disorders service. However, the coordination of care for the patient did improve.*

In this case, the consultant was acting entirely for the patient's benefit and the management acted out of hand because they felt criticised. This story highlights the tensions consultants can face when views about the kinds of clinical decisions that reflect their patients' best interests are not shared with service managers. This reflects a significant change in recent times, before which consultants were seen as leaders of services. Our view is that consultants are in the best position to act as health advocates, their priority always being the welfare of that patient, not what is convenient to the institution.

Where the opinion of the consultant and the service manager differs, it can be the duty of the consultant to challenge the manager, especially if patient welfare is at stake, as the following example shows:

> *A consultant psychiatrist in an eating disorders unit recommended that a patient should be discharged within a few days, to continue treatment as a community patient. The manager had other ideas and delayed the patient's discharge to keep the bed occupied and funded because there was no patient on the waiting list who was ready to take it. The consultant challenged the manager and the patient was discharged.*

The consultant psychiatrist as trusted doctor

For patients with more severe eating difficulties, a medically trained person who can monitor physical risk and provide support can be very helpful. This is especially the case where people may have had prolonged periods of illness, or where health can deteriorate dangerously. General practitioners often provide this function, seeking advice and assessment from the consultant psychiatrist when needing to decide whether a hospital admission may be necessary to save life.

> *"I've got a very, very good consultant, who has given me boundaries to cope with ... he knows my limitations and I know mine and we have come to some ... agreements ... and how I can stay out of hospital as long as I maintain my weight and keep very good contact ... my weight needs to be checked regularly ... it means that I can stay out of hospital."*
> Male patient seeing a consultant in the clinic (Robinson *et al*, 2015).

Sometimes, the role of the consultant is to be a long-term presence, albeit intermittently, in the patient's treatment:

> *A patient had been in a general psychiatric ward for 12 months, with little change in her weight, even though she had a naso-gastric tube. She was 39 and had struggled with eating difficulties since 18. A consultant psychiatrist in eating disorders was asked to assess her and he thought that her risk level was acceptable for the naso-gastric tube to be removed and for her to become an outpatient. He agreed to take over her care and saw her as an outpatient for four years, every two to three months. Over this period her health remained the same. However, in the fourth year she started to improve, and over the course of a year she regained a normal weight.*

The lessons here are 'never give up' and 'hang in there'. Even for someone who has had an eating difficulty such as anorexia nervosa for over 20 years, recovery is not impossible (Robinson, 2019). Moreover, in this case, no specific therapeutic technique was used other than encouraging the patient to improve her quality of life gently over time.

At times however, the consultant psychiatrist has to act very firmly in order to save the patient's life:

An 18-year-old patient was very malnourished and being monitored regularly in case she needed hospital admission. For five weeks her weight steadily increased and her muscle power (SUSS test (Etemadi et al, 2021)) remained satisfactory. After that time, although her apparent weight increased, she was unable to sit up from lying flat. In spite of further weight gain, she was admitted reluctantly to the eating disorders ward. On the day of admission she told staff she had been 'water-loading' over the previous two weeks (taking in excess water to disguise weight loss). She commented, 'I was so relieved to be sectioned. I could not have drunk any more.'

In this case, whilst the patient was seeing the doctor regularly, her deteriorating health was concealed by drinking water to appear heavier than she was. This was only discovered because of the muscle strength test. The right test at the right time proved a lifesaving moment, and was made possible by the good rapport she had with the consultant.

Overall, the consultant psychiatrist's role in relation to the individual patient is to establish a trusting relationship, to maintain communication, to adequately monitor physical state, to act without hesitation if risk becomes high, and never to give up hope.

Professor Robinson: Why I like working with eating difficulties

My own route into eating difficulties was a strong medical background, with five postgraduate years as a white-coated hospital doctor, and landing in a research post into eating difficulties during psychiatric training. The medical background meant that I was not scared of the severe medical problems experienced by some patients (as some of my psychiatric trainee peers were), and an interest in research led me to investigate various aspects of the science of eating difficulties.

When I tell people about my job, people (especially other doctors) often say, "I could never do that!" I think this response stems from a number of sources. One of them is stigma. The prejudice against anyone with psychiatric disorder is well known. However, even within psychiatry you can encounter somewhat of a spectrum between conditions in which the patient is not significantly blamed, such as dementia, schizophrenia and bipolar disorder, to those in which blaming the patient is part of both public and professional attitudes.

Eating difficulties fall at the latter that end of the spectrum – with borderline personality disorder further along and drug and alcohol misuse right at the far end. Eating difficulties are too often seen as self-inflicted, even a lifestyle choice. They are often viewed as feminine, whereas problematic behaviour we associate with men is often excused. No wonder our patients are not popular, as they may discover when they arrive in the emergency department or in a medical ward. Even in a psychiatric ward they can be stigmatised –"I've got a ward full of people with real illness, and she's occupying 50% of my time" (consultant adult psychiatrist.)

We all have our own drives and wishes, and many are not that rational. I came to see that patients struggling with eating difficulties do not, in fact, have a choice over their drives. They are often wrestling with irresistible compulsions and compelling behaviours without the support that's required to recover. That view has helped me communicate to patients that I do not criticise them for their behaviour, but that I *do* believe that with therapy, support and effort, they can make changes as long as they can see a better life ahead. When they do, this is extremely rewarding.

James: the nature of eating difficulties means trained psychiatrists are essential

I've been in and out of various eating disorders services over the years, having struggled with a range of eating problems since my teens. Looking back, there were times I saw the psychiatrists often, especially as a child, but they were not specialists in eating difficulties. There were many more tines when I could hardly ever see a psychiatrist because there wasn't one in the eating disorders team, or they were there one day a week.

As a result, a lot of things went missing. Eating difficulties often occur alongside other problems – be they mental or physical health problems – and they aren't all the same. I had a lot of unexplained physical symptoms, from chronic pain to severe digestive problems, and was in and out of hospital with the high medical risks that come from an extremely low weight. Mentally, I was unable to stick to anything, dropping out of many jobs and education courses, including medical school. This was all attributed to an eating disorder, and non-specialists struggled to see the bigger picture.

In my 30s I was diagnosed by a consultant psychiatrist with Attention Deficit Hyperactivity Disorder (ADHD) and suspected Ehlers Danlos Syndrome, a genetic hypermobility condition affecting connective tissues throughout the body. This was later confirmed by a genetics specialist. It shouldn't have taken so long to have someone piece together the pieces and help me to understand what I had been experiencing for decades, including how this related to my struggles with eating. The consultant psychiatrist role is the only one which integrates knowledge of all systems of the body in relation to the specific presentation of an individual with eating difficulties like me.

Without access to this uniquely comprehensive approach, I was left in the dark with physical problems I didn't understand. I could never establish an adequate baseline to engage with psychological therapies, and was given irrelevant information and inappropriate advice.

For me, the case is clear – psychiatrists with specialist knowledge of eating difficulties are an essential part of patient-centred and holistic care. No team is complete without them. All patients should be entitled to the individually specific formulation and treatment plan that I finally received, which was only achieved through working with a highly trained consultant psychiatrist.

A changing landscape

Healthcare is changing. The status of the medical consultant in every specialty has been redefined, and we do not have the influence we once had. In the history of psychiatry, the Medical Superintendent of Friern hospital in 1851 was responsible for up to 2,500 patients (London Metropolitan Archives, 1993). Friern has since closed and community care has largely replaced it, in our view for the better.

Services for people with eating difficulties developed in the 1960s thanks to Gerald Russell, Peter Dally and Arthur Crisp, among others, and methods of treatment have improved since then. The specialty within psychiatry has been recognized by the establishment of the Faculty of Eating Disorders within the Royal College of Psychiatrists.

While treatment of general psychiatric problems such as schizophrenia and bipolar disorder has largely become a matter of community care, the field of eating difficulties has rather lagged behind that example. Too many patients who could be treated at home are still admitted to hospital, sometimes for long periods. We hope that the models of community care that have been established for eating difficulties can be made more widely available in the coming years.

Psychiatry of eating difficulties as a career

There is a tendency to establish services for people with eating difficulties without a psychiatrist, relying on the medical backup of the patients' general practitioners. This is partly because of a lack of specialized psychiatrists but, for whatever reasons, it is a dangerous trend. Eating difficulties have a substantial mortality and one of our aims is to reduce that. This means training a group of doctors who can recognize and deal with the myriad psychological and physical problems represented by eating difficulties.

No other specialist in the multidisciplinary team has the combination of training in physical medicine *and* psychiatry that the psychiatrist possesses. This is relevant because of the coalescence of psychological and physical determinants in eating difficulties. We only need to consider one of our examples above to see this in action. The patient who is psychologically terrified of weight gain and drinks excessive amounts of water to avoid hospital admission is at risk of dangerously low sodium levels, which can lead to convulsions that can last for hours or days and which can be fatal. The origin is psychological, the mediation is behavioural, and the outcome in medical terms can be fatal.

The combination of training required – across physiology, medicine, psychology and psychiatry – is one of the most demanding in psychiatry, and at the same time is extremely rewarding. We hope that more medical students will choose to be psychiatrists with a specialty in eating difficulties, not only for the hugely stimulating work and personal reward, but so we can improve both the physical and psychological treatment for people in need of care.

Learning point 3

Take a moment to think about your experiences in relation to supporting people with eating difficulties, supporting someone personally, or navigating your own personal difficulties. You may want to imagine you are a member of a team treating patients with eating difficulties.

- Write down some of the challenges – what might be difficult about trying to help someone? What barriers might you face?
- What about the rewards? Write down what you think might be the benefits of working with people with eating difficulties. What might you learn?
- Do these rewards and challenges balance?
- If given the opportunity to work in this field, would you take it?

References

Etemadi S Xiaoliai Sun G, Leung S-P, Siddique A, Cooper S, Nwabunma Christiana Ezenwa NC, Treasure J, Robinson PH (2021) The Sit Up Squat Stand Test and Hand Grip Strength: What is the role of tests of muscle power in risk assessment in Anorexia Nervosa? *Eur Eat Disord Rev* **29** (4) 670-679.

London Metropolitan Archives 1993. Available at: https://search.lma.gov.uk/scripts/mwimain.dll/144/LMA_OPAC/web_detail/REFD+H12~2FCH?SESSIONSEARCH (accessed September 2021).

The Royal College of Physicians and Surgeons of Canada (2015) *CanMEDS: Better standards, better physicians, better care* [online]. Available at: www.royalcollege.ca/rcsite/canmeds/canmeds-framework-e (accessed September 2021).

Robinson PH, Kukucska R, Guidetti G, Leavey G (2015) Severe and enduring anorexia nervosa (SEED-AN): a qualitative study of patients with 20+ years of anorexia nervosa. *Eur Eat Disord Rev* **23** (4) 318-326.

Robinson PH (2019) Severe and Enduring Eating Disorders: Concepts and Management. In: Himmerich ed Eating Disorders, publ Intech Open. Available at: www.intechopen.com/chapters/68319 (accessed September 2021).

18. Inpatient and residential treatment of eating difficulties for children and young people

By Reid Robison, MD MBA

Chapter summary

Eating difficulties can be difficult to treat, and sometimes a higher level of care is needed in order to meet the medical, nutritional and mental healthcare needs of individuals with these conditions. Residential treatment is designed for those who are medically stable, but are unable to manage behaviours outside of a 24-hour care setting. Additionally, residential treatment aims at providing individuals with additional psychological treatment with the goal of mapping out a sustainable path towards recovery that can be maintained after stepping down to less-intensive levels of care. When an individual with an eating diffuculty has serious medical concerns, inpatient hospitalization is often considered to provide short-term medical stabilization. In this chapter, we will look at the reasons for considering residential treatment or in-patient hospitalization; criteria for when to consider around-the-clock care; what to expect during admission to a 24-hour care facility; and current outcomes of residential treatment. A case study approach will illustrate the various decision points in a typical trajectory for inpatient admission for a young person.

Introduction

Sometimes a higher level of care is needed along the road to recovery. When it comes to treating eating difficulties, early intervention is especially key as malnutrition can occur at any weight. In the case study provided after this introduction, a residential treatment program allowed the young person, Sasha, to begin her healing journey while maintaining the 24-hour support she needed to remain medically stable.

The continuum of care for eating diffulties is broken up into five levels (see Table 18.1). The first three levels are outpatient treatment, intensive outpatient (IOP), and partial hospitalization (PHP). At these levels of care, individuals are able to reside in their own home or with their family while they complete their treatment.

Table 18.1 : Levels of care in eating difficulty treatment of children and adolescents

Level of Care	Level 1: Outpatient	Level 2: Intensive Outpatient	Level 3: Partial Hospitalisation	Level 4: Residential Treatment Center	Level 5: Inpatient Hospitalisation
Medical Status	Medically Stable	Medically Stable	Medically Stable	IV, feeding tubes, daily lab tests not needed	Vital sign abnormalities (such as low heart rate or low blood pressure), electrolyte disturbances.
Suicidality	No	No	No	No	Yes
Weight (as percentage of healthy body weight) (Generally)	> 85%	> 80%	> 80%	< 85%	< 85%
Motivation to Recover	Fair-to-good	Fair	Partial	Poor-to-fair	Very Poor
Structure Needed for Eating/Gaining Weight	Self-sufficient	Self-sufficient	Needs some structure	Needs supervision at all meals	Needs supervision during/after meals
Control Over Compulsive Exercising	Can manage with self-control	Can manage with self-control	Can manage with self-control	Additional structure needed	Additional structure needed
Purging Behaviour	Reduced/No Incidents	Reduced/No Incidents	Reduced/No Incidents	Asks for support to inhibit purging	Needs supervision during and after all meals/ bathroom
Environmental Stress	Environment provides support/ structure	Environment provides support/ structure	Environment provides at least limited support/ structure	Severe family conflict/ problems/ absence of family/no support system	Severe family conflict/problems/ absence of family/ no support system
Geographic Availability	Located near treatment	Located near treatment	Located near treatment	Patient unable to participate in treatment from home	Patient unable to participate in treatment from home

(American Psychiatric Association, 2006, pp37-39)

In this chapter, we will focus on Levels 4 and 5, or residential and inpatient treatment respectively. For those struggling with an eating difficulty, residential treatment centres offer a stable 24-hour care setting combined with in-clinic psychological treatment. The aim of this treatment is to provide individuals with the support and tools needed to sustain their healing even as they progress to lower levels of care.

When an individual with an eating difficulty has serious medical concerns, inpatient hospitalization is often considered to provide short-term medical stabilization. Inpatient treatment typically involves a shorter stay than residential, although this varies widely by individual needs. The goals of inpatient care are focused on attaining initial medical and psychiatric stability which will enable them to enter a lower level of care in order to complete their treatment.

When considering treatment options for eating difficulties, it may be difficult to decide which level of care is needed for an individual. A useful guide is to consider the level of care which will offer the least restriction, while still providing the safety required for a stable recovery (Santucci, 2018).

Case study: When more help is needed

Sasha is a 16-year old Caucasian female. She's a runner for her high-school cross country team and a straight-A student. For the past six months Sasha has been on a 'health food kick' and losing weight quickly. Outsiders compliment her. Certain family members tell her that she looks great. Sasha's healthy eating progresses into increasingly rigid food rules as she continues to lose weight and further restrict her eating behaviour.

Sasha stops menstruating. She complains about getting full quickly. She begins to voice concerns that she might be lactose intolerant and then gluten intolerant. She complains about constipation. Due to her weight loss, Sasha's parents bring her to her primary care physician. She has a heart rate of 42, which is extremely low. "It's probably because she's a runner," the doctor explains. Sasha's labs come back within normal limits. Because a detailed exam isn't completed, Sasha's lanugo (fine hair on the arms) and pale and cool hands are not picked up and an eating disorder diagnosis is missed. Her doctor concludes that everything looks fine. Sasha, after all, is, "thriving as a 16-year old. She has good grades, she's athletic, and she's health-conscious," her doctor says.

After her appointment, Sasha's weight continues to decrease. One day, her blood pressure falls, and she loses consciousness (syncope). She is admitted to a nearby children's hospital. A psychiatric consultation is obtained and a diagnosis of Anorexia Nervosa is established.

The consulting child-adolescent psychiatrist recommends a transfer to an inpatient eating disorder unit for further medical stabilization and initial weight restoration.

Further laboratory assessments are done upon admission to the eating disorder inpatient unit, along with an EKG. A meal plan for nutritional rehabilitation is initiated and titrated upwards according to unit protocol and as tolerated. After a two week stay at the inpatient unit for medical stabilization, based on careful assessment by the treatment team members and discussion with Sasha's parents, the decision is made to transfer her to an adolescent residential unit for additional treatment.

Learning point 1

Before continuing this chapter, consider the following questions:

1. What are the various levels of care in eating difficulty treatment for children and adolescents?
2. When should 24-hour care (such as residential and inpatient treatment) be considered for children and adolescents with eating difficulties?

Case study: What to expect during inpatient and residential treatment

While in residential treatment, Sasha received intensive dietary and behavioral interventions through group and individual formats, along with meeting medical and psychiatric prescribers for ongoing assessment and management of eating difficulty-related health issues and any comorbid conditions. Her treatment team's goals for her residential stay included psychoeducation, ongoing weight restoration and maintenance, body acceptance, meal planning and improved relationship with food, and strengthening family relationships to support the recovery path and transition back to the home environment. After four weeks in the residential unit, Sasha is ready and motivated to discharge home to her family and step down to a partial hospitalisation program (PHP, or day treatment) while residing at home. After four weeks of day treatment, she is transitioned to three days per week of intensive out-patient (IOP) and monitored closely by her treatment team for ongoing progress.

When the need Arises for 24-hour care, the overall goal is to help the child or adolescent replace their eating difficulty with adaptive skills in order to avoid repeating patterns of thoughts and behaviours. It is also important that the individual develops a deep understanding of how to live their life in a way that still reflects their individuality in the absence of disordered eating.

For children and adolescents with eating difficulties, there are a number of unique considerations when it comes to 24-hour care treatment. Clear expectations, consistency, compassion, and a clearly delineated structure are essential in order to define how a patient can progress to the next level of care. It is also important to look at an individual's care as training (rather than merely treatment). The structured and supportive environment of inpatient and residential care presents an opportunity for challenges, which are ideally coupled with reasonable freedom and naturalistic consequences for deleterious behaviours.

Inpatient treatment

While the primary aim of 24-hour care is to medically and psychologically stabilize the client so they can resume treatment on an outpatient basis, these two levels of care differ slightly in the specificity of their goals when it comes to medical, dietary, and behavioural factors. For inpatient care, an individual's medical goals focus on stabilising their labs and vital signs. Nutritional rehabilitation (the beginning stages of weight restoration) is also a main focus at this stage. If a feeding tube is required for adequate caloric intake, this is generally an intervention done in an inpatient setting and represents one of the common criteria used to determine level of care needs.

The length of stay of inpatient treatment is typically (although not always) shorter in duration than residential care, given the focus on initial stabilization. Group and individual therapy are typically a part of inpatient care, although the focus is generally more geared towards initial psychoeducation and motivation towards recovery to prepare for the subsequent levels of care. While not all levels of care are needed for every individual, a typical course of treatment moves from more to less structured as the individual progresses along the path to full recovery.

Residential treatment

At the residential level of care, individuals will focus on continued weight restoration and maintenance, meal planning, food variety and food exposure. A decreasing meal plan structure can be implemented as an individual progresses toward attuned, intuitive and mindful eating. In both individual and group formats there is also a focus on deeper psychotherapeutic work while on the residential unit. After initial medical stabilization, clinicians can consider adding other therapies if needed. These may include dialectical behavioural therapy (DBT), addressing emotion regulation, exposure and response prevention (ERP), aimed at treating anorexia and obsessive-compulsive disorder (OCD), and other adolescent therapy focused on treating comorbid anxiety, depression, self-esteem, or interpersonal difficulties.

Therapy focuses on preparing the individual to transition back to their home environment with new awareness, insight and skills in order to navigate eating difficulty thoughts and urges and avoid the recurrence of significant deleterious behaviour patterns.

The length of stay in residential treatment depends on a variety of factors and covers a large range (anywhere from a few weeks to a year, in some cases). Treatment is usually slightly longer for those with anorexia nervosa as opposed to bulimia nervosa. While each residential treatment program is structured differently, many of them include a variety of therapies, along with group activities such as ropes courses, meal prep, yoga, art and exercise. Some programs also provide meditation and music exercises (Peckmezian & Paxton, 2020).

Residential treatment centers also vary in the level of autonomy which individuals are given. Some programs opt to involve patients in normal day-to-day activities as they progress through treatment, such as outings with family members. This allows a smoother transition for individuals when they return home following their treatment (Costin, 2007, p268).

A team-based approach

When treating eating difficulties in a 24-hour care center, communication between outside providers and treatment team members is another way to leverage a positive treatment outcome. This multidisciplinary team approach often includes specialists in psych, medicine, therapy, dietary and others as needed. Team members coordinate treatment goals, monitor progress towards both weight restoration and behavioural changes, and set guidelines for when to transition to other levels of care.

Family and caregiver involvement

Another unique component of inpatient and residential care for children and adolescents is the involvement of parents, family members and other caregivers. While caregiver support is thought to improve outcomes of individuals of any age, it is a necessity for medical decision making when a minor is in treatment (Treasure & Nazar, 2016, p16). Beyond medicolegal reasons, active involvement in inpatient and residential treatment by caregivers may reduce the likelihood of problematic relational patterns that could interfere with treatment goals and successful outcomes (Dennhag *et al*, 2019, pp1-17; Murray *et al*, 2015, pp. 302-314).

Caregivers, including parents and other family members, represent an often-untapped resource for enhancing change in individuals who struggle with eating difficulties. Aside from the fact that caregivers know their loved ones best, there are numerous practical reasons for the involvement of caregivers. First, those who struggle with behavioural or mental health issues often live at home, with a spouse or partner, or are dependent on their families in some way. Therefore, it is sensible to equip these individuals with evidence-based support skills for use in day-to-day interactions. When caregivers can offer support in the real-world settings where their loved one is most likely to struggle, outcomes also improve. Providing the caregiver with an active role in the service of their loved one's healing also decreases their feelings of powerlessness and paralysis, which can lead to burn-out, relationship strain, and the possible maintenance of their loved one's symptoms. There is strong data relating to the cost-effectiveness and the efficacy of structured family involvement and yet the treatment offered to many is individually focused, especially among adolescent and adult populations (Le *et al*, 2017, pp1356-1366).

Empathetic and compassionate caregivers are those who are committed to healing the whole family alongside the individual. Clear communication paired with consistent involvement of the family in treatment goal discussions, meal planning and dietary counseling allows each individual to fully integrate their training into their post-treatment life. Involvement of the family also allows providers to assess the relationship with food and body image that exists within the family.

Learning point 2

Before continuing this chapter, pause and think about your own family's relationship with food.

1. Describe the family food philosophy from each family member's perspective.
2. How do you view food and dining experiences within your family?
3. Do you have personal and/or family food patterns? Rules? Expectations?

Case study: Treatment outcomes

Sasha is now in stable outpatient treatment, meeting weekly with a therapist and dietitian as well as monthly with a psychiatrist and primary care provider. She still has occasional eating difficulty thoughts and urges, but has been able to abstain from most of the previous deleterious behaviour patterns. Sasha has an open and honest ongoing dialogue with her therapist and dietitian who support her in self-correcting when needed. With the help of supportive caregivers and an active treatment team, she has been able to maintain progress on an outpatient basis.

Learning point 3

After finishing this chapter, take a moment and think about the following questions:

1. How would you define success in eating difficulty treatment at various levels of care?
2. What are some of the expected outcomes of both residential and inpatient treatment for eating difficulties?

Conclusion

Inpatient and residential treatment are sometimes a crucial step in the healing process for those struggling with severe eating difficulties. While continued research is needed, residential and inpatient settings consistently show positive outcomes in disordered eating behaviours, motivation to change, psychological flexibility, quality of life, body weight, body image attitudes and co-occurring conditions such as depression and anxiety (Peckmezian & Paxton, 2020, pp246-259; Smith, 2016, p35).

While some form of outpatient treatment is still required following care in a 24-hour facility, inpatient and residential treatment can still provide the foundation for an individual to continue to the next level of treatment with a greater level of autonomy.

References

Dennhag I, Henje E & Nilsson K (2019) Parental caregiver burden and recovery of adolescent anorexia nervosa after multi-family therapy. *Eating disorders*, pp. 1–17 [advanced online publication].

Le LK, Barendregt JJ, Hay P, Sawyer SM, Hughes EK & Mihalopoulos C (2017) The modeled cost-effectiveness of family-based and adolescent-focused treatment for anorexia nervosa. *The International Journal of Eating Disorders* **50** (12) pp1356–1366.

Murray SB, Anderson LK, Rockwell R, Griffiths S, Le Grange D & Kaye WH (2015) Adapting Family-Based Treatment for Adolescent Anorexia Nervosa Across Higher Levels of Patient Care. *Eating Disorders* **23** (4) pp302-14.

Peckmezian T & Paxton SJ (2020) A systematic review of outcomes following residential treatment for eating disorders. *European Eating Disorders Review: the Journal of the Eating Disorders Association* **28** (3) pp246–259.

Santucci P (2017) *Treatment Centers and Levels of Care* [online]. Available at: https://anad.org/levels-of-care/ (Accessed October 2021).

Smith K, Lesser J, Brandenburg B, Lesser A, Cici J, Juenneman R, Beadle A, Eckhardt S, Lantz E, Lock J, Le Grange D (2016) Outcomes of an inpatient refeeding protocol in youth with Anorexia Nervosa and atypical Anorexia Nervosa at Children's Hospitals and Clinics of Minnesota. *Journal of Eating Disorders* **4**, p35.

Treasure J & Nazar BP (2016) Interventions for the Carers of Patients With Eating Disorders. *Current Psychiatry Reports* **18** (2) 16.

Yager J, Devlin MJ, Halmi KA, Herzog DB, Mitchell JE & Powers P Zerbe KJ (2014) Guideline Watch: Practice Guideline for the Treatment of Patients With Eating Disorders 3rd Edition. *Focus* **12** (4) pp416-431.

19. A paediatrician's guide

Dr Simon Chapman

Summary

Young people who are underweight with eating difficulties only see doctors when they are in crisis. Frail and vulnerable, they are scared when they are brought in by their parents to hospital. To understand how being underweight can lead to this, one needs to understand the biology of malnutrition.

For those with eating difficulties, understanding the biology and recognising the signs can be key to knowing when to worry and when to reach out for help. Anorexia nervosa carries with it a 10% lifetime risk of mortality. About half of this risk is related to the physical complications of being underweight. It is the most dangerous of all mental health conditions.

This chapter explains how the body handles calorie restriction, and how starvation affects how people feel. It explains the risks, and how these can be identified and reduced. It provides guidance on the steps that a young person might go through if they need medical help.

The biology of starvation

Starvation begins in a part of the brain known as the hypothalamus. Like a thermostat, the hypothalamus takes a central role in coordinating the body's response to energy deficiency. Any decisions it makes are mediated through the pituitary, a gland which sits just underneath, releasing hormones that control metabolism, growth, water balance, stress response and fertility. The process by which these are kept stable is known as homeostasis. The body's internal environment is maintained by a series of feedback loops, in the same way that a thermostat controls the temperature in the house around a set point by adjusting the radiators. The body will usually tolerate a narrow range of normal and defend this. For example, if the body temperature drops below normal (36 degrees celsius), a series of physiological responses occur to bring the temperature back up, such as constricting the vessels in the skin to divert the blood to the core, and causing the muscles to shiver to generate heat, and change behaviour to seek shelter/covering.

In starvation, the body is in a 'catabolic state' – that is, the intake does not meet the energy demand, and survival can only be guaranteed by reducing the demand. It does this in three ways:

1. 'Switching over' – Metabolic adaptation
2. 'Switching down' – Slowing metabolism
3. 'Switching off' – non-essential processes (growth, fertility)

'Switching over': metabolic adaptation

In a nourished state, the fuel of the body is largely provided by glucose. Glucose can be derived from all food groups and is broken down easily and used readily. In the fed state it is responsible for most activity – 100% of the brain fuel in the fed state is derived from glucose.

In the starved state, however, glucose intake falls and glucose stores dwindle. The liver and muscles only have capacity to store one to two days' worth of glucose in the form of glycogen, so other forms of energy have to be sought. These exist in the form of fat and protein, the latter found principally as muscle. Fat provides more than twice the amount of energy per gram as glucose (9kcal/g vs 4 kcal/g) but it is not so readily accessible. Glucose can be thought of as the liquid cash of the human metabolic economy – transient, easily earned and spent, whereas fat is like tying cash up in investments which give a good return, but are not easy to access in a hurry.

When fat is broken down, it releases glycerol (a sugar which can be broken down in the same way as glucose) and fatty acid chains. These fatty acid chains are long, and can be broken down slowly, each time releasing energy in the form of ketones. In high concentrations ketoacids can be smelt on the breath as pear drops. Ketones are remarkable chemicals, as they can be also used as fuel by the heart and the brain, sparing the limited glucose supply for other organs which cannot choose; evolution has provided a back-up fuel supply for the two most important organs of the body. The effect is that up to 80% of the brain's fuel can be derived from ketones.

'Switching down'

In a bid to reduce energy expenditure, cellular work declines. Heart cells in particular beat more slowly – going from 70bpm sometimes down to 40bpm. This is a consequence of 'vagal tone', a message from the brain to the heart's natural pacemaker to slow down. A slow pulse leads to low blood pressure, in turn causing dizziness on standing. This symptom is common.

It is not just the heart rate that slows; in fact, all cells do. Hair and skin cells divide more slowly, leading to hair loss and delayed healing; neutrophils, part of the body's white blood cell immune defences, slow down leading to a reduced capacity to fight infection. Gut cells, too; waves of muscle contractions which normally push stool round the colon reduce in number, leading to a slower 'transit time', harder stools, and 'delayed gastric emptying'. It is a paradox that, in starvation, appetite is often diminished, a consequence of this delay is for the stomach to empty and for there to be a high level of ketones, which can be experienced as nausea.

'Switching off'

Growth and fertility can be seen as expensive extras in this context. Fertility, particularly in girls and women, is demanding of energy, preparing for ovulation and then replacing iron and blood cells following menstruation. Growth, similarly, drains precious resources. The hypothalamus can control this by stopping production of all the hormones that control growth and fertility in the pituitary. When periods stop, it is known as 'amenorrhoea', and should be seen as the body prioritising survival over health. In large part this is reversible with weight restoration and only very rarely does it lead to longer term consequences.

Cognitive impact

It is now known that starvation has a significant psychological impact. As the body slows down, cognitive function also becomes affected. Psychological symptoms of low mood or anxiety can develop as a consequence of malnutrition.

Learning point 1

- Regular eating is not just for physical health. It affects negative thoughts too.
- In the early stages of recovery it is normal to feel full for longer – it can take some weeks for appetite to return once regular eating is re-established.
- Constipation can be uncomfortable and affect appetite. While medicine in the short term can help, regular eating, particularly of food rich in fibre, will improve constipation.

Signs and symptoms

At medical school, students are taught that symptoms are what patients describe; signs are what doctors find when they examine them. Starvation is a slow, gradually declining state, so symptoms come on gradually, and are often explained away. Dizziness and feeling cold are quite subjective symptoms, and are common in the general population and easily dismissed. When you consider them together, however, the picture becomes clearer.

Symptoms

There is often a quality to the sensation of **feeling cold**: layers and radiators cannot take the feeling away.

- **Tolerance for activity** is much diminished, though often masked by nervous energy.
- **Dizziness** is commonly reported, particularly when standing from a sitting or a lying position. Some people momentarily lose their vision or see spots and lines. This is called 'presyncope'.
- **Abdominal pain** is often a consequence of constipation, loss of appetite (from delayed gastric emptying and ketosis) and marked anxiety around mealtimes are common themes.
- A common effect is a **change in mood** – people often describe losing their 'spark', feeling low and unhappy, or anxious and worried. This can be due to malnutrition alone.
- **Loss of periods** (amenorrhoea) or **pubertal arrest** manifest by delay in pubertal milestones.
- For those who purge – **heartburn**, **halitosis** and **dental erosions** are common symptoms.
- **Disrupted sleep** can be a consequence of anxiety.

Signs

Measurements: Height and weight are measured to calculate a body mass index (BMI) (weight divided by height in metres squared). In children and young people, where height and body shape change over time, BMI is only meaningful if compared to others on a growth chart. Clinicians often refer to the 'percent median BMI' (%mBMI) or 'weight for height' (WfH). This compares the young person's BMI with the median value for all young people the same age and sex, expressed as a percentage. The lower the %mBMI, the greater the level of physical risk.

General signs: These include *muscle wasting*: this can be very prominent and manifests as visible tendons in the hands, muscle loss in the upper arms and thighs, prominent jaw bones and sunken eyes, visible ribs and pelvic bones, Hands may often be red or purple, with 'delayed capillary refill time' (time taken for the nail bed to turn from white to red on depressing it for five seconds and then releasing.) *Lanugo hair* is often seen – fine downy hair on the back and abdomen, occasionally the face. It exists only in starvation states, an evolutionary throwback to our primate ancestors whose fur coats would thicken in a low temperature.

Specific vitamin deficiencies: This depends on the vitamin in question. A sore red tongue (glossitis), broken skin in the corners of the mouth (angular cheilitis) or pigmented rashes on the skin can all be indicative of specific deficiencies. All are treatable. Thiamine deficiency rarely can cause behavioural change and confusion.

Bradycardia and hypotension: these are medical terms for slow heart rate and low blood pressure. A pulse below 60 bpm would be considered slow. The rare very fit individual would have a pulse in the 50s, but for most it is much higher. A pulse of 40bpm at rest would likely be much slower when asleep.

Dehydration: many young people who restrict their calories also unwittingly restrict their fluids. A substantial amount of our daily fluid intake comes from our food, which is often not made up for when fasting. A doctor can assess a degree of dehydration on the basis of skin elasticity, dryness of mucosa (lips/eyes), pulse and rate of breathing (often fast), as well as asking about urine output.

Muscle strength: As muscles waste, muscle strength is diminished. A doctor may test this by seeing if a young person can sit up from lying, or stand up from squatting without using their hands. Reflexes may also be reduced or absent.

MaRSiPAN (Medically At Risk Sick Patients with Anorexia Nervosa)

Since 2012, doctors have developed a risk assessment tool known as MaRSiPAN. This looks at a young person's signs and symptoms in a structured way and attributes a traffic light colour risk. The introduction of MaRSiPAN principles has improved the way physical and mental health clinicians work together to support young people with eating difficulties.

Case study

At 14 years of age Mary had resolved to make some changes. She was in year 9, her first year in a new private school. She was bright and doing well, but had not yet quite found her friendship group. She did well in subjects, particularly the sciences and music, and played for her local football team at the weekends. Not everything was going well though – her grandmother had recently died unexpectedly, and family life recently was uncomfortable. Her father's job was under threat, leading him to drink every night after work and argue with her mother.

A few months ago, in an offhand way, a friend of her closest friend joked that she had big cheeks. Stung by the comment she did not react. Over the following weeks she decided to change her lifestyle.

Initially she stopped helping herself to the snacks in the kitchen, or eating crisps or sweets, making only 'healthy choices'. As the weeks went by, she developed little rules which became increasingly rigid – she would not allow herself to eat more than the day before, and she could not eat before 4pm.

Every morning when she awoke she would feel light-headed when she stood up. She fainted at school leaving her classroom, but the teachers did not see and her friend caught her and helped her to a chair. Her friends were worried about her and told her so. She was cold all the time, in a way that she had never been before. At home she would wrap herself up in layers with a hot water bottle which left red marks on her skin. She didn't sleep. She didn't feel tired, but she would be breathless walking upstairs or between lessons. After two months her periods, which had always been irregular, got lighter and then stopped. She looked increasingly frail until one Monday evening her parents told her that the teacher had noticed she was looking unwell. They had noticed too and had not known what to do. They had booked an appointment with the GP.

The GP looked very worried. She said her pulse was slow, her blood pressure was low and she showed the family a list of all her risks which were red and amber. She organized an urgent referral to the child and adolescent eating disorders team.

Learning point 2

1. What aspects was Mary's GP considering when she saw her?
2. How might Mary have felt on hearing how the GP had assessed her?
3. What symptoms were clues to her being underweight?
4. When the GP examined her, what signs might she have found?

Nutrition and refeeding

Recovery from an eating difficulty cannot occur without eating. In severe states of starvation, reintroducing food is medicalized due to the risk of the 'refeeding syndrome'. In this rare situation, a person who is in a state of extreme starvation may develop serious electrolyte shifts when nutrition is reintroduced. With careful medical supervision and prescribed meal plans in the early days of refeeding, this can be avoided.

Once beyond the first few days, the challenge then is to restore weight to recovery. Many services provide personalized meal plans for young people to follow, with support from their families or carers. Meal plans are usually devised by specialist dieticians to ensure that the correct food groups and vitamins are replaced. Medical support is provided alongside the psychological support.

Recovery

It is hard to define recovery from an eating problem. It is easier to define physical recovery. Restoration of physical health comprises of at least four of the following elements:

1. Absence of symptoms of malnutrition
2. Absence of signs of malnutrition
3. Normal growth
4. Normal puberty/fertility
5. Recovered bone health (hard to measure)

Recovery of puberty or fertility in girls and women may represent return of the menstrual cycle (typically three consecutive periods). However, it is important this is not the only sign of recovery. And of course this cannot be used in boys. For those who have yet to start their periods, or those who are still in puberty, recovery can be defined as progression of pubertal milestones, defined as the Tanner stages. A paediatrician would need to make this assessment[1].

Conclusion

Understanding the biology of being underweight allows people with eating difficulties and their families to understand their symptoms. When young people are underweight, it is common for them to feel cold all the time, to become easily tired and feel lightheaded on standing. Likewise, many feel full after eating, have abdominal discomfort and are often constipated. Being underweight can affect mood and concentration too. Finally, those who have periods see them becoming lighter and stopping; those who don't, see their pubertal milestones arrest. This can all be explained when one understands how the body uses its resources and adapts to reduced calorie intake. Restoring regular eating can reverse all of these symptoms, often without consequence. A paediatrician, using the MaRSiPAN framework, assesses a young person's physical risk in a systematic way, to help guide the therapeutic team in how they support a young person who has difficulties with their eating.

References

Royal College of Psychiatry (2012) *Junior MaRSiPAN, Management of Really Sick Patients with Anorexia Nervosa.*

Cahill G (1970) Starvation in Man. *New England Journal of Medicine* (**282**) 668-675.

Benedict F (1915) *A study of prolonged Starvation.* Carnegie Institution of Washington.

1 https://childgrowthfoundation.org/wp-content/uploads/2020/03/Puberty-and-Tanner-Stages_v2.0.pdf (accessed November 2021).

20. Understanding eating difficulties (EDs) in Autistic Spectrum Conditions: Implications for diagnosis and management

By Clive Kelly & Rachael Raw

Introduction

Autistic Spectrum Conditions (ASC) have significant comorbidities, prominent among which are eating difficulties (EDs). Although previously regarded as a male-dominated condition, ASC are now known to be present in a high percentage of those who experience EDs. The diagnosis of ASC may be delayed in such people, especially in females who often learn to mask their symptoms and copy their neurotypical peers. This can have adverse consequences if the underlying diagnosis of ASC is delayed, as standard therapeutic approaches to the management of EDs are often ineffective at achieving complete recovery in those with ASC, even among those whose weight is restored. This chapter explores the link between EDs and ASC and highlights the importance of recognising and treating comorbidities that contribute towards EDs. We highlight important new research in this area while also providing practical suggestions for self-management.

The link between eating difficulties and Autistic Spectrum Conditions

ASC are neurodevelopmental conditions leading to difficulties with social interaction, communication and behaviour. Many of the features that characterize ASC are also present in people with eating difficulties EDs such as repetitive and rigid eating patterns, avoidance of social situations (especially those centred around food), and difficulty in communicating emotions. Anorexia nervosa (AN) is particularly prevalent, with up to 52% of those with AN meeting the diagnostic criteria for ASC (Westwood and Tchanturia, 2017). However, the relationship between ASC and EDs is not straightforward. While both conditions tend to be diagnosed during youth, there is a stark gender discrepancy between the two, with girls tending to show signs of EDs like AN most often and ASC traditionally considered dominated by the male gender.

The temporal relationship between ASC and EDs is also interesting. Does a delayed diagnosis of ASC render someone more vulnerable to developing later EDs, or do the neurodevelopmental issues seen in ASC foster a character more prone to abnormal patterns of eating? There are also several other psychiatric conditions that can co-occur in people with ASC and EDs, which may further complicate the situation. These include Body Dysmorphic Disorder (BDD), Obsessive-Compulsive Disorder (OCD), depression, anxiety and Attention Deficit and Hyperactivity Disorder (ADHD) (Westwood and Tchanturia, 2017). Arguably these other conditions can serve to reinforce EDs in ASC, for example through their promotion of rigidity/ritual (i.e. OCD), fear (i.e. anxiety), lack of motivation to change (i.e. depression) and excessive exercising (i.e. ADHD).

The co-occurrence of EDs and ASC makes the diagnosis of either condition quite challenging. There are already concerns about the over-representation of male characteristics in diagnostic tools for ASC (Westwood and Tchanturia, 2017). Although historically ASC was a male-associated condition, it is now increasingly diagnosed in females, albeit with a slightly different presentation. Females can hide their differences through masking and mimicry and may slip through the diagnostic nets for ASC. If EDs co-occur, they risk being labelled as having an ED without having their ASC acknowledged. This is worrisome because difficulties in the social, emotional and cognitive domains can all contribute to worsening outcomes in EDs.

Some effort has been made to adapt long-standing diagnostic tools to distinguish ASC from AN features: including a new section in the Autism Diagnostic Observational Schedule 2nd Edition (ADOS-2). The ADOS-2 is able to detect ASC traits in people with AN and, importantly, does so without being affected by the presence of other psychological symptoms such as those found in AN, depression and anxiety (Sedgewick *et al*, 2019). This is key, especially because the physiological implications of prolonged extreme starvation can induce ASC-like symptoms (as well as feelings of low mood) and hence confuse the situation further. Ultimately, an awareness of the tendency for EDs to occur in ASC (or vice versa) is critical because it affects how persons with both conditions will be managed and in turn, how well they are likely to 'recover'.

Learning point 1

- A strong link exists between ASC and EDs, though the association is made difficult to understand by other psychiatric conditions that commonly co-occur.
- Being aware of the co-occurrence of ASC and EDs has implications for how both conditions are assessed and treated.

Types of eating difficulties EDs associated with Autistic Spectrum Conditions

The most common ED in ASC is anorexia nervosa (Baron-Cohen *et al*, 2013, Westwood and Tchanturia, 2017; Sedgewick *et al*, 2019; Solmi *et al*, 2020). People with AN display cognitive profiles and patterns of emotional intelligence typical of ASC, specifically a highly systematic approach to thinking (with reduced empathy) and difficulties with recognising and responding to emotions (Baron-Cohen *et al* 2013). This might provide some clues to as to which difficulty Arises first. For example, ASC might manifest as a preoccupation with food and/or exercise, leading to various EDs. Accordingly, ASC traits demonstrated as early as seven-years-old can predict EDs arising during adolescence (Solmi *et al*, 2020). This suggests that the cognitive, emotional and social difficulties in ASC act as major risk factors for disordered eating further down the line. Traits specific to ASC can also mediate the type of EDs that later Arise.

While AN prevails in ASC, 'Eating Disorders Not Otherwise Specified' (ED-NOS) is also recognized. The range of EDs in ASC is so vast that some have argued for a 'spectrum' approach, suggesting that, like autistic features, EDs can range from mild to extreme, with different types of food-related focus (Solmi *et al* 2020). The ritualistic and rigid behaviours associated with ASC lend themselves to an equally inflexible attitude towards food and eating. People with ASC may find social gatherings, commonly driven by food-related activities, particularly difficult. They may also become preoccupied with specific food groups and refuse to eat outside of their predetermined list of acceptable items.

The more recently termed 'orthorexia' is a fixation with health food. It can lead to restrictive patterns of eating which focus on the source of food and added ingredients (Dell'Osso *et al*, 2016). Orthorexia, when taken to the extreme, can indeed lead to an anorexic presentation, which might explain why so many people with ASC who have a food-related focus can end up meeting the criteria for AN. Equally, a person with ASC who takes up excessive exercise (possibly as a means of releasing unspent energy in co-morbid ADHD) can lose too much weight as a by-product of this ritual. Such patterns of EDs in ASC imply that the difficulty is less to do with weight or body image and more due to a need for routine/control. This would explain why ED behaviours in people with ASC often persist even after weight gain (in the case of restricting types such as anorexia) has been achieved through treatment (Karjailainen *et al*, 2019).

Learning point 2

- There is a spectrum of EDs in ASC, ranging from textbook anorexia to more individualised ED-NOS behaviours.
- Eating difficulties in ASC may be less to do with body image and more about maintaining routine/control.

Sensory and gastrointestinal issues seen in Autistic Spectrum Condition

Much work has been done to understand the reasons for gut symptoms reported by young people with ASC. Pain, bloating and constipation are the most common gastrointestinal complaints: these symptoms are associated with considerable stress in children and their parents (Lezanska-Toma, 2018). As youngsters with ASC eat a narrower range of foods than other children, a restrictive, repetitive eating pattern is typical and may be associated with later malnutrition, increased risk of fracture and premature osteoporosis (Neumeyer *et al*, 2018). Specific gut diseases such as reflux, coeliac disease and food allergies are frequently reported and an association with colitis has been confirmed (Mannion, 2014). Sensory aversions contribute to, or result from, highly selective eating and most people with ASC report hypersensitivity to foods, most often relating to texture and taste, although appearance and smell may also feature (Leader *et al*, 2020).

Foods avoided by people with ASC may include carbohydrates such as bread, rice and potatoes. This is often justified by texture or gluten sensitivity. Avoidance of these foods may contribute to weight loss. Many people with ASC ultimately adopt a vegetarian or vegan diet, avoiding meat, fish and often dairy produce, which places them at risk of nutritional deficiencies. As such, supplemental intake of vitamins B and D are required. Highly selective eating is often accompanied by rigidity or ritualization around mealtimes. Food may be prepared and consumed at a fixed time and location, sometimes in isolation. Interference with this process can cause genuine distress. Such people prefer to be alone during food preparation and consumption and may report sensory overload if obliged to eat with others. This can exacerbate both adverse physical consequences from inadequate food intake and pre-existing social isolation as family and friends may struggle to understand. Mutual rejection may result making future attempts at support more difficult to initiate and receive.

Learning point 3

- Food sensitivities and gastrointestinal symptoms are common in ASC and may contribute to EDs.
- This may produce both adverse physical and social consequences for the individual.

Cognitive, emotional and hyperactive aspects influencing EDs in Autism Spectrum Conditions

The idea that 'anorexia is just a symptom, and the cause is autism' hints at the central part that ASC can play in EDs (Brede *et al*, 2020). Reduced central coherence (i.e. the ability to 'see the bigger picture') and increased rigidity are demonstrated in both conditions. EDs in ASC are less about body image and more likely a result of inner cognitive issues (Brede *et al*, 2020). Early onset or long-lasting EDs may be mediated by defects in cognition and coherence in ASC. The prognosis for recovery from EDs also appears to be adversely affected by the presence of ASC, with a higher probability that highly selective eating will persist (Saure *et al*, 2020).

General and social anxiety is overrepresented among people with ASC. This can extend to issues with food, and anxiety may be precipitated or exacerbated if individuals are obliged to consume items outside of their normal diet, routine or company. If this is a regular challenge, food intake may be reduced or even stopped until they are able to resume their usual arrangements. Although people with ASC are often perceived by others as lacking empathy, they can indeed feel emotions very strongly. Nevertheless, their ability to understand and process their own emotions is frequently reduced and they may struggle to describe their feelings in any detail. This can lead to complex relationship issues and may even precipitate self-harm if the individual finds it difficult to handle the conflict caused internally or externally. This lack of 'emotional intelligence' is often termed 'alexithymia' and incorporates very genuine challenges in recognising and responding to the emotional needs and expressions of others. Alexithymia is found in as many as 50% of people with ASC and in a similar proportion of those with EDs. It has been proposed as a unifying feature and a potential cause of EDs in ASC (Hobson *et al*, 2020).

Hyperactivity and obsessive behaviours are also regularly comorbid with ASC (Westwood and Tchanturia, 2017). Both may contribute to unintended weight loss. A compunction to exercise excessively every day is rarely primarily driven by a desire for weight loss in ASC. It is rather typically the consequence of a perceived obligation to develop and maintain an exercise routine which often consumes more calories than are replaced, and/or an attempt at nervous system or sensory regulation. Such routines are often complex and even perfectionist in their execution. Similar structural changes in the brain are evident on imaging in both those with ASC and those with EDs. Reduced volume and associated grey matter changes in specific areas of the brain also associate with rigid thinking and difficulties with social integration, with both implications and opportunities for therapeutic intervention (Bjornsdotter *et al*, 2017).

Learning point 4

- Cognitive difficulties, especially reduced central coherence, may play a central role in EDs in ASC.
- Anxiety relating to changes in the eating environment may precipitate weight loss.
- Alexithymia (difficulty in recognising emotions) links ASC and EDs.
- A perceived obligation and/or compulsion to excessively exercise may contribute to weight loss.

Treatment options for EDs in those with Autistic Spectrum Conditions

Treatment approaches to EDs must consider the additional challenges faced by individuals with coexisting ASC. People with ASC and EDs possess several barriers to classical treatment pathways such as reduced central coherence, difficulty in understanding/expressing emotions, communication difficulties and varying degrees of physiological symptoms relating to food intake. Issues such as delays in ASC diagnosis and poor education on the part of the clinician can also further hinder the pathway to recovery (Kinnaird *et al*, 2019).

Although research on specific treatment approaches is currently in its infancy, a few pilot studies have attempted to address these additional layers of need. One such approach is 'Cognitive Remediation Therapy' (CRT) which focuses on improving cognitive coherence in the context of EDs. Results of this method are promising: repeat sessions of one-on-one CRT can improve cognitive skills in people with comorbid AN and ASC (Dandil *et al*, 2020). However, no study has yet examined whether improved central coherence following CRT then translates to reduced EDs and appropriate weight gain in those who require it.

Importantly, CRT only really addresses the cognitive element of EDs in ASC and may neglect the emotional, communicative and sensory elements that also interplay. Accordingly, the more recent 'PEACE Pathway' intervention also embodies important additional elements comprising CRT, 'Cognitive Remediation and Emotion Skills Training' (CREST- to address alexithymia), a sensory screening tool and specialized 'PEACE Menus'. The latter are formulated with specialized dieticians, while specific educational resources are provided for the clinician, carers and the person themselves (Tchanturia *et al*, 2020). We do not yet know if this multifaceted approach improves EDs outcomes in ASC but it certainly seems to contain all the ingredients of a holistic approach.

Outside of formalized treatment interventions there are a few practical tips which may help people with ASC and EDs. Firstly, we recommend that you tell trusted others how you feel about food and why. Explain which foods you like and those that you try to avoid. Explain your preferences around food preparation and consumption. Once other people understand, you may then be able to both negotiate having the kitchen to yourself and avoid the challenges of feeling obliged to eat in company. Next, collect recipes that you enjoy – either of your own or from others and online. Ensure a good variety of foods including plenty of fruits/vegetables and an adequate daily energy intake. If you are vegan, eat plenty of nuts, beans and pulses to provide daily protein requirements. Explain to the manager of the shop you frequent exactly what you need so that they can make sure that it is always available for you. Try to include the full range of vitamins in your diet or at least supplement your food intake with vitamins B12 and D. Be cautious with alcohol, as it may lead you astray, make your EDs worse, or even lead to an addiction. Exercise daily if you wish, but always try to replace the calories expended. Weightbearing and core muscle strengthening are particularly good options to include in your exercise routine. Above all, be open and honest with yourself and with others.

Learning point 5

- Treatment interventions for co-occurring ASC and EDs should be modified to account for the unique challenges these individuals face.
- Practical examples of how to approach treatment of EDs in ASC include sharing your food preferences with others, advance planning, and ensuring a varied diet.

Summary

Autism Spectrum Conditions and EDs commonly co-exist, which can prevent diagnosis and treatment of both conditions. EDs in ASC fall on a spectrum from classic anorexia nervosa (Baron-Cohen *et al*, 2013, Westwood and Tchanturia, 2017; Sedgewick *et al*, 2019; Solmi *et al*, 2020) to fixations on specific food groups (e.g. orthorexia) (Solmi *et al*, 2020).

In ASC, EDs are likely to be less to do with body image and more to be a consequence of rigid/ritualistic behaviour patterns driven by the ASC (Dell'Osso *et al*, 2016). Food sensitivity (Lezanska-Toma, 2018; Neumeyer *et al*, 2018; Karjailainen *et al*, 2019; Leader *et al*, 2020), poor central coherence (Brede *et al*, 2020; Saure *et al*, 2020), the inability to understand or express emotions (Hobson *et al*, 2020), social anxiety, and hyperactivity (Bjornsdotter *et al*, 2017) may also contribute to the development of EDs in ASC. Treatment approaches must account for the unique challenges faced by this group. Cognitive Remediation Therapy, CREST, dietitian-led interventions and clinician/carer/patient education have been proposed but have not been trialled extensively (Kinnaird *et al*, 2019; Dandil *et al*, 2020; Tchanturia *et al*, 2020). Meanwhile, practical examples for how to manage EDs in ASC could include open discussions with others about food preferences with a view to fostering an environment of mutual understanding in the context of eating.

References

Baron-Cohen S, Jaffa T, Davies S et al (2013) Do girls with anorexia nervosa have elevated autistic traits? *Molecular autism* **4** 24, 1-8.

Bjornsdotter M, Davidovic M, Karjalainen L et al (2018) Grey matter correlates of autistic traits in women with anorexia nervosa. *J Psychiatry Neurosci* **43** (2) 79-86.

Brede J, Babb C, Elliott M et al (2020) 'For me the anorexia is just a symptom and the cause is autism' Investigating restrictive eating disorders in autistic women. *J Autism Dev Dis* **50** S1-803.

Dandil Y, Smith K, Adamson J & Tchanturia K (2020) Individual cognitive remediation therapy benefits for patients with anorexia nervosa and high autistic features. *Eur Eat Dis Review* **28** 87-91.

Dell'Osso L, Abelli , Carpita B et al (2016) Historical evolution of the concept of anorexia nervosa and relationships with orthorexia nervosa, autism and obsessive-compulsive disorder. *Neuropsychiatr Dis Treat* **12** 1651-1660.

Hobson H, Westwood H, Conway J et al. (2020) Alexithymia and autism diagnostic assessment; evidence from twins at genetic risk of autism and adults with anorexia nervosa. *Res Autism Spectr Disord* **73** 101531.

Karjailainen L, Rastam M, Paulson-Karlsson & Wentz E (2019) Do autism spectrum disorder and anorexia nervosa have some eating disturbances in common? *Europ Child Adoles Psychiatry* **28** 69-78.

Kinnaird E, Norton C, Stewart C & Tchanturia K. (2019) Same behaviours, different reasons: what do patients with concurring anorexia and autism want from treatment? *Int Rev Psych* **31** (4) 308-317.

Leader G, Tuohy E, Chen J, Mannion A & Gilroy S (2020) Feeding problems, gastrointestinal symptoms, challenging behaviour and sensory issues in children and adolescents with autism spectrum disorder. *J Autism Dev Dis* **50** 1401-1410.

Lezanska-Toma A (2018) Gastrointestinal Abnormalities in Children with Autism Spectrum Disorder and Typical Development. An Irish Perspective.

Mannion A (2014) Gastrointestinal Symptoms in Autism Spectrum Disorder: A Literature review. *J Autism Dev Disord* **1** 11-17.

Neumeyer AM, Sokoloff NC, McDonnell EI et al (2018) Nutrition and Bone Density in Boys with Autism Spectrum Disorder. *J Acad Nutr Diet* **118** (5) 865-977.

Saure E, Laasonen M, Lepisto-Paisley T et al (2020) Characteristics of autism spectrum disorders are associated with longer duration of anorexia nervosa. *Int J Eating Dis* **53** 1056-1079.

Sedgewick F, Kerr-Gafney J, Leppanen J & Tchanturia K (2019) Anorexia Nervosa, Autism, and the ADOS: How Appropriate Is the New Algorithm in Identifying Cases? *Frontiers in Psychiatry* **10** Article 507.

Solmi F, Bentivegna F, Bould H et al (2020) Trajectories of autistic social traits in childhood and adolescence and disordered eating behaviours at age 14: a UK population cohort study. *J Child Psychol Psychiatry*. https://doi.org/10.1111.jcpp.13258.

Tchanturia K, Smith K, Glennon D & Burhouse A (2020) Towards an improved understanding of the anorexia nervosa and autism spectrum comorbidity: PEACE pathway. *Frontiers in Psychiatry* **11** (640) 1-7.

Westwood H & Tchanturia K (2017) Autism spectrum disorder in anorexia nervosa: an updated literature review. *Curr Psychiatry Rep* **19** 41.

21. Meal planning: understanding the different approaches

By Sarah Fuller

Introduction

When someone who has experienced eating difficulties is re-establishing regular nutrition, a variety of approaches can be used. Some treatment models for children and young people, for example, advocate no meal plans and focus on parents knowing what their child needs to eat and having the confidence to manage this. However, in reality, many parents are able to feed their family but as soon as one member has an eating difficulty, they can feel disempowered and will say, 'Yes I can feed our other children, but not one with an eating difficulties'. They ask for more guidance.

An adult patient, on the other hand, may reflect that they 'just don't know what to eat' and are stuck in a vicious cycle of overthinking and not being able to make any decisions around their eating. Meal planning can be supportive, but many different strategies are available. Depending on who you are and where you are currently with your eating difficulty, one strategy may be more appropriate than another. For example, an 11-year-old who is presenting with restricted eating versus someone who is 25 years old, is living independently and is learning to manage their eating difficulty, will benefit from very different approaches. No one size fits all. This chapter is designed to give an overview of the more common strategies, allowing you to identify the pros and cons of each and, hopefully, to find one that personally suits you, your loved one or your client.

Meal plans can be helpful to many people with eating difficulties as they provide a structure for eating, give permission to eat and take away guilty feelings and many of the difficult decisions regarding what, when and how much to eat. Furthermore, if they are made in collaboration with someone who is seeking help and the professional supporting them, it can feel like the professional is alongside the patient when they are at home, outside of the clinic.

Whichever approach you follow, it is important to note that meals plans are not supposed to be rigid. Rather, they should be flexible and amended at different stages of treatment with a gradual progression to more variety of foods/meals and more flexibility in eating patterns (Grave, 2005). Identifying the aim of the meal plan is important: whether it is to help someone restore regular eating, weight restoration and/or expand the variety of foods managed. Therefore, it is important to ensure that the meal plan is reviewed regularly by a member of the treatment team (it is vital not to become stuck on the same plan for years!). This is especially true for children and young people as the nutritional demands of growth and puberty mean that if a 14-year-old old is still on the meal plan they were placed on at 12 years old, the chances are this will not be sufficient to meet their nutritional requirements and would result in poor weight gain or even weight loss.

Guiding principles

Before we consider the different strategies more commonly used in meal planning, it is important to note that regardless of which one you choose, there are some guiding principles of all plans that need to be acknowledged.

1. **Re-establishing regular eating:** Many people with eating difficulties will have engaged in aberrant eating behaviours such as irregular or delayed eating. Not going longer than three or four hours without nutrition is key to recovery as this will keep blood sugars stable and prevent episodes of bingeing. This likely means that someone will need to eat three meals and three snacks in a day. This perhaps seems like a very 'mechanical' approach to eating, yet the approach is endorsed by many eating disorder therapists. It will be helpful to set times for these meals or snacks as most people with eating difficulties either cannot tell if they are hungry or have become adept at ignoring these signals (Herbert & Pollatos, 2018). Regular eating is important as it helps to regulate blood sugar levels, which in turn can help to stabilise mood. Eating every three to four hours is key to preventing the body from switching into 'starvation mode' as well as reducing the chance that someone will develop sharp hunger signals which could lead to them bingeing.
2. **Plan ahead:** Use a set time to plan meals a few days ahead, or up to a week. This reduces the opportunity for negotiation and last-minute changes. If someone is in the early stages of recovery and have a sense of a lot of choice around what to eat, nine times out of ten the person may feel unable to make the food choice that they actually want. An eating difficulty will tend to lead a person to choose the 'safest' meal, i.e. the one lower in calories, carbohydrates or fat etc. However, this can also lead the person to feel totally paralysed by choice. For example, if someone is given the choice between spaghetti bolognaise and lasagne, the spaghetti bolognaise may have more carbohydrates than the lasagne, but the lasagne may have more

cheese. Which one is the 'right' one? This 'eating disorder maths' can be paralysing. The person may end up choosing to have neither and perhaps substituting the meal with a 'safer' (and usually less nutritionally equivalent) meal. Planning ahead removes the dilemma of choice. The solution, for example, might be to have lasagne tonight and spaghetti bolognaise tomorrow.

Another area that will require planning ahead is food shopping. If you are supporting a child or young person with an eating difficulty, it may be not be appropriate for them to be involved in shopping for food. However, if you are an adult, you may need support in food shopping. Being faced with all the choice that a supermarket provides can be overwhelming and may result in only 'safe' foods being purchased. Planning a shopping list, ordering exactly what is needed online or shopping with someone who can support you are all practical ideas that can help many people ensure that the food they need is in the house.

3. **Focusing initially on meeting calorific requirements:** Many people with restrictive eating difficulties will have a small number of safe foods and this can often mean they have inadvertently excluded entire food groups along the way (Izquierdo *et al*, 2019; James *et al*, 2017). Having to suddenly reintroduce these foods into their diet may feel very scary. Focusing on increasing the total amount of nutrition/calories someone is having in a day, therefore, is more important than getting the balance right. The balance of the overall diet can be worked on later. In the meantime, if someone is not able to eat a balanced diet, an A-Z vitamin and mineral supplement can be used to ensure there are no nutritional deficiencies.

4. **Incorporating feared foods:** Many people with eating difficulties will fear and therefore avoid specific foods. These may be the 'social foods', such as cake, biscuits, chocolate and sweets. Foods that are deemed by the person to be 'too high' in fat/carbohydrates etc. may also be feared. Either way, it is common for people with eating difficulties to have feared foods. A good meal plan, once well established, will use this structure to challenge many of these feared foods and incorporate them into the diet, thus challenging the belief that these foods are to be avoided. Once a feared food is successfully reintroduced, it is important that this challenge is repeated a number of times and for it to become routine within the normal diet again.

5. **Consider the role of 'diet' foods:** This is a tricky one. Depending on what stage of recovery you are at, the advice may change. If the goal is to increase your total amount of daily nutrition, it could be argued that using foods that feel 'safe', for example diet yoghurts or low-calorie cereal bars, can be appropriate. However, this may give a mixed message, especially if someone needs to gain weight. Ideally, with time, diet products should be removed from the meal plan and swapped for equivalent foods.

6. **Be aware of things which are counterproductive:** Sadly, the poorly regulated diet and wellness industry often markets specific foods, drinks and tablets they claim will 'boost metabolism' or 'aid weight loss' etc. If it were true that food X helped speed up your metabolism, drink Y would help you lose weight, or tablet Z would reduce your appetite, the health service would be promoting these (and probably giving them out for free) given the obesity crisis that faces many Western countries today. However, many people with eating difficulties will consume these items hoping they will lose weight as a result. If someone is on a meal plan and still consuming these items, this will likely be counterproductive from a psychological perspective.
7. **Seek help from an expert if stuck:** Some people may not need much guidance regarding establishing a meal plan. However, if you become stuck it will be sensible to seek help from a dietitian with training and expertise in eating difficulties who will be able to go through the available options with you and help you to choose the option most likely to help.

> **Learning point 1**
>
> Following some key guiding principles can support people with eating difficulties to create helpful and recovery-promoting and sustaining meal plans.

Portion exchange plans

The idea with portion exchange plans is that the meal plan is organized around a series of food group exchanges. Each exchange is of the same food group and of nutritional value. Exchanges are for carbohydrates, fruits, vegetables, dairy, proteins, fats and social foods. There are a total number of exchanges to aim for each day; this allows for all items to be treated equally. For example, one portion of rice is equivalent to one portion of pasta; therefore, these can be used interchangeably when meal planning. It is important to note, however, that some people struggle with this concept as the portion sizes used may not reflect socially perceived 'normal' portions of foods. For example, a sandwich may require two portions of bread, a portion of protein and a portion of fats, and some people may struggle with the idea of having two portions of something, i.e. bread, in a meal.

The 'entrée and sides' system

This is a similar approach to the exchange-based meal plan outlined above, but takes a more generalised approach to portion sizes. Instead of breaking a meal down into various exchanges (such as the sandwich example) there are only two categories, namely entrées and sides. The main meals, or entrées, are supported by a specific number of snacks and nourishing drinks each day. This is a simple model of meal planning to follow and can be used successfully in family-based approaches to eating difficulties. However, this approach arguably lacks the precision some people require when their eating difficulty is very entrenched.

The 'plate by plate' approach

This approach to meal planning requires a 10-inch (~25cm) plate. The idea is simple: to fill the plate in specific proportions. If a person needs to gain weight, the plate should be half filled with carbohydrates, a quarter filled with protein and a quarter filled with vegetables/salad/fruits, with a side portion of dairy and or fats. If a person needs to maintain their weight, for example as is often the case in bulimia nervosa or binge eating disorder, these proportions can be adjusted to one third carbohydrate, one third protein and one third vegetables/salad. This approach provides structure to meals without the need to calorie count. However, it can be harder to achieve with 'mixed meals' such as a cottage pie or paella.

Calorie counted, or calorie ranged, plans

Some professionals working in the field of eating difficulties would advise against using a calorie-counted meal plan, through a concern that calorie-counting developed as part of the eating difficulty and may therefore keep it going (for example, see Romano *et al*, 2018). Calorie-counted plans, however, have their place – but perhaps only if someone is already calorie-counting (so as not to ignite a new eating difficulty safety behaviour). This may be a simple approach of someone needing to eat X number of calories each day. However, this approach may still allow for food to be delayed and a 'food traffic jam', where there are many remaining calories to eat within a short timeframe, to occur at the end of the day (which is often when people report it is hardest to eat). Another approach could be to set a calorie limit to meals and snacks and to work out different options for each, for example:

- Breakfast: 400kcal
- Snacks: 3 x 250kcal
- Lunch: 500kcal
- Evening meal: 500kcal main and 200kcal pudding

This approach means that no meal or snack would be avoided based on its nutritional content and therefore can promote variety. It may be helpful to advocate starting with one or two breakfast options, three snack options, two or three lunch options and four or five evening meals etc. However, this approach may mean that some meals or snacks could be artificially small or large in order to make up the required amount. Furthermore, it is important to ensure that the plan progresses and more variety is added is over time.

> **Learning point 2**
>
> No meal-planning system should stagnate for extended periods. The aim should always be to add flexibility and diversity incrementally over time.

Nourishing drinks and prescriptible supplements

Many people, especially in the early stages of nutritional restoration, will report that drinking is easier than eating. Therefore, nourishing drinks such as fruit juices, smoothies and milkshakes can help someone to meet their nutritional requirements (Garber *et al*, 2012). These nourishing drinks can be shop-bought or homemade. It is often easier to incorporate more calories into a homemade drink. Smoothies, for example, can easily be made to contain 400kcal with the addition of ingredients such as bananas, whole milk, oats, ice cream and seeds. It is important to note that, in some cases, the volume of nourishing drinks required may go over some national healthy eating guidelines e.g. recommended 150ml portions for fruit juices. However, these guidelines are designed for the general population, i.e. for those who need to maintain a healthy weight and may be at risk of being overweight, rather than people with restrictive eating difficulties.

As with all meal planning, the role of nourishing drinks can vary. Some people may be worried about teaching themselves to over-eat and therefore feel they can better manage a 2,000kcal/day meal plan and have nourishing drinks as the additional nutrition they require to promote physical health restoration (weight gain). Others, who may be struggling to establish any form of meal plan, may find that nourishing drinks can help bridge the gap between what they need to eat and what they can manage.

In some circumstances, a medical professional/GP can prescribe supplement drinks that are high in calories but small in volume, e.g. 300kcal in 125ml. Taking the stance that these products are 'medicine' rather than food can be especially helpful for some people who are struggling to establish an appropriate number of calories. However, this approach runs the risk of food not being eaten in favour of drinks and of a person becoming reliant on these products.

And finally... a warning regarding 'mindful' or 'intuitive' eating

The idea behind mindful and/or intuitive eating is simple: that people are able to learn to be in tune with their body by eating what they want when their body signals that it is hungry and to stop eating when they are full (e.g. Tribole & Resch,

1995). Many people who have struggled with eating difficulties strive, though find it very difficult, to achieve this. This is in part due to differential interoceptive awareness present in the eating difficulties population (differences in the way internal signals are felt and processed, such as hunger and fullness signals) (Fassino *et al*, 2004).

It is also important to remember that the majority of people have their days structured around external factors such as education or work. It is simply not practical to start eating a meal halfway through a lesson or meeting, for example. Furthermore, many people who report recovery from eating difficulties say that, while they are currently managing it well, difficult thoughts related to food and eating are still present and need to be fought against. Some people, sadly, slip back into their eating difficulties after they have moved away from structured eating and tried to focus on mindful/initiative eating (especially those who have experienced restrictive eating difficulties, as even in a starved state they may not feel hungry). In reality, I would recommend that only those who feel they are significantly recovered with the presence of sharp hunger and fullness signals should attempt to follow these intuitive eating patterns.

Learning point 3

Intuitive or mindful eating approaches may be more appropriate for people who are further along in their recovery journey.

Concluding

There is no 'one size fits all' approach to meal planning. This chapter has highlighted some of the routine approaches used in clinical practice. Meal plans can be helpful to many people with eating difficulties as they provide a structure to daily eating which can help to normalize both eating and eating behaviours. With time, flexibility around food and eating should be worked towards, even if this remains within a structured approach.

Sources of further information

The 'entrée and sides' system: *'Assessment of eating disorders'* by JE Mitchell and CB Pearson.

Plate by plate approach: *'How to Nourish Your Child Through an Eating Disorder: A Simple, Plate-By-Plate Approach to Rebuilding a Healthy Relationship with Food'* by Casey Crosbie

'REAL food guide': http://cbt-t.group.shef.ac.uk/wp-content/uploads/2019/05/REAL-Food-Guide-Appendix-5.pdf

Mindful eating: *'Savor: Mindful Eating, Mindful Life'* by Thich Nhat Hanh and Dr Lilian Cheung.

References

Fassino S, Pierò A, Gramaglia C & Abbate-Daga G (2004) Clinical, psychopathological and personality correlates of interoceptive awareness in anorexia nervosa, bulimia nervosa and obesity. *Psychopathology* **37** (4) 168-174.

Garber AK, Michihata N, Hetnal K, Shafer MA & Moscicki AB (2012) A prospective examination of weight gain in hospitalized adolescents with anorexia nervosa on a recommended refeeding protocol. *Journal of Adolescent Health* **50** (1) 24-29.

Grave RD (2005) A multi-step cognitive behaviour therapy for eating disorders. *European Eating Disorders Review: The Professional Journal of the Eating Disorders Association* **13** (6) 373-382.

Herbert BM & Pollatos O (2018) The relevance of interoception for eating behavior and eating disorders. *The Interoceptive Mind: From Homeostasis to Awareness* **4** (4) 165.

Izquierdo A, Plessow F, Becker KR, Mancuso CJ, Slattery M, Murray HB & Thomas JJ (2019) Implicit attitudes toward dieting and thinness distinguish fat-phobic and non-fat-phobic anorexia nervosa from avoidant/restrictive food intake disorder in adolescents. *International Journal of Eating Disorders* **52** (4) 419-427.

James C, Harrison A, Seixas A, Powell M, Pengpid S & Peltzer K (2017) "Safe Foods" or "Fear Foods": the implications of food avoidance in college students from low-and middle-income countries. *Eating and Weight Disorders-Studies on Anorexia, Bulimia and Obesity* **22** (3) 407-419.

Romano KA, Becker MAS, Colgary CD & Magnuson A (2018) Helpful or harmful? The comparative value of self-weighing and calorie counting versus intuitive eating on the eating disorder symptomology of college students. *Eating and Weight Disorders-Studies on Anorexia, Bulimia and Obesity* **23** (6) 841-848.

Tribole E & Resch E (1995) *Intuitive eating: a recovery book for the chronic dieter: rediscover the pleasures of eating and rebuild your body image.*

22. Type 1 diabetes and disordered eating (T1DE)

By Dr Sarah Brewster, Dr Helen Partridge, Dr Carla Figueiredo, Michelle Bennett, Claire Pinder, Lindsey Rouse, Jacqueline Ryder, Nicola Stacey, Sarah Alicea

Chapter summary

Imagine being able to eat whatever you want and still lose weight. All you have to do is stop giving yourself regular injections of insulin. People with Type 1 Diabetes are faced with this temptation every day. It is no wonder that eating difficulties (ED) are more common in this group.

Early mortality in type 1 diabetes is already higher than people without diabetes, and EDs have the highest mortality rate of any mental illness. No surprise then that where these two conditions coexist, mortality is high. Enabling specialist diabetes and ED services to work together is essential to support people to cope and manage their condition in a society in which having control of your weight is valued so highly.

In this chapter we aim to increase understanding, insight and empathy so that people struggling with these conditions can talk openly and without fear of blame. There will also be suggestions as to how supportive services may work together.

Introduction: What makes people with type 1 diabetes more at risk of ED and how is it different?

Type 1 diabetes is a complex, long-term health condition. Its management relies on a number of self-care practices, which when combined with the biological and psychological consequences of living with diabetes, can inherently increase the risk of the development and maintenance of eating difficulties (Treasure *et al*, 2013). The reasons for this association include, but are not limited to, those listed in Box 22.1.

Box 22.1: Risk factors for people with type 1 diabetes developing an eating difficulty

- The need to carefully read food labels.
- The focus on weight and food intake at diabetes clinic appointments.
- The need to eat to treat hypoglycaemia, which can cause weight gain and can sometimes be counterintuitive (e.g. having to eat when not hungry), contributing to feelings of guilt.
- An increased awareness of the body through the need for self-monitoring of weight and glucose levels.
- A constant awareness of carbohydrates or calories in food in order to match insulin requirements for meals.
- The effort put into diabetes self-management does not always equate to the outcomes of these efforts causing frustration, guilt and shame, which may be influenced and reinforced by health care professionals' (HCPs) responses to diabetes data.
- Unrealistic expectations set by healthcare providers regarding blood glucose levels.
- The language of diabetes which can be polarised e.g. good versus poor control; in range versus out of range.
- A heavy focus on numbers and the assumptions about the link between numbers and effort or value/self-worth.
- Difficulty maintaining a desired weight.
- Weight loss prior to diagnosis and regain on starting insulin, cementing an association between insulin and weight gain.
- Others' scrutiny of and assumptions about diet and diabetes management e.g. family, friends and colleagues.

While there will be similarities with other EDs, weight and shape concerns that develop within the context of type 1 diabetes are particularly complex. The unique ability to control weight and shape by omitting insulin exposes the individual to additional risks. These include higher rates of short-term complications such as hyperglycaemia and elevated ketones, dehydration and diabetic ketoacidosis (DKA) and the impact hyperglycaemia has on cognition. Long-term complications include an increased susceptibility to developing retinopathy, neuropathy, nephropathy, gastroparesis and cardiovascular disease. The increased risk of short- and long-term complications are linked to a reduced quality of life and life expectancy (Diabetes UK, 2020).

It is increasingly recognized that optimum management of type 1 diabetes requires support for physical and mental health, and yet individuals are often managed in silos with little joined-up working between physical and mental health teams.

Challenges defining and diagnosing eating difficulties in type 1 diabetes

Despite recognising an increased risk of ED co-existing with type 1 diabetes, there is no recognized diagnostic criteria or nomenclature. The term 'diabulimia' has been used colloquially but is not recommended in medical literature. For the purposes of this document the term 'Type 1 Diabetes and Disordered Eating (T1DE)' is used to describe the presence of an ED in the context of type 1 diabetes.

Despite NICE guidance for treatment of ED recommending routine screening for eating difficulties in people with type 1 diabetes, no consensus exists regarding what measures should be used (NICE, 2017). Furthermore, routine screening tools for ED are not valid in the context of type 1 diabetes due to the inherent focus on food that having type 1 diabetes entails. These tools therefore have the tendency to overestimate the frequency of eating difficulties in this cohort (Powers *et al*, 2016).

Some screening tools specifically looking at eating difficulties in type 1 diabetes do exist (Powers, 2016; Markowitz *et a*l, 2010; Zuijdwijk *et al*, 2014) but these are challenging to incorporate routinely into busy diabetes consultations. Diabetes clinicians may feel concerned about whether they have the necessary skills to open up this area of conversation (Brewster *et al*, 2020). Red flags that may suggest a risk of T1DE can be seen in Box 22.2 below and have been suggested by Partridge *et al* (2020).

Box 22.2: Red flags for T1DE

- Increase in HbA1c or erratic blood glucose levels.
- Multiple diabetic ketoacidosis (DKA) or near DKA episodes.
- Dietary restriction or binge eating.
- Secrecy about diabetes management.
- Weight loss history or fear of weight gain.
- Disengagement from services.
- Diabetes distress.
- Fear of hypoglycaemia.
- Depression and anxiety.
- Concerns about body image.

If red flags are identified, Partridge *et al* (2020) proposed the following working criteria to help establish a diagnosis of T1DE:

Box 22.3: Working criteria of T1DE

People with type 1 diabetes who present with all three criteria:

1. Disturbance in the way in which one's body weight or shape is experienced or intense fear of gaining weight or of becoming overweight.
2. Recurrent inappropriate direct or indirect* restriction of insulin (and/or other compensatory behaviour**) in order to prevent weight gain.
3. Person must present with a degree of insulin restriction, eating or compensatory behaviours that cause at least one of the following:
   - Harm to health
   - Clinically significant diabetes distress
   - Impairment in areas of functioning.

*Indirect restriction of insulin refers to reduced insulin need/use due to dietary restriction.
**Self-induced vomiting, laxative use, dietary restriction, excessive exercise.

Case study

A 20-year-old female with a history of anorexia developed type 1 diabetes three years ago. She lost a lot of weight on initial diagnosis but on starting insulin and learning how to manage her diabetes, she independently put the weight back on. She found this distressing and noticed that by reducing her recommended insulin doses, she was able to maintain then reduce her weight. It was noted at successive diabetes appointments her weight was dropping and her average blood glucose levels were increasing. She felt unable to discuss reasons for this and started to miss appointments.

Learning point 1

- How could her HCP try to re-engage with this young lady? What could be the drivers stopping her attending clinic?
- How could we approach a discussion about concerns/risks and start to develop realistic, achievable, patient-centred goals?

Prevention

Acknowledging the impact of aspects of diabetes that predispose individuals to T1DE, and addressing those that can be modified within diabetes healthcare, could act as a preventative measure for future development of T1DE. For example, attention to the language used in diabetes consultations, the expectations set at diagnosis about management of glucose levels, the focus on weighing and the messages communicated in relation to weight. In order to minimise the potential for triggering previous ED, it is recommended that healthcare professionals ask those newly diagnosed with type 1 diabetes about previous ED experiences. Educating healthcare professionals who may be involved in the care pathway of those with type 1 diabetes (e.g. emergency department workers, those working in acute medicine, podiatrists, dietitians) is important to facilitate this approach and to help identify red flags at an early stage.

Case study: Healthcare professional awareness of T1DE

A 24-year-old male with a known history of type 1 diabetes had three admissions to the emergency department in six months with hyperglycaemia but no ketosis. He was discharged from the emergency department each time with no follow up organized. He was unknown to the specialist team, having been a non-attender following his transition from paediatric services six years before. A further presentation with DKA resulted in admission to the acute medical ward and the diabetes team were made aware of his admission. On enquiry he admitted to purging, bingeing and over-exercise.

Learning point 2

- Whose responsibility is it to try engaging with this man to enquire into any thoughts or feelings driving his behaviours?
- Were there opportunities following earlier presentations to the emergency department for intervention?
- What questions could have been asked to identify his needs?

Assessment

When an individual is suspected of having a T1DE diagnosis, a bespoke service with a multi-specialist team should be involved. Where possible, this should include a consultant diabetologist and psychiatrist, a diabetes nurse specialist, specialist dietitian, diabetes clinical psychologist and ED specialist practitioner. Initial assessments should be conducted jointly by two members of the team to allow the assessment of both psychological and physical health. Physical comorbidities such as gastroparesis (delayed gastric emptying secondary to altered stomach motility) or retinopathy (damage to the backs of the eyes which can affect vision) can also greatly influence the treatment pathway and should be considered.

Fortnightly clinical multidisciplinary meetings are advised to discuss new referrals, assessments and suitability for the service, as well as to follow progress, address individual concerns/needs and to review care plans. Physical and mental health risk, along with patient engagement should be reviewed, with escalation plans for assertive outreach agreed, if needed.

Case study: A multi-disciplinary team approach

A 32-year-old female with type 1 diabetes since adolescence was diagnosed with gastroparesis. She had poor glycaemic control and described experiencing diabetes distress and periods of burnout alongside a significant fear of needles. Conversations with the diabetes team revealed a history of insulin restriction for fear of gaining weight as well as guilt and shame attached to eating carbohydrates, depression and anxiety.

Learning point 3

- Which health care professionals likely need to be involved in providing care to this person?
- Who offers what?
- Which specialist teams might they come from and how might this impact upon communication and record keeping?
- How would those healthcare professionals make sure they are offering treatment in a joined-up way and how will this be communicated to the patient?
- In what order are treatments offered?
- How would it be best to track progress and the needs of the patient as treatment progresses?

Approach

A nominated care co-ordinator is integral to the process. They act as a single point of contact for the person with T1DE and facilitate effective communication between the individual and the rest of the treating multidisciplinary team. All decisions and plans should be influenced by the strengths, values and goals of the individual, their personal preferences for intervention (where possible) and their therapeutic fit with team members.

Psychological interventions

There is an emerging but limited evidence base regarding the psychological interventions effective in treating T1DE (Banting *et al*, 2018). NICE guidance proposes that further research is needed regarding treatments for eating difficulties in people with comorbidities (NICE, 2017). Specifically, it notes the potential to investigate the effectiveness of a modified ED therapy for those with a long-term health condition addressing both conditions and avoiding the need for two different interventions (in parallel or one after the other).

Key elements of the psychological treatments suggested by Partridge *et al* are summArised in Box 22.4. It is suggested that treatment sessions are initially delivered weekly to complement the other interventions offered to address nutrition and diabetes management. Where practical, psychological interventions should be delivered by an eating disorder clinician jointly with a specialist diabetes practitioner so as to bring both aspects of eating difficulties and diabetes into the therapy and facilitate learning between specialists.

Box 22.4: Key components of psychological interventions

- Developing a picture of how the problems have developed and are being maintained (capturing the interplay between the ED and psychological difficulties of living with diabetes).
- Psychoeducation.
- Enhancing self-efficacy.
- Building sense of importance and confidence around making changes.
- Cognitive restructuring (e.g. body image and diabetes management).
- Mood regulation, including understanding and coping with strong emotions.
- Developing compassion for oneself.
- Building acceptance (e.g. of diabetes as a long-term health condition).
- Identifying and living in line with personal values.
- Understanding and planning for high-risk situations as part of relapse prevention work.

In addition to formal 1:1 psychological therapies, an overarching psychological approach to all contacts the person with diabetes has with the team should include a focus on:

- Building engagement (seek to understand the difficulties from the person's perspective and come alongside them to envisage what change might look like).
- Having empathy (validate the emotions of the person with diabetes, believing the person is doing the best they can, while also holding hope, offering encouragement and assisting the person to take the next steps needed).
- Developing realistic expectations and working at the individual's pace (while supporting staff to contain their anxieties about this) and conceptualising slips back as just that (rather than indicating failure).
- Noticing progress and celebrating effort.
- Keeping the person connected with their values and why they feel it is important for them to make a change.
- Building a life beyond ED with space for diabetes within it.

Risks

Each treatment plan must be personalized and based on the processes that appears to be maintaining the eating problem and taking into account the identified risks. Physical health risks include diabetes parameters (HbA1c, ketosis), biochemical parameters and the risk of refeeding syndrome (in the context of starvation and the inability to utilize macronutrients in the absence of physiologic insulin). Mental health risks centre around harm to self or others, self-neglect, vulnerability and disengagement from services.

Family and peer support

There has been significant work in the field of eating difficulties looking at the role of the family, with current thinking being that the family has a crucial role in supporting recovery (Treasure *et al*, 2016; Langley *et al*, 2019). This would seem to be no less true in those with T1DE. Educating family members can create an environment which is conducive and enabling for the individual. Supporting someone who is working on challenging their eating difficulty alongside managing diabetes requires insight, understanding, empathy and patience.

Peer support also has an important place in the recovery journey of someone with T1DE. There are online communities for people with diabetes and concomitant ED in existence nationally and internationally.

Insulin management

Cohesive protocols for both outpatient and inpatient care to support personalized, documented insulin re-introduction algorithms that are developed collaboratively between the person with diabetes and the team, need to be introduced prior to the commencement of psychological intervention within the team. Discussions are encouraged around speed of insulin increase and appropriate sick day rules, with an emphasis around the emotional needs of the individual, particularly as insulin re-introduction can be associated with an initial deterioration in mental health that may accompany improvements in physical health and weight restoration.

Special attention should be paid to the risk of insulin oedema, distress linked to pseudohypoglycaemia (symptoms of hypoglycaemia at higher blood glucose levels), refeeding syndrome and the emergence of alternative compensatory behaviours such as excessive exercise, vomiting and laxative and diuretic abuse.

An immediate focus on ideals of near normal glycaemic management are unreasonable and unsafe. Instead, an emphasis on small incremental steps that are attainable and in line with a harm reduction approach that prioritises reducing the risk of diabetic ketoacidosis is encouraged. While it may feel uncomfortable for the healthcare professional to accept high blood glucose and ketone levels, it is a temporary measure with the aim of working with the person at their own pace to gradually increase the regularity and amount of insulin dosing and monitoring, moving towards recommended targets.

Nutrition

Dietetic assessment may highlight a range of compensatory dietary strategies, for example:

- Restriction of total energy intake.
- Selective restriction of carbohydrate intake.
- Unrestricted eating of carbohydrate in a deliberate attempt to keep blood glucose and ketones raised to achieve weight loss.

Once any risks associated with re-feeding have been managed, dietary counselling should aim to work with the person with diabetes to gradually move towards a normalized pattern of balanced eating in line with mainstream nutrition recommendations for type 1 diabetes. As with changes to insulin doses, a gradual stepped approach to change should be supported. There may be benefit for some people with T1DE temporarily leaving to one side carbohydrate counting, instead taking a more generalised dietary approach alongside fixed doses of insulin.

Conclusion

T1DE is a complex condition. Recognition, identification and management are still emergent, but steps are being taken to improve understanding. Increased recognition of the condition, particularly among healthcare professionals involved in the care pathway of those with type 1 diabetes, is important to allow for early identification and referral to specialist services as necessary. Services involved in the treatment of T1DE should include a multidisciplinary specialized team including those with expertise in diabetes and ED. A person-centred approach that includes their family is advised with realistic, shared and acceptable goals for progress.

References

Banting R & Randle-Phillips C (2018) A systematic review of psychological interventions for comorbid type 1 diabetes mellitus and eating disorders. *Diabetes Management* **8** (1) 1-18.

Brewster et al (2020) Healthcare professional awareness of eating disorders in people with type 1 diabetes: a staff survey. *The British Journal of Diabetes 20* (2) doi: 10.15277/bjd.2020.507

Diabetes UK (2020) *Our position statement on diabulimia* [online]. Available from: www.diabetes.org.uk/professionals/news--updates/our-new-position-statement-on-diabulimia (accessed August 2021).

Langley J et al (2018) *Caring for a Loved One with an Eating Disorder.* Routledge.

Markowitz JT et al (2010) Brief screening tool for disordered eating in diabetes: internal consistency and external validity in a contemporary sample of paediatric patients with type 1 diabetes. *Diabetes Care* **33** (3) 495–500.

National Institute for Health and Care Excellence (2017), *Eating disorders: recognition and treatment: NICE Guideline [NG69]* [online]. Available at: www.nice.org.uk/guidance/ng69 (accessed August 2021).

Partridge et al (2020) Type 1 diabetes and disordered eating (T1DE): the ComPASSION Project – Wessex. *Practical Diabetes* **37** (4) doi: 10.1002/pdi.2286.

Powers MA et al (2016) Development and validation of the Screen for Early Eating Disorder Signs (SEEDS) in persons with type 1 diabetes. *Eating Disorders* **24** (3) 271–88.

Powers MA et al (2016) Determining the influence of type 1 diabetes on two common eating disorders questionnaires. *Diabetes Education* **39** (3) 387–96.

Treasure J & Schmidt U (2013) The cognitive-interpersonal maintenance model of anorexia nervosa revisited: A summary of the evidence for cognitive, socio-emotional and interpersonal predisposing and perpetuating factors. *Journal of Eating Disorders* **1** 13.

Treasure J & Palazzo Nazar B (2016) Interventions for the carers of patients with eating disorders. *Current Psychiatry Rep* **18** (2) 16. doi: 10.1007/s11920-015-0652-3.

Zuijdwijk CS et al (2014) The mSCOFF for screening disordered eating in paediatric type 1 diabetes. *Diabetes Care* **37** (2) e26–7.

23. How the dental team supports individuals with eating difficulties

By Nicola Murdoch

Summary

All people deserve to have a comfortable mouth that allows them to speak, eat, smile and laugh with confidence. Eating difficulties have characteristic effects on the mouth and teeth and evidence of this can become apparent soon after onset. As a result, members of the dental team are often the first healthcare professionals to suspect that an individual may be struggling with eating difficulties and are in a position to encourage them to seek support. Potential pain, sensitivity and aesthetic issues may have a detrimental effect on quality of life and add to the psychological burden and feelings of low self-esteem that may be experienced by those with eating difficulties. Visiting a dental surgery and discussing concerns related to food and eating can be daunting, especially for those who are anxious about dental treatment.

Fortunately, early care from the dental team and adopting a tailored preventive and treatment strategy can minimise damage to the mouth and teeth and restore the smile. There are strategies available to help with dental anxiety and to overcome barriers to seeking and accessing dental care. This process is likely to be most effective with the support and understanding of families, carers and other healthcare professionals.

Visiting the dentist and prioritising oral health can be a positive step in self-care and recovery for those with eating difficulties.

Eating difficulties in the context of oral health

Oral signs of eating difficulties and clinical eating disorders follow characteristic patterns and can be seen in as little as six months following development of an eating disorder (Douglas, 2015). Dental professionals are trained to recognize these potential early clinical signs (Patel, 2019). For example, 47-93% of people who experience bulimia show signs of thinning of the tooth enamel (Uhlen *et al*, 2014).

Members of the oral healthcare team including dentists, hygienists and therapists, are ideally placed to support individuals with eating difficulties, and to offer advice to the wider healthcare community involved in their care. The dental team may be the only healthcare professionals that the individual has seen on a regular basis during their younger years and with whom they already have a trusting relationship. Of all under 18s in England, 58.6% went for a dental check-up in the 12 months prior to December 1st 2018 (NHS Digital).

The article (RDH, 2020) entitled *Confronting Eating Disorders in the Dental Chair: Advice from a survivor* honestly describes one individual's journey from the perspective of their oral health and illustrates how important the relationship with a dentist can be.

> *'Ultimately, it was a dental professional who prompted me to seek mental health and medical services for my eating disorder, and in doing so helped end my long years of suffering. For much of the time I struggled with the disorder, particularly during my college years, the only medical professionals I came in to contact with were dentists or hygienists.'*

Oral health and eating difficulties

Eating difficulties can have characteristic effects on the mouth that vary in pattern depending on the type and duration of experiences (Patel, 2019). These can include:

- High levels of dental decay due to frequent consumption of foods and beverages with a high sugar content.
- Increased thinning, chipping and sensitivity of the teeth due to loss of the tooth surface (tooth wear). This can either be due to acids dissolving the tooth surface through frequent vomiting or a high acidic food and beverage intake (dental erosion), and/or brushing the teeth immediately following vomiting (dental abrasion).
- Dry mouth and oral thrush as a result of reduced salivary flow.
- Mouth ulcers, a sore mouth and tongue, and gum disease due to nutritional deficiencies.
- Enlarged salivary glands due to frequent vomiting, the so-called 'chipmunk cheek'.
- A bad taste in the mouth and bad breath.

Understandably, these effects may add to the psychological burden and feeling of low self-esteem that eating difficulties may already have caused (RDH, 2020).

Fortunately, accessing early care and support from the dental team and adopting a tailored preventive strategy can reduce the progression of these issues. A co-ordinated approach involving the dental team, family members, carers, GPs, dietitians and other healthcare professionals to prioritise oral health is to be encouraged (Johnson *et al*, 2017). It is important to increase awareness of the oral health implications of eating difficulties in order to support and encourage prevention of dental disease.

Learning point 1

Before you continue reading, think about your own mouth and teeth, or ask the person you care for about their own experiences.

- How do you feel about how your mouth looks and feels when smiling, eating and speaking?
- Do you notice any impact of eating difficulties on your mouth and teeth? Do you feel informed about oral health, or know where to go for more information?

Overcoming barriers to visiting the dentist

Some individuals may be particularly apprehensive about visiting the dentist, especially if they are nervous, have had experiences which have not been positive in the past, have been an irregular dental attender, or are embarrassed or uncomfortable discussing their eating difficulties (Willumsen & Graugaard, 2005). This may be a particular problem if the dental professional has known their family well for many years and they are concerned that family members will be told about the dentist's concerns.

Dentists are trained to help patients who may be anxious about dental care and are generally very understanding (NHS 2018). Initially, if possible, it could help to discuss these concerns with a trusted family member, friend or another healthcare professional. Taking another person to dental appointments for support and reassurance may also help.

Often, medical history forms and those asking for details of current dental problems are completed before the visit. This can be a good way of making the dentist aware of any eating difficulties, formal diagnosis of an eating disorder, anxieties about treatment and any particular oral health problems that are being experienced. Explaining which parts of the dental visit are of particular concern can aid in discussions about the best way in which care can be delivered by the dental team.

If the individual needs to find a new dentist, asking for someone to be recommended by friends or family and looking at the practice's website or online reviews to see how they treat nervous patients can be a useful first step. Emailing or calling the dental practice before the first appointment to explain any particular concerns can ensure that enough time is allocated and that the dentist is prepared to discuss supportive strategies that can be put in place.

There are a number of techniques available to help with dental anxiety or phobia (Rafique *et al*, 2008). These range from listening to music and distraction techniques to CBT and hypnotherapy, desensitization techniques and conscious sedation.

Legally, discussions between the dental practice, dental professional and patient, and the written records, are confidential and can only be shared with the permission of the individual (GDC, 2013). This means that any information about eating difficulties shared during dental care cannot be revealed to any third parties without permission, including family members and other healthcare professionals.

> *"My dentist was incredibly supportive and encouraging of me through this process, but he also made clear that I had to acknowledge my eating disorder to receive continued help. For the first time, I knew someone believed in me and that I could conquer my habits. It didn't happen overnight, but he didn't get annoyed with me, reject me, or give up on me. It made all of the difference."* (RDH, 2019)

A dental surgery is a safe place to discuss eating problems. This is how I approach the discussion with a patient when I suspect a potential eating difficulty.

> *"When clinical examination leads me to suspect that a patient may experiencing eating difficulties, I gently but clearly describe the findings of my examination and that this particular pattern of conditions may be caused by an eating disorder amongst other possible causes. I then allow time for discussion of behaviours that may be causing this appearance. I understand that admitting to or revealing eating problems may not be easy and that it may take several visits before the patient feels they are able to talk about this, so I aim to be kind and patient, develop a trusting rapport and give plenty of time for disclosure and discussion. I signpost them to other healthcare providers who will be able to give additional mental and physical support and advise that I can refer them directly if they prefer. For patients already undergoing treatment for eating difficulties, I may also ask permission to contact their GP or any specialist services they may be accessing to ensure that they are aware of the oral health issues the patient is experiencing and measures they can undertake to help support their oral health during treatment."*

Learning point 2

Before you continue reading, think about your experiences and feelings about visiting members of the dental team or ask the person you are caring for about their experiences.

- How do you feel about visiting the dentist? Do you have any reasons to feel apprehensive or anxious?
- How might you find a new dentist and make them aware of your eating difficulties, oral health concerns and anxieties related to dental care?
- Which techniques are available to help with dental anxiety or phobia?

Prevention strategies

The following measures are recommended to minimise damage to the teeth and soft tissues of the mouth caused by eating difficulties. For other healthcare professionals, this advice must be taken in context as there must be a balance between oral disease prevention and the essential nutritional and psychological rehabilitation that the people being cared for may require. As treatment progresses, and the patient's nutritional demands are stabilized, the advice given should be reviewed and moderated in line with national oral health guidelines.

Key oral healthcare advice for patients with eating difficulties and their carers

(From Ashcroft & Milosevic, 2008; Levine & Stillman-Lowe, 2019; Lussi & Jaeggi, 2008)

- Get regular examinations by a dentist including an open discussion about oral symptoms and any eating disorder diagnosis.
- Limit the consumption of high sugar foods/drinks/feeds to mealtimes (three or four times per day) if possible and practical.
- Drink only water between meals if possible and practical.
- Reduce the amount and frequency of intake of acidic drinks.
- Drink acidic drinks such as fruit juices/smoothies and carbonated drinks through a straw placed at the back of the mouth.
- Use a fluoride containing toothpaste twice a day (containing at least 1,350ppm fluoride), and a fluoride containing mouth-rinse (0.05% NaF) once a day at a different time to brushing. Fluoride strengthens the surface of the tooth and makes it more resistant to tooth decay and erosion.
- Use a desensitising toothpaste if the teeth are sensitive.

- Do not brush your teeth immediately before or after vomiting or consuming acidic food or drinks. The surface of the tooth is softened by stomach or dietary acids and can be further damaged by the toothbrush removing the softened tooth. Wait at least an hour before toothbrushing. Rinsing with water, chewing sugar free gum, or using a fluoride mouth-rinse following these episodes is a preferred option.

The positive psychological effects of dental care for those experiencing eating difficulties cannot be underestimated. A recent study has shown that individuals with eating difficulties who visited a dentist regularly were significantly more likely to feel that their teeth and mouth had a positive effect on how they looked to themselves and others, and on kissing and romantic relationships compared to those who did not (Silverstein *et al*, 2019).

Learning point 3

Before you continue reading, think about how you care for your mouth and how often you have sugary or acidic foods or drinks, or ask the person you are caring for about their habits and experiences.

- Which oral hygiene measures can you use to look after your mouth and minimise the effects of eating difficulties?
- What effect can high sugar and acidic foods and drinks have on your teeth?
- What happens to your teeth if you brush immediately after vomiting and how can you minimise damage?

Dental treatment for the oral effects of eating difficulties

Often, a regular monitoring and a preventive strategy is all the dental care that is required. If the damage to the teeth is causing aesthetic issues, pain or problems with function (biting and chewing), dental treatment may be required (Mehta *et al*, 2012). The treatment plan produced by the dental team will aim to repair, cover and protect damaged tooth surfaces, reduce pain and sensitivity, improve the aesthetics of the teeth and treat soft tissue lesions.

Simple treatments may be carried out easily in general dental practice. For more extensive or complex plans, referral to a specialist in treatment of tooth wear either in general practice or within a hospital setting may be required.

The positive physical, psychological and quality of life benefits of a healthy and comfortable mouth for those with eating difficulties cannot be underestimated. Using the strategies described in this chapter and the support of the dental health team, families, carers and other healthcare professionals to improve oral health can be a valuable step in self-care and recovery.

Further resources

- www.nationaleatingdisorders.org-dental-complications-eating-disorders
- Eatingdisorders.co.uk
- www.bodywhys.ie
- https://www.dentalphobia.co.uk

Further resources for healthcare professionals

- Oral Health Foundation – dentalhealth.org
- Delivering better oral health: an evidence-based toolkit for prevention – PHE/DOH
- www.nhs.uk/live-well/eat-well/how-to-cut-down-on-sugar-in-your-diet/

References

Ashcroft A & Milosevic A (2008) The Eating Disorders: 2. Behavioural and Dental Management. *Dental Update* **34** (10).

Douglas L (2015) Caring for dental patients with eating disorders. *BDJ Team* **1** 15009.

GDC (2013) Standards for Dental Professionals. London: General Dental Council.

Johnson LB, Boyd LD, Rainchuso L, Rothman A & Mayer B (2017) Eating disorder professionals' perceptions of oral health knowledge. *International Journal of Dental Hygiene* **15** (3) 164-171.

Levine R & Stillman-Lowe C (2019) The Scientific Basis of Oral Health Education. 8th ed. Springer Nature.

Lussi A & Jaeggi T (2008) Erosion -- diagnosis and risk factors. *Clinical Oral Investigations*. **12** (Suppl 1): p. S5-13.

Mehta SB, Banerji S, Millar BJ & Suarez-Feito JM (2012) Current concepts on the management of tooth wear: part 1. Assessment, treatment planning and strategies for the prevention and the passive management of tooth wear. *British Dental Journal* **212** (1) 17-27.

NHS (2018) *Fear of the Dentist* [online]. London: NHS. Available at www.nhs.uk/live-well/healthy-body/fear-of-the-dentist-help/ (accessed August 2021).

NHS Digital (2019) NHS Dental Statistics for England, 2018-19, Second Quarterly Report. London: NHS [online]. Available at: digital.nhs.uk (accessed 2021).

Patel N & Milward M (2019) The Oral Implications of Mental Health Disorders Part 1: Eating Disorders. *Dental Update* **46** 49-52.

Rafique S, Banerjee A & Fiske J (2008) Management of the petrified dental patient. *Dental Update* **35** (3) 196-8.

RdhMag (2019) Confronting eating disorders in the dental chair: Advice from a survivor [online]. Available at: www.rdhmag.com (accessed August 2021).

Silverstein LS, Haggerty C, Sams L, Phillips C & Roberts MW (2019) Impact of an oral health education intervention among a group of patients with eating disorders (anorexia nervosa and bulimia nervosa). *Journal of Eating Disorders* **5** 7:29.

Uhlen MM, Tveit AB, Stenhagen KR & Mulic A (2014) Self-induced vomiting and dental erosion--a clinical study. *BMC Oral Health* **29**; 14-92.

Willumsen T & Graugaard PK (2005) Dental fear, regularity of dental attendance and subjective evaluation of dental erosion in women with eating disorders. *European Journal of Oral Sciences* **113** (4) 297–302.

24. Starving to conceive: infertility and eating difficulties

By Kate B Daigle

Introduction

There is insufficient research on the intersection of eating difficulties with fertility issues, yet research has shown that 20.7% of patients struggling with infertility have experienced eating difficulties (Easter *et al*, 2011). Psychotherapy with this population can reveal shame rooted in unexpected difficulties in conception, pregnancy or early motherhood. The lack of open discussion around these topics increases internalised judgment and self-criticism.

This chapter will focus on the challenges related to conceiving a healthy pregnancy and the emotional, physical and relational impact that infertility can have on a woman with eating difficulties. Discussion will examine research linking the presence of anorexia nervosa, bulimia nervosa or binge eating disorder to fertility issues. Experiential exercises exploring how to process this with clients are outlined. This chapter will be a guide to addressing, working with, and healing from emotional struggles related to fertility and eating difficulties.

Infertility and eating difficulties

Infertility and eating difficulties are two topics that are shrouded in secrecy, shame and struggle. How are they interconnected? And how can we help heal the shame that women with these issues feel?

Many women who have struggled with eating difficulties since their teenage years, who then reach childbearing age and are financially and emotionally ready to begin a family, find it difficult to conceive. Adding insult to injury, this can leave a woman experiencing feelings of shame and loss, compounding the suffering she has already experienced for many years.

Eating difficulties also affect many women of a childbearing age. Research suggests that eating disorders affect 5.2-6.5% of young females (Sadeh-Sharvit, 2016) but often go undetected in healthcare. The number could be even higher. This may be due to an atypical eating disorder not being recognized for what it is or hesitancy on the part of the client to admit she is struggling.

A common misconception in the medical community regarding infertility it is that primarily women who are underweight and who restrict their food intake are those who will experience fertility issues. While it is true that insufficient body fat can have an impact on fertility, this overlooks women living in bodies in higher body mass indexes (BMIs) who also struggle with eating difficulties and fertility. This can lead a woman going through fertility issues to feel 'invisibilised' or not seen for the severity of their eating difficulties. Furthermore, atypical representations of eating difficulties are common across the spectrum of the clinical eating disorders.

Learning point 1

Women of all weights, including those with body mass indexes falling within the average ranges, can experience fertility issues on account of eating difficulties.

Research tells us that as many as 75-80% of women will go on to conceive after being successfully treated for an eating disorder and that there is no reason for her history of eating difficulties to affect fertility if she is in sustained physical and emotional recovery (Linna *et al*, 2013). This is to say that there can be medical and emotional factors which can complicate the conception process, but these are independent of eating difficulty factors in sustained recovery.

Reflection points

Before you continue reading, consider:

- What you have known about infertility and eating difficulties before this point.
- Why you think someone with infertility issues might feel uncomfortable sharing their eating difficulties with their medical team.
- Your own experience with nourishing your body and whether you have ever ignored its signals.

The medical impact of eating difficulties on the reproductive system

Many of the physical complications of anorexia nervosa are due to effects of starvation. A major marker of anorexia is amenorrhea, or the loss of a woman's menstrual cycle. Primary amenorrhea occurs when a woman aged 15 or older has never had a menstrual period and secondary amenorrhea occurs in a woman who has had regular periods but loses her period for a time span of three months or more. The loss of menstruation prohibits egg production and shuts down the reproductive system. Hypothalamic amenorrhea, a component of secondary amenorrhea, is common in people with anorexia and occurs when the hypothalamus, which controls reproduction, stops producing gonadotropin-releasing hormone (GnRH). This is the hormone which starts the menstrual cycle and can stop it if it does not sense sustainability. This can be due to low body weight, which may or may not be connected to an eating disorder.

When the body is forced into starvation as occurs in anorexia, the brain attempts to protect itself. This reaction can be called our 'caveman brain': events are not processed mindfully and slowly but, rather, the brain senses danger and potential death and thus acts on its most primal instinct. This stems from the days of our ancestors where threats to our survival were plentiful.

In this state of 'fight, flight, freeze or fawn', our bodies feel stressed and compelled to preserve as many internal resources as they possibly can, while recognising that this is not a time suitable for procreation. When a person is dealing with severe anorexia, the brain can go into this same self-protection and fear mindset. It may sense that death could be imminent as there is very little or inconsistent fuel coming into the body to sustain it. Thus, the brain shuts down 'non-essential' organs to preserve what little energy it does have and reverts to prepubescent times.

When starved, a mature female brain will shut down sex hormones, shrink the ovaries and eliminate menstruation until it is deemed 'safe' enough to revert to their normal state. Safe in these terms would mean sustained nutrition for an extended period of time and enough body fat to sustain a pregnancy. For some women, it can take up to a year of recovery from anorexia for her to get her period back and for her hormones to become regulated.

Learning point 2

For a woman desiring to have a family, the most important thing she can do is dedicate herself to full recovery from her eating disorder before trying to conceive.

Menstrual irregularities are also common in females with bulimia nervosa, though it is not certain whether these disturbances are related to weight fluctuations, nutritional deficiencies, hormonal imbalances, emotional stress or a combination of these factors. Bingeing and purging behaviours can flush the body of needed nutrients, cause dehydration and electrolyte disturbances, and result in hormonal imbalances. People struggling with bulimia are at risk of potassium deficiency from purging which can lead to an irregular heartbeat and other cardiac issues. The body is sustained at a high rate of stress during bulimic episodes and can shut down hormone production: most importantly estrogen production which is needed for reproduction. There are significant risks to a pregnancy if a woman is actively bingeing and purging while she is carrying a child.

Menstrual irregularities are also common in binge eating disorder, especially if a woman is overweight or obese. Obesity in women can result in high levels of androgens, or male hormones, which can lead to abnormal menstrual cycles and block ovulation.

It is important to remember, however, that contrary to popular belief, many women with eating difficulties become pregnant despite significant menstrual irregularities. An increasing number of women diagnosed with anorexia and bulimia are reporting unintended pregnancies (Reba-Harrelson *et al*, 2010). While the bodies of many women with anorexia will halt all egg production due to nutritional restriction, some women have intermittent egg production, meaning that they release an egg 'from time to time' rather than each month. Women may not think they can become pregnant when they have anorexia and therefore fail to use contraception. However, they can be mistaken.

Learning point 3

Women with eating difficulties can and do become pregnant. Both the woman themselves, and those supporting them (i.e. medical professionals) can be taken by surprise by conception, particularly if the women is not experiencing regular menstruation.

Reflection points

Imagine the emotional and physical distress a woman in this population may be experiencing. How would you help her to navigate harm reduction with her difficult eating behaviours?

What other implications do you think eating difficulties have on a woman's life if she is trying to conceive?

Impact on relationships

Over one million couples worldwide go through fertility treatments every year in an attempt to have a child. Upwards of one-third of these couples are told they have 'unexplained' or idiopathic infertility, which translates as the doctors being unable to find anything wrong with the male's sperm or the female's fallopian tubes or uterus (Galhardo *et al*, 2011). This is devastating for so many of these couples.

Andrea, aged 33, and her husband Travis (pseudonyms) have been trying to conceive a child for three years. Andrea struggled with anorexia beginning in her sophomore year of high school and all through college. She received outpatient therapy, intensive outpatient treatment and several hospitalizations. Andrea began to recover at the end of her senior year of college and has not had any eating difficulties since that time. She now says, "I am starting to question if the narrative of 'recovered' works for me (due to her recent challenges with getting pregnant)".

Andrea shares: "I have been trying to conceive for the past three-and-a-half years. I have never been pregnant. I have tried medication (clomid cycles) and have had two failed intrauterine inseminations (IUIs) and have undergone three rounds of IVF. It was found that my egg quality was poor and we have gone through two failed embryo transfers. My infertility is diagnosed as 'unexplained.' However, during my eating disorder I lost my period for several years. I have a distinct memory of a therapist asking me, "Do you ever want to have kids, or do you want to be skinny?" I said I wanted to be skinny. Now I carry a lot of guilt about that. I know the research is inconclusive about long-term amenorrhea and its connection to infertility, but I *firmly* believe that a decade of living well below my set-point (natural range of body weight without nutritional restriction) has had a negative effect on my fertility. I have now paused all fertility treatments for the foreseeable future. I fear that I may be a hopeless case."

Andrea continues: "I carry shame from the question posed to me years ago by my therapist. I have had fearful thoughts of my infertility being fate intervening because perhaps I would pass an eating disorder to my child, would make an unfit mother, or pregnancy would cause a relapse for me. I sought out a support group, but there are none in my area. Currently I am searching for a therapist who specializes in infertility, but this has also been a struggle. I would say that leaning on my husband and family members has been the most helpful approach I have taken thus far". Andrea is now a psychologist, and although she doesn't work with people with eating disorders or fertility issues, she feels that her past and current struggles have influenced her to want to help others who suffer from mental and physical health issues.

Learning point 4

The desire to have something within one's control is often a maintaining factor of an eating disorder. The experience of infertility is, perhaps, the utmost definition of loss of control.

Clinical tools for working with individuals or couples experiencing infertility

1.) Treasure map of the infertility journey

Create a treasure map of the infertility journey. Other journeys may converge with this one, including children from a previous relationship, eating disorder recovery, learning about infertility before relationship, etc.

Support the client to consider what mountains they have climbed, cliffs they have fallen from, rivers they've waded across, places they have rested, stormy seas they have weathered, hidden treasures they have found etc.

2.) Weaving a nest (can be undertaken in group setting, couples, or individual)

The individual/group weaves a 'nest' of yarn together as they share difficult feelings. Each person weaves their yarn as they talk, then they pass it onto the next person. Once the nest is completed, so many things can be done with it. Individuals or couples can write on strips of paper words which depict the grief and shame they feel regarding the infertility, or any emotions or intentions they want to share. The nest can be kept in the therapist's office or elsewhere as a resource for healing and processing.

3.) Shame container

Creating a 'shame container' can sometimes help clients to access and heal shame. The therapist provides small boxes (matchboxes, tea containers, shoe boxes, etc.) and asks the client to decorate the outside of the box with collage or drawing/ painting imagery etc. to represent how they show their shame (or hide it away) to the outside world. On the inside, the client can use imagery and collage, as well as writing, objects, photographs, etc. to depict what their shame feels like inside.

4.) Building on mindfulness and guided imagery

Therapists can guide clients to a state of mindfulness through guided imagery or journaling that gently and empathetically puts them in touch with their shame. The next step is then to guide them to locate/describe/image what this shame experience feels like (in a way that builds empathy). They can then be guided to make the connection with how their eating difficulty experiences have informed and/or impacted on this shame. The therapist may then guide the client in becoming a parent and caregiver to that part of themselves that is experiencing shame, supporting them to offer compassion to that part of themselves.

5.) Re-imagining the 'reproductive story'

This exercise can be done with an individual or with a couple. The aim is to support the couple or individual to process their 'reproductive story', which starts from when they were young, including the story they imagined about themselves ultimately becoming a parent one day. It can be supportive to take time to explore familial and cultural influences etc. Accompanying this with breathwork and soothing guided visualizations can help to ground clients in their bodies as part of this process. Once they feel grounded, they can start trying on 'new stories', thus allowing them to fantasise about what possible changes or new choices in the story could look and feel like. This involves considerable acceptance work and self-compassion. These stories might be very different from the original stories they have been telling themselves about reproduction, fertility and so on.

Miscarriage and pregnancy loss: another form of infertility

Miscarriage and pregnancy loss are often referred to as 'silent' losses, yet there is nothing silent about them. These losses can occur for many reasons, and frequently doctors do not know why a miscarriage or stillbirth takes place. A woman may most commonly miscarry due to chromosome defects in the embryo which would make the pregnancy unsustainable in the long term. Other medical complications and factors can also influence the sustainability of a pregnancy.

The term 'miscarriage' unjustly and pejoratively implies that the woman mis-carried the child, arguably suggesting that she is at fault and possibly prompting further internalization of the stigma and shame that can come with experiencing a miscarriage. I believe that this is one of the reasons why miscarriages, like eating difficulties, are not often talked about. It would be incredibly reparative for all women (and their partners) in this population if we could come up with a less blaming word to describe this type of loss.

While it can be healing for women who have experienced pregnancy loss to hear from others about their own journeys with miscarriage, it would appear that many women wait periods of time, sometimes years (or decades), to open up about their loss. Beth (pseudonym), aged 37, who has struggled with fertility issues shares, "I think [women opening up about their fertility struggles] is happening more and more often. I also think that people open up gradually over time, and not in the early days because the experience is so intense and so raw – it's not that you want to be private, it's just that you can't keep coming emotionally undone every little second. Wanting a child and not being able to conceive is a vulnerable and powerless feeling unlike any other – it's just such a primal impulse to want to bear a child. And losing a child that you feel so hopeful about is so very isolating. I extend so much love to all the women struggling."

For some women who are active in their eating difficulties while pregnant, the lack of sustained nutrition, dehydration and weight fluctuations (some of them significant) can affect their growing fetus. A growing fetus needs more fat, carbs and complex nutrition than a woman's body would have previously required to be healthy before becoming pregnant. Eating disorder behaviours during pregnancy, such as chronic restriction, bingeing and purging, laxative abuse or excessive exercise, can put the baby at risk of not getting the sustained nutrition it requires to develop into a healthy and sustainable child (Kimmel *et al*, 2015).

Learning point 5

It is of the utmost importance to clinically and medically support pregnant women to understand and sustain the nutritional demands of a growing fetus.

We know that our 'caveman brain' wants to protect the body by any means possible if it perceives a risk of starvation or death. Eating difficulties can threaten the health of the body and if it feels there are not enough resources to grow a baby and keep the woman alive, it may terminate the pregnancy so the women's body can survive. This is a devastating trade-off but one stemming from our ancestors to preserve the future of the human species. The stress of an eating disorder on the body can also override the equilibrium of the physiological system and put the woman at risk for her body rejecting the pregnancy (Priel *et al*, 2000).

Perhaps surprising is the high rate of miscarriage and pregnancy loss in women with binge eating disorder (BED) (Kimmel *et al*, 2015). In their 2013 study of women who had eating difficulties and were pregnant, researchers found that 50% of the participants who had BED suffered a miscarriage, which is almost twice the rate of non-ED miscarriages. Lashen *et al*. (2004) have suggested that perhaps the effects of polycystic ovarian syndrome PCOS, diabetes, endometriosis, oocyte abnormality and/or high insulin, which are all associated with obesity, may have detrimental effects on a woman's pregnancy. Other complications such as elevated stress hormones related to binge eating, abnormalities in leptin and adiponectin production (protein hormones which help regulate glucose levels and break down fatty acids), dietary factors, hypertension and cardiovascular disease may also contribute to fertility issues.

Reflection points

Pause to consider:

1. What should be included when assessing a woman's mental health if she has an eating disorder and is pregnant or wants to get pregnant?
2. As important as collaborative care is, what are the factors that may prohibit a pregnant mother from disclosing to her medical team that she has an active/recent ED and how do you as her mental health therapist navigate that situation?

3. What factors would you consider if assessing a client who has an eating disorder and presents for therapy saying that she wants to try to get pregnant?
4. What biases, assumptions or countertransference may show up for you in working with a woman who is pregnant who has an ED?
5. What are the top three clinical needs to be addressed in working with a woman who has been dealing with infertility?

Conclusion

There is still so much to learn about the intersection of eating difficulties and infertility. What is certain is the level of shame and loss these women and couples typically experience. Supporting women to realise that infertility is not their fault and helping them to continue to take care of themselves physically and emotionally appears to be the most effective approach. A team of non-pathologising medical professionals is necessary in treating and supporting this population.

References

Easter A, Treasure J & Micali N (2011) Fertility and prenatal attitudes towards pregnancy in women with eating disorders: results from the Avon Longitudinal Study of Parents and Children. *BJOG: An International Journal of Obstetrics & Gynaecology* **118** (12) 1491-1498.

Galhardo A, Pinto-Gouveia J, Cunha M & Matos M (2011) The impact of shame and self-judgment on psychopathology in infertile patients. *Human reproduction* **26** (9) 2408-2414.

Kimmel MC, Ferguson EH, Zerwas S, Bulik CM & Meltzer-Brody S (2016) Obstetric and gynecologic problems associated with eating disorders. *International Journal of Eating Disorders* **49** (3) 260-275.

Lashen H, Fear K, Sturdee DW. (2004) Obesity is associated with increased risk of first trimester and recurrent miscarriage: matched case-control study. Hum Reprod., 19(7):1644-6. doi: 10.1093/humrep/deh277. Epub 2004 May 13. PMID: 15142995.

Linna MS, Raevuori A, Haukka J, Suvisaari JM, Suokas JT & Gissler M (2013) Reproductive health outcomes in eating disorders. *International Journal of Eating Disorders* **46** (8) 826-833.

Priel B & Besser AVI (2000) Adult attachment styles, early relationships, antenatal attachment, and perceptions of infant temperament: A study of first-time mothers. *Personal relationships* **7** (3) 291-310.

Reba-Harrelson L, Von Holle A, Hamer RM, Torgersen L, Reichborn-Kjennerud T & Bulik CM (2010) Patterns of maternal feeding and child eating associated with eating disorders in the Norwegian Mother and Child Cohort Study (MoBa). *Eating behaviors* **11** (1) 54-61.

Sadeh-Sharvit S, Levy-Shiff R, Arnow KD & Lock JD (2016) The interactions of mothers with eating disorders with their toddlers: identifying broader risk factors. *Attachment & human development* **18** (4) 418-428.

25. Eating difficulties and pregnancy

By Amanda Bye, Abigail Easter, Christina Wilson, Victoria Mountford

Introduction

Pregnancy and early motherhood can be challenging for some women with eating difficulties. Some may have an increased risk of several adverse pregnancy and birth outcomes. Men and same-sex partners can also be affected by eating difficulties, however there has been a lack of research on their experience in parenthood. This chapter will focus on the experiences of women and new mums with eating difficulties. It outlines the considerations for women during and following pregnancy and describes how best to identify and support women. A written account and a poem illustrate an example of lived experience. We include several learning points to provide opportunities for women to reflect on their experience and health professionals to reflect on their clinical practice.

Prevalence of eating difficulties during pregnancy

Eating difficulties are not uncommon during and following pregnancy. Prevalence studies show that around 15% of pregnant women are likely to have had a history of a diagnosed eating disorder and around 7.5% are affected during the course of their pregnancy (Bye *et al*, 2020; Easter *et al*, 2013; Watson *et al*, 2013). Eating difficulties may range in type and severity, and intersect with the wider physical, psychological and social challenges of this period of great change. As a result, those expereincing eating difficulties deserve the attention and care of health professionals both during and after pregnancy.

Psychological wellbeing during pregnancy

Pregnancy can be a challenging time for some women with eating difficulties, particularly in the early stages. Most women will adjust as their pregnancy progresses and embrace their new pregnant identity (Fogarty *et al*, 2018). Among pregnant women with current eating difficulties, symptoms such as purging usually improve during this time, although binge eating and anxiety about body image and gestational weight gain may persist (Micali *et al*, 2007; Watson *et al*, 2013). Women with a history of eating difficulties may find symptoms resurface (Easter *et al*, 2015) and in rare cases women may develop symptoms for the first time during pregnancy (Watson *et al*, 2013). Anxiety, depression and self-harm may also be experienced by some women (Bye *et al*, 2020; Easter *et al*, 2015).

There is particular concern for women actively engaging in behaviours such as purging, restrictive eating or binge eating during pregnancy as this can increase the risk of complications. Women may feel shame or guilt about their eating difficulties, especially if they have been unable to stop engaging in behaviours during pregnancy (Fogarty *et al*, 2018). They may be reluctant to talk to others due to fears of being judged negatively as a mother or stigmatised (Bye *et al*, 2018). It is important, therefore, that women are provided with a safe and non-judgemental space to discuss their concerns during pregnancy. Health professionals may consider asking about eating difficulties as part of their routine assessment of mental wellbeing (see Box 25.1 for questions which may encourage such a discussion). Identifying eating difficulties in pregnant women can be difficult because of the fluctuations in symptoms and the likely overlap with common pregnancy symptoms. Pregnancy symptoms such as nausea and vomiting and changes in appetite can pose additional challenges for some women as they may find it difficult to know whether their symptoms are related to the pregnancy or their pre-existing eating difficulties (Easter *et al*, 2013). Asking women about symptoms prior to pregnancy and changes during pregnancy may provide a better understanding.

Box 25.1: Questions developed with women and health professionals which aim to encourage a discussion about a woman's eating difficulties during and following pregnancy

- How would you describe your eating on a typical day before you became pregnant? And how is your eating now?
- Have you or has anyone else ever had any concerns about your eating or weight?
- Have you ever eaten an excessive amount of food and felt like you could not stop yourself? How did you feel about that?
- How are you currently managing your eating and weight?
- How are you feeling about the changes to your body shape or weight?
- Have you ever received any treatment for an eating difficulty?

Given the typical changes in symptoms during pregnancy, women with diagnosable eating disorders should be monitored throughout pregnancy so that any deterioration in wellbeing is quickly recognized (National Institute for Health and Care Excellence, 2014). A nominated health professional (e.g., a general practitioner, midwife or health visitor) can provide the continuity needed for ongoing monitoring and support during and following pregnancy (NICE, 2017), building a rapport so the individual feels comfortable to discuss any concerns she may have about nutrition, changes in weight and managing symptoms during pregnancy[1]. These discussions need to be sensitive to a woman's anxieties, so she feels supported and empowered. Health professionals may wish to consider a referral to a perinatal mental health team or eating disorders service and/or signposting to voluntary organizations for online and local peer support. Good communication between all those involved in a woman's care and working together as a multidisciplinary team is essential for developing an integrated care plan.

Considerations for pregnancy

Pregnant women with eating difficulties may be more likely to experience certain adverse pregnancy and birth outcomes, particularly when experiencing severe difficulties during the current pregnancy. However, the risks vary according to type of eating difficulty, duration and severity, nutrition and gestational weight gain.

Some evidence suggests that women with eating difficulties may be more likely to experience an unplanned pregnancy (Easter *et al*, 2011), may be at greater risk of hyperemesis during pregnancy (Mantel *et al*, 2020), and at risk of having a pre-term birth and baby who is small for their gestational age (Charbonneau & Seabrook, 2019). Anorexia nervosa is associated with lower infant birth weight; bulimia nervosa may increase the chance of miscarriage; and binge eating disorder can be associated with having a baby who is large for gestational age (Charbonneau & Seabrook, 2019).

Some women will experience pregnancy or birth complications which may or may not be related to their eating difficulty, while many women will have healthy pregnancies. It is important that information about possible risks is not used as a tool to scare women as this can be counterproductive to women accessing support (Holmes, 2018). Instead, health professionals should provide monitoring and support according to a woman's particular healthcare needs, including assessing the need for fetal growth scans to monitor the growth of the unborn baby.

Case study of lived experience

Christina Wilson writes about her struggle with eating difficulties and how they affected her during her pregnancies:

I was 29 years old when I became unexpectedly pregnant with my first child. The month previously I had been re-prescribed anti-depressants and had the results of a scan stating that I had osteopenia (low bone density; the early stages of osteoporosis).

1 See www.eatingdisordersandpregnancy.co.uk for resources on nutrition and weight gain

I quickly found my eating difficulties increased in severity and was desperately worried about the impact this might have on the baby. At the antenatal booking appointment, I cried to the midwife and explained how worried I was. I was reassured that I looked fine and was provided with leaflets about healthy eating and foods to avoid during pregnancy. The advice felt so catastrophically simple, dismissive and alienating.

Morning sickness complicated things further. I found it distressing not knowing what was real or what was acceptable; what was a pregnancy symptom and what related to my relationship with food. I increasingly distrusted myself and my body. I was also terrified about the reality of having a baby. I had deep fears about my capacity to love and feared the likelihood of postnatal depression. Since I believed I was not looking after my baby in the womb, I was convinced that I would be a selfish and incompetent mother. I saw a different midwife for every visit and tried to tell them I was worried but felt silenced; there was little space for my fears among all the physical health checks. I was initially referred to a community mental health team, and then on to a specialist eating disorder inpatient service in a different area. It felt like I was my own care coordinator, as if my mental and physical health were separated and I had to try to negotiate communications between the different teams.

My subsequent two pregnancies were planned. I believed for each one that I would manage better but each time my mood plummeted and my eating deteriorated. I was admitted for inpatient treatment and felt guilty and ashamed. I received conflicting and damaging opinions. For example, I was told by one professional that women who experience famine conditions manage fine with a limited diet and by another that my eating was endangering my baby and would cause my body to abort my child. One sonographer told me that because I was small, having a baby measuring small was no problem, while another told me that my baby was alarmingly small. One health visitor told me I just needed to 'eat some stodge' and 'fatten myself up', which both terrified me and made me feel incompetent. The language people use is powerful; it really does matter.

There were times when I felt supported including during midwifery appointments where I was listened to with compassion, not judgement, and where extra time was given for me to listen to the baby's heartbeat because I was so afraid. There were times I was given space to talk about my fears, encouraged to be honest about my behaviours and shown how to find my own voice in among the conflicting thoughts in my head. I needed acknowledgment of the difficulties I was experiencing, space and time for complexity to be in the room and to feel heard rather than denied. I was fortunate to be given reassurance from some professionals, family and friends that I was a good mother and that my struggle with eating was not an indication of my capacity to love or my capability as a mother. The greatest gift of support I received was compassion: a counterbalance to the internal judgement, conflict and criticism I was overwhelmed by. The power of compassion and hope cannot be overestimated.

Learning point 1

Having a named midwife (rather than seeing a different midwife for each visit) for the duration of the pregnancy, or being under consultant-led care, may be particularly beneficial for women experiencing eating difficulties or who have experienced such difficulties in the past.

Reflection points for those with lived experience

Before reading further, think about your experience of eating difficulties and consider the following questions:

- How do you think your body and sense of self may change during pregnancy and early motherhood?
- How do you think you will feel about these possible changes?
- Do you think there may be concerns about your health and the health of an unborn baby if you were to become pregnant?

Reflection points for health professionals to reflect on their clinical practice

Before reading further, you may like to consider the following questions or ask them of a woman with experience of eating difficulties:

- How do you think a woman may feel about the prospect of her body and sense of self changing during pregnancy and motherhood?
- What concerns might you have about the health of a pregnant woman and her unborn baby?

Nutrition and gestational weight gain

A recent review of studies has shown that women with certain types of eating difficulties may gain more weight during pregnancy than other women (Martínez-Olcina *et al*, 2020). Gestational weight gain can be positive for women who were underweight before pregnancy as it appears to protect them from some of the potential pregnancy risks. Conversely, excessive gestational weight gain among women diagnosed with bulimia nervosa or binge eating disorder may increase the risk of complications. The findings on postnatal weight loss are mixed, with some studies indicating that women with eating difficulties may lose weight faster than other women, whereas others find the opposite. This likely reflects the array of eating difficulties women may experience.

These findings highlight the importance of health professionals having informed discussions with women about healthy nutrition and weight changes during and following pregnancy. These discussions need to be sensitive to women's anxieties about eating and weight and considerate of the stigma around weight. Similarly, it is important to be sensitive when weighing women as part of their care, acknowledging that for some women being weighed can be distressing. Asking a woman beforehand about how she feels about being weighed can be a useful starting point. Good communication between all those involved in a woman's care can help avoid repeated, unnecessary and potentially harmful weighing. The emphasis should be on the importance of healthy nutrition for the growth and development of the unborn baby and for postnatal recovery and breastfeeding, rather than focusing on changes in weight. Some women may also benefit from seeing a dietitian.

Learning point 2

Women with eating difficulties benefit from sensitive and compassionate discussions about nutritional requirements and weight and body shape changes during pregnancy.

Experiences during the postnatal period

The early postnatal period can be another challenging time for women with eating difficulties. Without the same motivation to eat well as when they were pregnant, women may find that their symptoms return as they try to adjust and identify with their new postnatal body and the challenges of motherhood (Fogarty *et al*, 2018). Women with eating difficulties may also be at increased risk of developing postnatal depression (Morgan *et al*, 2006).

Women with eating difficulties may experience certain challenges with infant feeding (Martini *et al*, 2020). Findings indicate that women may be more or just as likely to start breastfeeding as other women but may experience challenges with continuation of breastfeeding, and benefit from additional support. They may find infant weaning and toddler feeding challenging; for example, an infant's refusal to eat solids, slow feeding or a poorly established feeding routine.

Given the risk of relapse and postnatal depression, it is important for new mums to be monitored for signs of declining mental wellbeing so that appropriate support can be provided (NICE, 2014). This period is another opportunity to identify women who have not previously felt able to speak to health professionals about their eating difficulties. Again, it is important to build a rapport with a new mum so she feels comfortable talking about concerns she may have with her eating, weight or feeding her baby. She may need practical and tailored advice on how to eat healthily postnatally[2]. New mums will need sensitive and consistent advice and support with infant feeding and weaning. This should include discussions on the benefits of breastfeeding and, depending on how a woman decides to feed her baby, how to breastfeed or make up a feed (NICE, 2008). Women with eating difficulties may need more time, advice and support for these discussions and to explore any arising difficulties or concerns. Health professionals may want to consider other options for support, such as referring to a Specialist Health Visitor in Perinatal & Infant Mental Health (PIMH) or a local children's centre, or signposting her to national or local peer support for new mums.

Breastfeeding as a Corset

A poem by Christina Wilson

They said I was letting him drink the life out of me, they said
I had to think about what he needed: a mother, not just milk.
I knew his bleats and little bird squeaks, his cries, but
even after our first few hours they said, *use a bottle*.
Without words I put their bottle and its faded yellow teat
on the overbed table, swung it to my left and squeezed
gold out of my breasts, watched each globule swell round,
drop glistening into syringes, wrote his name on the side,
lifted him from his jelly bed, held him in my heat as baubles
hung suspended from each pipette, dropped onto his lips, trickling
down his tongue like dew. He swallowed, then sucked, slept, sucked,
swallowed, sucked, bleated, sucked, grew, slept, grew, sucked.
They told me I was being pulled in, too tight,
told me breastfeeding was not about losing
calories, plotted our little bodies on graphs, my fingers
tightening strings that kept me upright. I hid my breasts,
pumping in secret, freezing milk to put in the bottle when
when they came to inspect us. They wrote reports, said
your legs are getting thin. And ever so gently I unlaced
our strings, wrapped bones in tissue paper, satisfied
their gaze. They left us, untethered, but he held my finger,
head soft on my chest. I was mother, I was milk.

2 See www.eatingdisordersandpregnancy.co.uk for resources on nutrition and weight gain.

Learning point 3

New mums with a history of eating difficulties should be monitored for signs of struggle and relapse to ensure timely support is provided.

Further reflections points for women with lived experience

Think about your experience of eating difficulties and consider the following questions:

- What could you do to help prepare for pregnancy and motherhood?
- What support might you need before, during and following pregnancy?
- Where could you access this support?
- What could be helpful for professionals responsible for your care and for family and friends to be considerate of?
- How open do you feel about discussing your eating difficulties and needs with professionals responsible for your care and with family and friends?

Further reflection points for health professionals to reflect on their clinical practice

You may like to consider the following questions or ask them of a woman with experience of eating difficulties:

- What support might a woman benefit from before, during and following pregnancy?
- How could you support a woman before, during and following pregnancy?
- How could you help a woman to feel comfortable about discussing her eating difficulties and needs with you?

Conclusion

Women with experience of eating difficulties may have particular needs during and following pregnancy. Pregnancy represents a unique opportunity for health professionals to talk to women about their eating difficulties and discuss options to support the best possible outcomes for her and her baby. Our hope is that this chapter will have helped you reflect on what support pregnant women may need and how it can be accessed.

References

Bye A, Nath S, Ryan E G, Bick D, Easter A, Howard LM & Micali N (2020) Prevalence and clinical characterisation of pregnant women with eating disorders *European Eating Disorders Review* **28** (2) https://doi org/10 1002/erv 2719.

Charbonneau KD & Seabrook JA (2019) Adverse birth outcomes associated with types of eating disorders: A review In *Canadian Journal of Dietetic Practice and Research* **80** (3) pp 131–136) Dietitians of Canada https://doi org/10 3148/cjdpr-2018-044.

Easter A, Bye A, Taborelli E Corfield F Schmidt U Treasure J & Micali N (2013) Recognising the Symptoms: How Common Are Eating Disorders in Pregnancy? *European Eating Disorders Review* **21**(4) 340–344 https://doi org/10 1002/erv 2229.

Easter A, Solmi F, Bye A, Taborelli E, Corfield F, Schmidt U, Treasure J & Micali N (2015) Antenatal and postnatal psychopathology among women with current and past eating disorders: longitudinal patterns European Eating Disorders Review : *The Journal of the Eating Disorders Association* **23** (1) 19–27 https://doi org/10 1002/erv 2328.

Easter A, Treasure J & Micali N (2011) Fertility and prenatal attitudes towards pregnancy in women with eating disorders: results from the Avon Longitudinal Study of Parents and Children *BJOG: An International Journal of Obstetrics & Gynaecology* **118** (12) 1491–1498 https://doi org/10 1111/j 1471-0528 2011 03077.

Fogarty S, Elmir R, Hay P & Schmied V (2018) The experience of women with an eating disorder in the perinatal period: a meta-ethnographic study *BMC Pregnancy and Childbirth* **18** (1) 121 https://doi org/10 1186/s12884-018-1762-9.

Holmes S (2018) Responses to warnings about the impact of eating disorders on fertility: a qualitative study *Sociology of Health & Illness* **40** (4) 670–686 https://doi org/10 1111/1467-9566 12676

Mantel Ä, Hirschberg AL & Stephansson O (2020) Association of Maternal Eating Disorders with Pregnancy and Neonatal Outcomes *JAMA Psychiatry* **77** (3) 285–293 https://doi org/10 1001/ jamapsychiatry 2019 3664.

Martínez-Olcina M, Rubio-Arias JA, Reche-García C, Leyva-Vela B, Hernández-García M, Hernández-Morante JJ & Martínez-Rodríguez A (2020) Eating disorders in pregnant and breastfeeding women: A systematic review In *Medicina (Lithuania)* **56** (7) pp 1–19. MDPI AG https://doi org/10 3390/ medicina56070352.

Martini MG, Barona-Martinez M & Micali N (2020) Eating disorders mothers and their children: a systematic review of the literature In *Archives of Women's Mental Health* **23** (4) pp449–467) Springer https://doi org/10 1007/s00737-020-01019-x

Micali N, Treasure J & Simonoff E (2007) Eating disorders symptoms in pregnancy: a longitudinal study of women with recent and past eating disorders and obesity. *Journal of Psychosomatic Research* **63** (3) 297–303 https://doi org/10 1016/j jpsychores 2007 05 003.

Morgan JF, Lacey JH & Chung E (2006) Risk of postnatal depression miscarriage and preterm birth in bulimia nervosa: retrospective controlled study. *Psychosomatic Medicine* **68** (3) 487–492 https://doi org/10 1097/01 psy 0000221265 43407 89

National Institute for Health and Care Excellence (2008) *Maternal and child nutrition: guidance (PH11)* [online]. London: NICE. Available at: www.nice.org.uk/Guidance/PH11 (accessed August 2021).

National Institute for Health and Care Excellence (2014) *Antenatal and postnatal mental health: clinical management and service guidance (CG192)* [online]. Available at: www.nice.org.uk/guidance/CG192 (acessed August 2021).

National Institute for Health and Care Excellence (2017) *Eating disorders: recognition and treatment (NG69)* [online]. Available at: www.nice.org.uk/guidance/ng69 (accessed August 2021).

Watson HJ, Von Holle A, Hamer RM, Knoph Berg C, Torgersen L, Magnus P, Stoltenberg C, Sullivan P, Reichborn-Kjennerud T & Bulik C M (2013) Remission continuation and incidence of eating disorders during early pregnancy: a validation study in a population-based birth cohort. *Psychological Medicine* **43** (8) 1723–1734 https://doi org/10 1017/S0033291712002516.

Websites

Eating Disorders and Pregnancy
Resources for women and health professionals
www.eatingdisordersandpregnancy.co.uk

Best Beginnings
Support and information for parents and health professionals
www.bestbeginnings.org.uk

Maternal Mental Health Alliance
Resources for women and health professionals
www.maternalmentalhealthalliance.org

Part 3: Therapies for eating difficulties

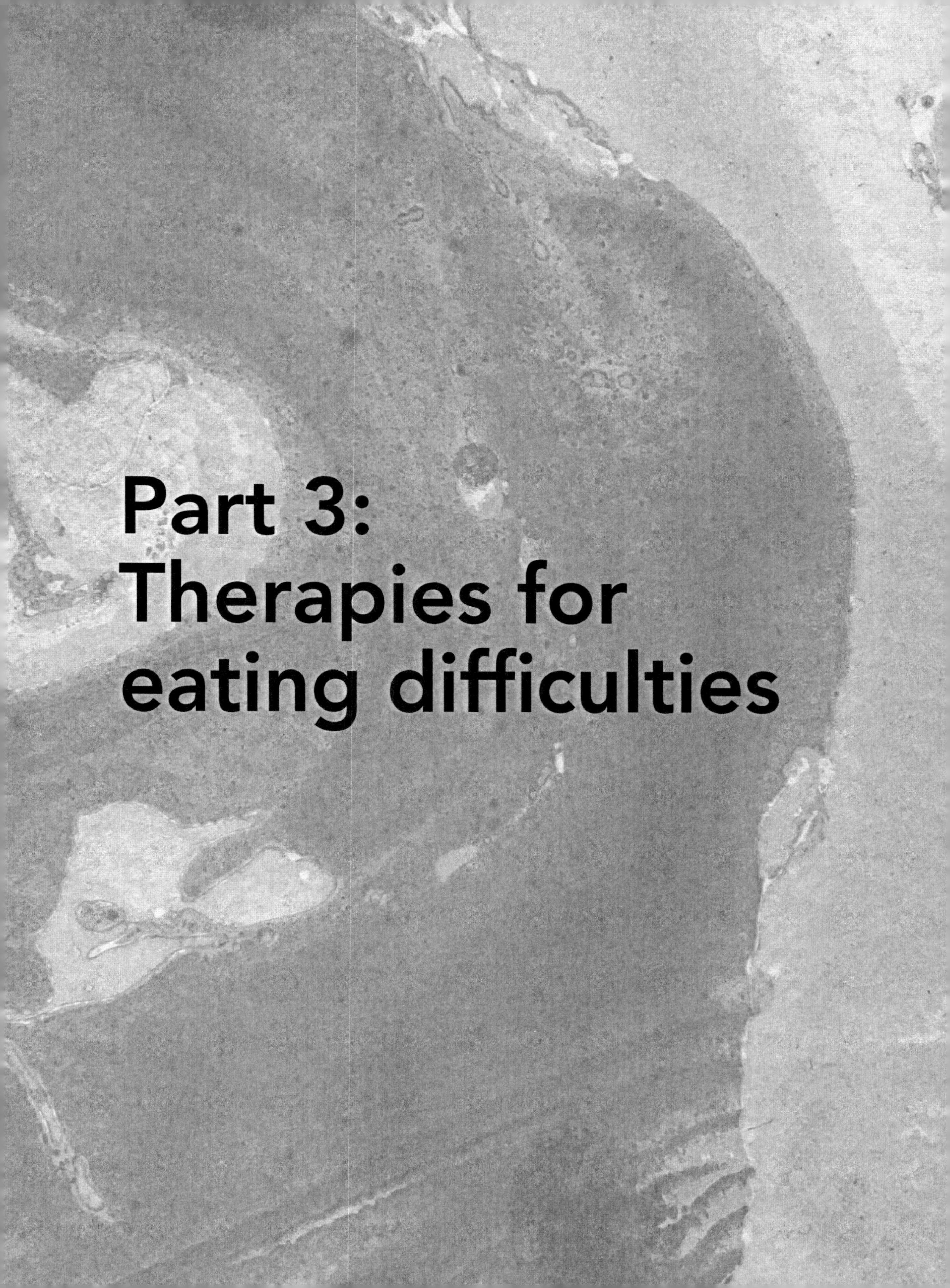

26. Practical considerations for trauma-informed care and practice in the treatment of eating difficulties

By Timothy D Brewerton

Chapter summary

This chapter briefly explains the principles of trauma-informed care and its relevance for individuals experiencing eating difficulties, including the systems of care that may support them. Clinical research evidence has demonstrated significantly higher rates of childhood maltreatment and other severe lifetime traumatic events in those with eating difficulties compared to those without, particularly among those experiencing binge eating and/or purging.

An array of adverse consequences from traumatic experiences, ranging from clinical diagnosis of post-traumatic stress disorder (PTSD) to trauma-related difficulties with mood, anxiety and substance use have been established. The rational, concurrent integration of existing evidence-based treatments for both eating difficulties and experiences of trauma are recommended, which move beyond sequentially delivered therapies, e.g. therapies with different goals delivered one after the other by different providers or programs. Although the need for such integrated treatment is clear, the roadblocks and obstacles to achieving such goals for individuals with eating difficulties and experiences of trauma are significant. Nevertheless, improved outcomes are anticipated where trauma-informed care and trauma-focused treatments are embraced by clinicians and treatment programs alike.

Understanding trauma

What is trauma anyway?

As described by the Substance Abuse Mental Health Services Association (SAMHSA), trauma is best described in light of the 'three E's', i.e. Events, Experiences and Effects (SAMHSA, 2014a). Psychiatric diagnoses (including eating disorders and related diagnoses) are the primary Effects of Events that are Experienced adversely. It is now widely accepted that traumatic experiences are nearly universal in the lives of individuals with one or more psychiatric diagnoses including eating disorders (Mitchell *et al*, 2012; Brewerton, 2018; Afifi *et al*, 2017). Therefore, the need to focus on trauma has progressively become viewed as an essential component of successful behavioural health assessment and treatment (SAMHSA, 2014b).

The relationship between trauma and eating difficulties

Learning point 1

Before reading further, take a moment to reflect on your own knowledge and understanding of eating difficulties.

Do you think considering trauma is relevant?

What are your views about whether health care providers should routinely inquire about traumatic experiences in individuals with eating difficulties?

Higher rates of traumatic events and subsequent PTSD are associated with eating difficulties as well as commonly co-occurring conditions that often accompany them, such as mood, anxiety, substance use, dissociative and obsessive-compulsive diagnoses, and attention deficit hyperactivity and personality disorders (Brewerton, 2018).

Trauma has increasingly appeared on the radar of mental health clinicians and researchers alike over the last two to three decades, yet more work needs to be done to increase awareness of the clinical science. Much evidence suggests that severity of eating problems and associated comorbidity are strongly linked to histories of trauma, particularly repeated and prolonged traumatic events and experiences that occur in high 'doses', and subsequent PTSD and complex PTSD (Brewerton, 2018; Brewerton *et al*, 2020a; Molendijk *et al*, 2017). Trauma and PTSD symptoms often go unrecognized, are minimised, unaddressed and/or untreated even by experts in eating disorders (Brewerton *et al*, 2019; Brewerton, 2018). Such reluctance or failures to address trauma-related issues can eventually lead to treatment refractoriness (lack of response), earlier and more likely relapse and chronicity, and even more concerning, increased morbidity and mortality, including suicide. Therefore, it is incumbent upon mental health clinicians of all disciplines to be conscious of the profound deleterious effects trauma can have on the course of eating difficulties.

What is trauma informed care and what does it mean for professionals and institutions involved in the assessment and treatment of eating difficulties?

Trauma informed care (TIC) seeks to increase awareness of the destructive effects of trauma – both short- and long-term – on people of all ages (see Table 26.1). It fosters resiliency at the individual, organizational and systemic levels to create safety and hope for everyone, including patients and staff, both clinical and non-clinical. TIC is deeply grounded in the understanding and recognition of the burdensome impacts on multiple levels, including neurobiological, psychological and social, that trauma can have on individuals, families and communities. Essentially, TIC strives to clearly recognize human suffering and vulnerability while simultaneously striving to identify and mobilise survivors' strengths, capacities and resources for healing and recovery. In addition, trauma-informed service organizations make concerted efforts to fully integrate knowledge about trauma into its policies, procedures and practices, and strive to vigorously resist re-traumatization (see Table 26.1).

TIC extends beyond following a prescribed set of procedures or practices but rather emphasizes six key values or ideologies (SAMHSA, 2014a; SAMHSA, 2014b), which include the following:

1. Safety
2. Trustworthiness and transparency
3. Peer support
4. Collaboration and mutuality
5. Empowerment, voice and choice
6. Cultural, historical and gender issues

Learning point 2

Reflecting on your own experiences – whether personal or professional – can you identify the role of trauma and its destructive effects in those experiences?

How might the values of TIC be something you could emphasise in your life and work?

TIC is distinct from trauma-specific or trauma-focused interventions or treatments that are designed specifically to address PTSD and other psychiatric consequences of trauma and to facilitate healing (Harris & Fallot, 2001a). TIC occurs when all components of any given service-provided system have been reconsidered and evaluated in the light of a basic understanding of the role violence plays in the lives of adults, children and adolescents and families or caregivers seeking mental health services.

As outlined in Table 26.1, a 'trauma informed' individual or system uses that understanding to design service systems that accommodate the vulnerabilities of trauma survivors and allows services to be provided in such a way that will avoid unintentional re-traumatization while expediting patient and caregiver participation in treatment. It also demands, as much as possible, closely knit collaborative relationships with other service systems assisting these patients and the local network of private practitioners with specific clinical expertise in trauma-related conditions and trauma recovery (Harris & Fallot, 2001b).

Can ED-PTSD be effectively treated? And if so, how?

Given the large body of research evidence supporting the premise that trauma often plays a significant role in predisposing toward, precipitating, and/or perpetuating, eating difficulties, it is imperative that trauma is recognized and incorporated into the comprehensive assessment and care of individuals with eating and related difficulties. There are a number of evidence-based, trauma-focused treatments for PTSD that have been shown to impact PTSD and related symptoms significantly and positively, e.g., depression and anxiety (Watkins *et al*, 2018). Integration of existing evidence-based treatments, including systemic family therapy, cognitive behavioural therapy (CBT) with prolonged exposure (PE), cognitive processing therapy (CPT), dialectical behaviour therapy (DBT), and eye movement desensitization reprocessing (EMDR) are recommended (Brewerton, 2018; Brewerton *et al*, 2020b).

Evidence suggests that eating disorder clinicians consider integrated treatment approaches for individuals with ED-PTSD to be important, yet tend to have numerous concerns about administering such a treatment, including worsening of symptoms (Trottier *et al*, 2017a). Guidelines for starting trauma treatment in traumatized eating disorder patients have been published elsewhere (Brewerton, 2004; Trim *et al*, 2017). It is recommended that assessment, diagnosis and treatment of trauma and related disorders, such as PTSD, begin concurrently with assessment and treatment of eating disorders, but with an initial emphasis on nutritional rehabilitation (ending restricting, binge eating, purging and compulsive exercising and initiating re-nourishment), psychoeducation and establishing the adaptive links between traumatic and eating disorder symptoms. Disordered eating behaviours often play a role in attempting to regulate trauma-related symptoms. As trauma-informed care and treatment is embraced by all clinicians and treatment programs that assess and treat eating and related difficulties, better outcomes are anticipated (Trottier *et al*, 2017b; Trottier *et al*, 2016).

Case study

Sally is a 17-year-old, single, white, cisgender woman who began to binge and purge when she was 13 years old following a sexual assault by an older boy in her school. She had gone to a party where she was introduced to alcohol for the first time, had too much to drink and passed out. During this time, she awakened in a stupor to find that she was being raped by a boy she hardly knew and another boy was watching. She became extremely distraught and was terribly ashamed, and did not tell anyone, including her parents, who were going through a divorce. Sally felt marked shame, depression and panic anxiety. She blamed herself, had thoughts of suicide, and began to eat more and more to comfort herself.

Sally told no one of her troubles, and began to gain weight, all the while hoarding and hiding food in her room. Her binge eating continued unabated until on one occasion she ate so much that she spontaneously vomited. She experienced brief relief, almost as if she were numbed, and this developed into a habitual pattern of behaviour over the ensuing months in an attempt to reverse her weight gain. Her mother noticed she had become very withdrawn and depressed, had gained weight, and that her grades dropped, so she brought her to her family doctor for an evaluation. Sally admitted to being depressed and eating more fast foods but did not disclose purging or her sexual assault at that time.

Sally was diagnosed with major depressive disorder and was treated with fluoxetine, a serotonin re-uptake inhibitor antidepressant. Although her depression improved slightly, she continued to binge and vomit regularly for several weeks until one day her mother caught her in the bathroom vomiting. Sally burst into tears and admitted her eating problems to her mother. Upon returning to her doctor, she was diagnosed with bulimia nervosa and referred to a counsellor for psychotherapy. However, no inquiries about the possibility of prior trauma were made, and she was not assessed for PTSD. The counsellor used a combination of family, psychodynamic and cognitive-behavioural therapies and referred her to a dietician, who developed a meal plan.

Sally engaged in the treatment plan, but remained depressed and anxious and continued to binge and purge almost daily, particularly at night when she would experience flashbacks of the rape followed by intense feelings of shame, guilt and self-deprecation. As the second anniversary of the rape approached, the frequency of her bingeing and purging increased and she also began to cut herself with razors on the inside of her thighs where she thought no one would notice. During a session with her counsellor Sally talked about wishing she was dead and threatened to overdose on her medication. She also disclosed that she had been cutting herself and showed her counsellor the deep cuts on her inner thighs.

The counsellor was so concerned that she called her mother and recommended she take her to the local emergency department. Her mother was upset to find out that Sally was cutting herself and had her admitted to an inpatient psychiatric hospital. When directly asked about sexual assault, Sally disclosed to the child psychiatrist that she had been raped but refused to say by whom. The psychiatrist also diagnosed PTSD and referred Sally to a trauma-informed residential treatment facility for eating disorders that also treated PTSD. It was only there that Sally began to make true progress. She stopped bingeing and purging and her PTSD symptoms were significantly reduced once she began to engage in cognitive processing therapy (CPT). CPT involves writing an impact statement about why the trauma occurred and how it has affected one's life. In addition to identifying related 'stuck points' or cognitive distortions, CPT is driven by the therapist's 'avoiding avoidance' and the use of Socratic questioning with a focus on the themes of safety, trust, power, intimacy and esteem (Resick *et al*, 2017). Rather than solely processing high impact events, CPT entails teaching skills for challenging distorted beliefs that can be employed post-therapy.

Conclusion

Taken together, trauma-informed care and practice for the treatment of eating difficulties is a timely and compassionate integration of available data and practices that promises to improve the treatment and outcomes of those suffering with severe eating difficulties.

Learning point 3

Having read this chapter, note any reflections you have on your understanding of eating difficulties from the perspective of trauma-informed care and practice.

Have any of your ideas about eating difficulties and the role of trauma changed?

How might you integrate the values and ideas of this chapter into your own personal or professional life?

Table 26.1. Key features of trauma-informed care and practice systems adapted for eating disorders (Fallot & Harris, 2001; Harris & Fallot, 2001b; Harris & Fallot, 2001a).

Individuals and systems without trauma sensitivity	Trauma-informed individuals and systems
Individuals are labeled and pathologized as 'manipulative', 'needy', 'attention-seeking'.	Are inclusive of the survivor's perspective and there is effort toward comprehensive views without reductionism and blaming.
Misapplication or abuse of power, e.g., rigid demeanor, involuntary commitment, forced feeding, weighing.	Realise coercive interventions cause traumatization/ re-traumatisation and are to be avoided. Utilises motivational interventions, readiness for change.
'Culture of secrecy' has no advocates, poorly monitors staff, is patriarchal and authoritarian.	Recognise high rates of PTSD/complex PTSD and trauma-related disorders in children and adults. Collaborative stance, 'do no harm'.
Staff are primarily rule enforcers and may engage in insensitive and intrusive behaviors, e.g., pat downs, strip searches, and use rigid weighing protocols.	Provide early and thoughtful diagnostic evaluation with focused consideration of trauma in people with complicated, treatment-resistant illness. Understand high punishment sensitivity in EDs.
Little use of 'least restrictive alternatives' other than medications.	Recognise that mental health treatment environments are often traumatising, both overtly and covertly.
Organisations that emphasise compliance rather than collaboration. Oppressive environments, cognitive rigidity of staff and administration.	Recognise that mental health staff are often uninformed about trauma, do not recognise it and do not treat it. Educate about and integrate trauma-informed care and practices.
Organisations that disempower/ devalue staff who then transmit that disrespect to service recipients. Perpetual culture of abuse.	Value consumers in all aspects of care and create safe, secure, compassionate and nurturing environments.
High rates of staff and recipient assault and injury resulting in retraumatisation.	Respond empathically, are objective and use supportive language. Compassionate witnessing.
Lower treatment adherence: poorer outcomes.	Offer individually flexible plans or approaches: better outcomes.
High rates of adult, child/family complaints: dissatisfaction, distress, trauma.	Avoid all shaming and humiliation: Enhanced self-esteem, self-efficacy.

Individuals and systems without trauma sensitivity	Trauma-informed individuals and systems
Higher rates of staff turnover and low morale: system negativity, inconsistent care.	Provide awareness and training on re-traumatising practices: integrated, consistent care.
Longer lengths of stay/increase in recidivism: no tracking of outcomes or transparency.	Are institutions that are open to outside parties, e.g., advocacy and clinical consultants: outcomes research with responsive, appropriate modifications.
Poor access to training and education: lack of nurture, inexperience, incompetence, repetition of ineffective practices.	Provide training and supervision in assessment and treatment of people with trauma histories: competent, integrated care, openness to learning.
Culture that focuses on symptoms and diagnoses without reference to a life journey: categorical, narrow perspective, weak central coherence.	Focusing on what happened to the client rather than what is 'wrong with you': continuous, 'big picture' perspective, strong central coherence.
Ignore/discourage disclosures of trauma and fail to address safety issues: inauthenticity, culture of deceit, failure to report abuse.	Ask questions about current and past abuse: authenticity, transparency, awareness, reports abuse to proper authorities as per local laws and ethics.
Doesn't take responsibility for how a person will cope once discharged from care: callous disregard, 'not my problem'.	Address the current risk and develop a safety plan for discharge: flexible, responsive maneuvers, communicates/collaborates with outside providers.
Avoid focus on experience of trauma and minimise importance of trauma on presentation: collusion with avoidance.	Presume that every person in a treatment setting may have been exposed to abuse, violence, neglect or other traumatic experiences: avoids avoidance.

References

Afifi TO, Sareen J, Fortier J, Taillieu T, Turner S, Cheung K & Henriksen CA (2017) Child maltreatment and eating disorders among men and women in adulthood: Results from a nationally representative United States sample. *International Journal of Eating Disorders* **50** 1281-1296.

Brewerton TD (2004) Eating disorders, victimisation, and comorbidity: Principles of treatment. In: BREWERTON, T. D. (ed.) *Clinical Handbook of Eating Disorders: An Integrated Approach*. New York: Marcel Decker.

Brewerton TD (2018) An overview of trauma-informed care and practice for eating disorders. *Journal of Aggression, Maltreatment & Trauma* **28** 445-462.

Brewerton TD, Alexander J & Schaefer J (2019) Trauma-informed care and practice for eating disorders: personal and professional perspectives of lived experiences. *Eat Weight Disord* **24** 329-338.

Brewerton TD, Perlman MM, Gavidia I, Suro G, Genet J & Bunnell DW (2020a) The association of traumatic events and posttraumatic stress disorder with greater eating disorder and comorbid symptom severity in residential eating disorder treatment centers. *International Journal of Eating Disorders* **53** 2061-2066.

Brewerton TD, Trottier K, Trim JG, Myers T & Wonderlich S (2020b) Integrating Evidence-Based Treatments for Eating Disorder Patients with Comorbid PTSD and Trauma-Related Disorders. In: Tortolani CC, Goldschmidt AB & Le Grange D (eds.) *Adapting Evidence-Based Treatments for Eating Disorders for Novel Populations and Settings: A Practical Guide.* New York, NY: Routledge.

Harris M & Fallot RD (2001a) Envisioning a trauma-informed service system: a vital paradigm shift. *New Dir Ment Health Serv* 3-22.

Harris M & Fallot RD (2001b) *Using Trauma Theory to Design Service Systems: New Directions for Mental Health Services*, San Francisco, Jossey-Bass.

Mitchell KS, Mazzeo SE, Schlesinger MR, Brewerton TD & Smith BN (2012) Comorbidity of partial and subthreshold PTSD among men and women with eating disorders in the National Comorbidity Survey-Replication Study. *International Journal of Eating Disorders* **45** 307-15.

Molendijk ML, Hoek HW, Brewerton TD & Elzinga BM (2017) Childhood maltreatment and eating disorder pathology: a systematic review and dose-response meta-analysis. *Psychol Med* **47** 1402-1416.

Resick PA, Monson CM & Chard KM (2017) *Cognitive Processing Therapy for PTSD: A Comprehensive Manual*, New York, The Guilford Press.

SAMHSA (2014a) SAMHSA's Concept of Trauma and Guidance for a Trauma-Informed Approach. In: SUBSTANCE ABUSE AND MENTAL HEALTH SERVICES ADMINISTRATION, O. O. P., PLANNING AND INNOVATION (ed.). Rockville, MD: U.S. Department of Health and Human Services.

SAMHSA (2014b) A Treatment Improvement Protocol (TIP 57): Trauma-informed Care in Behavioral Health Services. In: *Substance Abuse and Mental Health Services Administration, O. O. P., Planning And Innovation* (ed.). Rockville, MD: U.S Department of Health and Human Services.

Trim JG, Galovski T, Wagner A & Brewerton TD (2017) Treating Eating Disorder - PTSD Patients: A Synthesis of the Literature and New Treatment Directions. In: Anderson LK, Murray SB & Kaye WH (eds.) *Clinical Handbook of Complex and Atypical Eating Disorders.* New York: Oxford University Press.

Trottier K, Monson CM, Wonderlich SA, Macdonald DE & Olmsted MP (2017a) Frontline clinicians' perspectives on and utilization of trauma-focused therapy with individuals with eating disorders. *Eat Disord*, **25** 22-36.

Trottier K, Monson CM, Wonderlich SA & Olmsted MP (2017b) Initial Findings From Project Recover: Overcoming Co-Occurring Eating Disorders and Posttraumatic Stress Disorder Through Integrated Treatment. *J Trauma Stress* **30** 173-177.

Trottier K, Wonderlich SA, Monson CM, Crosby RD & Olmsted MP (2016) Investigating posttraumatic stress disorder as a psychological maintaining factor of eating disorders. *International Journal of Eating Disorders* **49** 455-7.

Watkins LE, Sprang KR & Rothbaum BO (2018) Treating PTSD: A Review of Evidence-Based Psychotherapy Interventions. *Front Behav Neurosci* **12** 258.

27. Open Dialogue and being dialogical: an eating difficulties perspective

By Adrienne Adams, Dr Sara Betteridge, Jennifer Danby, Mia Kurtti, Elina Löhönen, Cathy Thorley and Iseult Twamley.

Summary

This chapter is a collaboration between seven women with a passion for being dialogical and for working with people with eating difficulties and their families and networks. We begin by looking at what Open Dialogue and dialogical practice means and how this would look in an eating difficulty service. We then give a snapshot of dialogical approaches and family therapy in different contexts in Europe. We begin in western Lapland where Open Dialogue began. We then look at the perspectives of two practitioners from an Irish Open Dialogue service.

We then focus on the UK, where a family therapist will share her experiences of working in a specialist all-age eating difficulty service, a dialogical practitioner will share her perspective of working in an adult inpatient unit, and, finally, a family member (who is also a dialogical practitioner) will share some of her experiences.

How would an eating difficulty service look if it were an Open Dialogue service?

In Open Dialogue, practitioners that are first involved with the person with the eating difficulty and their network remain working with them for the life of the problem. If the person with the eating difficulty were to need an inpatient admission, for example, then the team would continue to work with the person while on the ward, and also when they are discharged from the ward into the community.

When a person is in crisis, there is an immediate response, and there is no sitting on a waiting list. The practitioner contacted would be responsible for asking who should join them for a meeting with one or two more practitioners. Where and when the meeting takes place and the length and frequency of these meetings would be up to the members of the network.

What is Open Dialogue and dialogical practice?

The term 'Open Dialogue' is used to describe both a way of organising mental health services, so that there is continuity, and of being together with a group of people when someone is considered to be in crisis.

Open Dialogue is an approach used to help people experiencing mental health problems and their social network to feel heard, respected and validated. It originated in western Lapland in Finland in the 1980s (Touri *et al*, 1998). Key to this approach is staff altering their response to the person in crisis, by including their network and other professionals in the process, with everyone present from the start coming together in network meetings.

These meetings are a cultural and paradigm shift for staff, service users, their families and the organization. They aim to be non-hierarchical, privileging collaboration with the person and their network as the key players. There is no set agenda; individuals in the network are each asked what they would like to talk about. It involves a slowing of pace and of deep listening, aiming to create a new joint language for those experiences that do not yet have words. Key values are transparency and openness. This is achieved by practitioners engaging in reflective conversations together during the network meetings where everyone is invited to listen and respond. Practitioners might speak of personal connections, resonances and embodied feelings. All decisions are made during the network meeting with the person and their network.

Tolerating uncertainty is the most challenging element when working dialogically. We are more used to helping relieve distress, having the 'right' answers and making decisions for individuals. However, by not rushing to solutions, meaning and new ways forward can emerge through the silences and the dialogue. The emphasis is on developing a relationship where all voices can be heard and sustaining the relationship for as long as is needed (Seikkula & Arnkil, 2017).

Learning point 1

An important aspect of being dialogical is listening and being present for the person, not rushing to find a solution. Can you think of a time when you felt truly heard? If you are a family member or an eating difficulties professional we would like to invite you to notice times when you sit with someone who is struggling and listen attentively without offering advice. If possible, have a conversation with them about how this feels.

Responding to eating difficulties in Western Lapland Health Care District Adolescent Clinic: Reflections from Mia Kurtti and Elina Löhönen

Eating difficulty services are part of mental health services in Western Lapland Healthcare District, Finland. One of the key elements is that people do not need a referral to access the service; they can refer themselves directly.

The eating difficulty is considered to be a crisis in the network. The professional team must react as soon as possible. A key value is gathering together the family, the social network, and the person who has called us, so that they can all meet together from the beginning. In addition to this, working closely with schools and school nurses is very important, with the voices of all the people in the network coming together and being listened to.

Resourcefulness is created in times of crisis, enabling people to get help at the early stages by using the existing networks and supportive relationships to increase the sense of owning their own stories and authority.

The two teams who work in adolescent services in the area and the staff in the schools have been collaborating for many years. When early signs of an eating difficulty are noticed in the school, the process of bringing the network together begins. A system has been created together where staff can find a way of responding to the worries and crisis.

Within a general hospital there is a child and adolescent ward. This is one of the key factors in creating shared arenas. Here, discussions take place about the work so that it is as integrated as possible. Together we decide with the person, the family and all the other agencies involved, how we will proceed in the process. This means that the therapeutic, nutritional and physical health perspectives would be present as essential voices and are aligned in a needs-adapted way. The working team needs to hold the therapeutic space for the person and family, and also reach out and collaborate with surrounding agencies and voices that need to be included in the dialogue. In order to do so, they need training in dialogical practices. The staff in mental health services have also received training from the Finnish eating disorders association, which is carried out mainly by people with their own lived experience. Training has given profound understanding to the staff and has been empowering and supportive.

Reflections from an Irish Open Dialogue service from Adrienne Adams and Iseult Twamley

Our service is a general adult Mental Health Service, with no access to specialist eating disorder services. Working with eating difficulties can be very challenging to staff. An Open Dialogue Clinic has been set up since 2016, where first referrals are seen from one sector of a catchment area. The Open Dialogue team was requested to support a person with an eating difficulty and their network, in a situation that was understood to have exhausted all external specialist treatment options.

The pain of anorexia is so powerful in the relational context. The never-ending struggle that is faced by the family and their loved ones on a daily basis, the fear of living and dying. Their loved one's constant battles, between two identities: that of the internal voice of anorexia that wants to be heard, that wants to control and dominate, and the identity of a beautiful person who wants to live.

It was also painful for the team to have a person fading away, where they are losing weight month by month, as the grip of anorexia is so powerful. In these settings practitioners are all just as frightened and just as miffed with the eating difficulty. Faced with knowing that all interventions offered to date had not changed the course of the issue, what had we to offer?

We offered a safe space where all voices were heard. The focus was on promoting dialogue, not for unanimous understanding, but for each person's voice(s) to be heard.

The family and their loved one decided what would be helpful to talk about in the sessions. The voice of anorexia was invited into the sessions. We witnessed and reflected on how hard the person was fighting, and the challenges for all concerned. One challenge was that of feeling isolated and alone.

Each week the practitioners met with the family and the person with an eating difficulty. Initially the practitioners were sent away, but they would return each week and offer the space. Now there is a deep trusting relationship between the family and the professionals. Dialogue takes place where there is mutual respect for everyone present.

The 'outcome' is still uncertain. Our client is more than a decade into an eating difficulty and is experiencing a constant threat to life due to their low weight. Working dialogically, we focus on being present with the person and family whatever the outcome. As a network, we sit with uncertainty, and facilitate authentic conversations, as we navigate this road together.

Learning point 2

Are you a person with an eating difficulty or a family member? Working dialogically, we believe that having and developing a social network can help us to feel a sense of belonging and connection. Are there individuals, communities, other family members, neighbours or friends, that you might take a fresh look at and reach out to, to be alongside you on your journey? We appreciate how hard this might feel. Is there someone you are already close to who could help to think through who you could contact and how you might go about it?

The curiosity about the potential value of Open Dialogue from a family therapy perspective: Jennifer Danby

Open Dialogue and dialogical practice has its roots in family therapy so is closely aligned. As a family therapist working in a specialist eating disorder service, I often find myself in awe of the network that I have the privilege of working with, especially the parents. For anyone who has experienced helping a loved one with eating difficulties (ED), they will appreciate how taking on the caring role is no simple feat – it requires courage, resilience and love.

Emerging from a history of what could crudely be referred to as a culture of 'parent blaming', there is now, finally, a collective acknowledgement that families are NOT the cause of eating difficulties. Rather, they can have an integral role to play in supporting the individual on their road to wellness. As practitioners we now commonly find ourselves telling parents "we need you", "you are essential in the treatment process", but almost in the same breath we are explaining the complex and life-threatening nature of the illness. For the parents of an unwell child, this must be very hard to hear. And yet, as professionals, we seemed surprised and frustrated when these parents seem to struggle to follow the advice that we have given them.

From my experience, the barriers to parental empowerment boil down to two main factors: fear and self-blame. Research has shown that these are the common culprits in preventing caregivers from having an effective role in their child's recovery (Stillar *et al*, 2016). And it is these emotions – fear and self-blame – that most professionals feel ill-equipped to handle, trying to placate (often ineffectively) with reassurance and/or avoidance. This stems from a desire to avoid going back to a culture of blame.

I personally have found the use of Emotion-Focused Family Therapy to be a powerful way of supporting carers to overcome the emotional obstacles of taking on the recovery tasks (Lafrance *et al*, 2020). It leans in-to, rather than away-from, these difficult emotions with the aim of freeing up the carer to do what they so desperately desire – to help their child towards wellness. Could Open Dialogue help create a safe space to explore these potentially toxic emotional states that can halt even the most motivated of parents in their tracks?

Perspectives on being dialogical in an in-patient unit from Sara Betteridge

My experience of using a dialogical approach within an adult inpatient ED unit has been incredibly rewarding but also difficult to do on my own. As I was unable to offer a full Open Dialogue service, I was often confused and sometimes conflicted about how to remain dialogical.

I think the greatest improvement Open Dialogue could add to any inpatient unit are the principles of a Social Network Perspective (actively involving clients' family and staff networks in their treatment), flexibility and mobility of practitioners in being open to where and when the meetings take place, and to have a non-hierarchical setting where the client has an equal part of the decision making and treatment process. More specifically, within an ED unit, these principles would also be applied to mealtimes and post-meal supervision. It is vital for clients to be able to feel heard and validated in moments when they are often left feeling highly anxious and vulnerable. The unit's main objective was weight gain, with therapy reserved for those who were motivated and gaining weight. Using the Open Dialogue approach would create a therapeutic experience for all clients throughout their admission, by focusing on their emotional and psychological experience, rather than just food, a point which clients regularly raised and complained about.

However, in my family therapy work I was able to incorporate more Open Dialogue by bringing members of the family network together, encouraging and enabling dialogue and polyphony, tolerating uncertainty, and using 11 of the 12 key elements (Olson *et al*, 2014). The element I could not use was working with two or more therapists in the meeting, and at times being on my own in a non-dialogical system made it harder to tolerate the uncertainty of the ED. This often led to me being more directive in sessions. I used the analogy of an iceberg and explained to families that the tip of the iceberg represented the ED (and all associated behaviours) and that the bulk of the iceberg was in fact below the surface of the water, which represented the client's internal world of thoughts, emotions and experiences. I would then say that our sessions would be focused on exploring what was below the surface of the water, and though this analogy was useful in providing a helpful frame for my sessions, it sometimes felt more directive than the Open Dialogue approach would necessarily suggest.

Another related conflict for me was that families benefitted (as did I) from the Emotion Focused Family Therapy (EFFT) model when dealing with ED behaviours at home. Given that I was working on my own, I focused on this more psychoeducational approach, and this meant that the family received a less dialogical experience. Essentially, setting the boundary of the iceberg and using EFFT were 'doing' rather than 'being', and I remained conflicted as to whether I should tolerate the uncertainty and hold the silence, or offer practical support.

Despite these conflicts, families overwhelmingly felt that the sessions were among the best 'help' that they had ever received from services (often with many years of experience), and I remain convinced that without my Open Dialogue training my family therapy experience with ED would not have been so meaningful for all of us involved.

Learning point 3

Are you working in an eating difficulty inpatient context? How about beginning to make ward community meetings involving staff and patients more dialogical? You could aim to be less hierarchical by asking to hear from each person there and inviting different ideas and feelings before any decisions are made.

When a client talks to you about any issues you could ask them about what other family or friends might say about it too, incorporating their network as much as possible.

A personal story from Cathy Thorley

Eating difficulties really took a hold in our house about 10 years ago, and seven years ago my son was admitted to an inpatient unit. I felt guilty and to blame and became very attuned to others' judgements, hunches and body language; the sideways looks. Around that time, some of my work involved working as a family therapist with adolescents with eating difficulties and their families. I rarely felt able to share that I had similar experiences, although I thought at times that it would help families and me to share it. I thought other workers would judge me, and so I kept this big part of our family's life a secret.

When on dialogical training on the outskirts of Helsinki, I shared some of my story with a small group. I felt listened to and heard on many levels, like I was being connected to, with not just my words but all of myself. I felt no judgement but that the group were alongside me. They felt some of what I felt and shared their own feelings and experiences from difficult times. Tears were shed and they did not just come from me. A little bit of healing happened that day.

On our family's journey, I wish that we could have been met by two or three dialogical practitioners when my son was in crisis and beyond, and that it could have included a person or family member with lived experience. Sadly, he was around 20 by then and deemed an adult, so his outpatient eating difficulty team never connected with us. When I received a call from an approved social worker to say that she wanted to bring two psychiatrists round to our house, I knew, because of my experience in mental health services, that my son was potentially going to be sectioned. This was the first we knew of it. It transpired that my son hadn't gone for a badly needed blood test. We explained that we didn't know this and that we would go with him to have one the next day. Had I not had more knowledge and power to intercede here, then my son would very likely have been taken away that day, perhaps against his will. We would all have had to deal with the trauma of this.

My son has read this and has generously agreed for me to share it.

Final thoughts

We have come together from different contexts to begin the conversation about Open Dialogue and eating difficulties. We have shared examples of how we are working in our different contexts. There have also been reflections from an Open Dialogue practitioner about how helpful this way of working could have been for her family. Our hopes are that Open Dialogue can develop in this area so that when someone has an eating difficulty and the person or family reach out, a response will be immediate and include people important to them from the start. We hope that the same professionals would meet with them for the life of the difficulty to build trusting therapeutic relationships where healing can happen. We look forward to making space for listening and responding to many more voices to develop our ability to be alongside each other on this difficult and meaningful journey.

Bibliography and references

Lafrance A, Katherine A, Henderson KA & Mayman S (2020) Emotion-Focused Family Therapy: A transdiagnostic model for caregiver-focused interventions. American Psychological Association.

Olson M, Seikkula, J & Ziedonis D (2014) The Key Elements of Dialogic Practice in Open Dialogue. The University of Massachusetts Medical school. Worcester, MA.

Parker J & Lea I (eds) (2014) There is life after disordered eating. 136 Context

Reed A (2011) Therapist attentiveness and negative capability in dialogical family meetings for psychosis. Journal of Family Therapy 35 (4) 227-240.

Seikkula J & Arnkil TE (2006) Dialogical Meetings in Social Networks. London: Karnac Books.

Seikkula J, Trimble D (2005) Healing elements of therapeutic conversation: dialogue as an embodiment of love. Family Process 44 (4) 461-475.

Stillar A, Strahan E, Nash P, Files N, Scarborough J, Mayman S, Henderson K, Gusella J, Connors L, Orr ES, Marchand P, Dolhanty J & Lafrance Robinson A (2016) The influence of carer fear and self-blame when supporting a loved one with an eating disorder. Eating Disorders 24 (2) 173-85.

Tuori T , Lehtinen V, Hakkarainen A, Jääskeläinen J, Kokkola A, Ojanen M, Pylkkänen K, Salokangas R, Solantaus J & Alanen Y (1998) The Finnish National Schizophrenia Project 1981-1987: 10-year evaluation of its results. Acta Psychiatrica Scandinavica 97 (1) pp10-17

Websites

Association of Family Therapy. www.aft.org.uk accessed March 2021

Emotion Focused Family Therapy. www.mentalheathfoundations.ca accessed Feb 2021

Finnish Eating Disorders Association. www.syomishairioliitto.fi accessed March 2021

28. Compassion Focused Therapy for people with an eating difficulty

By Ken Goss and Catherine Haynes

Summary

Sadly, our current therapies only help around 50% of people who seek eating disorder treatment. Therefore, we need to increase our understanding of why our current therapies have limited benefits and improve current treatment outcomes. This chapter will explore the role of shame and self-criticism in eating difficulties and how compassion can be key to recovery. We will outline Compassion Focused Therapy (CFT) and how it has been adapted for people with an eating difficulty (CFT-E2). We will provide some questions that will help you decide whether CFT-E2 could be helpful for your client and suggest ways you can learn more about this promising therapy. CFT-E2 is designed to be delivered by clinicians with training and supervision in assessing and working with people with an eating difficulty and in CFT.

The role of shame and self-criticism in eating difficulties

Shame and self-criticism affect treatment engagement and outcomes for people with an eating difficulty and often remain a problem even after symptoms have improved. Ongoing shame and self-criticism are also likely to trigger relapse. Shame involves both internal and external evaluative processes. In *internal shame*, our attention is directed inwards and we see ourselves as unworthy, bad and likely to be rejected. In *external shame*, our attention is directed outwards and we believe that others see us as inadequate, flawed or unattractive. Self-criticism is a key process in shame.

Learning point 1

- How would you notice if your client felt ashamed?
- How could shame and self-criticism make their recovery journey more difficult?

Key questions to ask clients:

- Do you feel ashamed of yourself, your body or the way you eat?
- Do you worry about what other people think about you, your body or what you eat?
- When things are difficult, do you beat yourself up?

Compassion is an antidote to shame. In CFT, compassion is defined as the ability to notice suffering and be motivated to do something about it. Compassion has several key competencies to allow us to engage with and address suffering, which are outlined in Diagram 1. Key to compassion is the ability to tolerate distress so that we can understand it and use our wisdom and courage to be helpful.

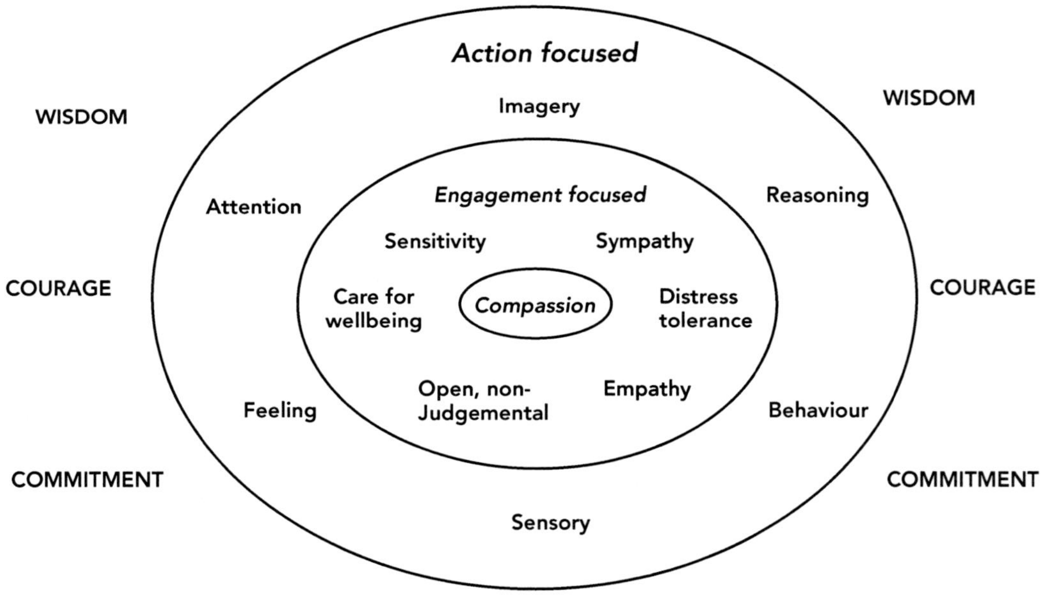

Figure 28.1: Adapted from Gilbert (2009) Compassionate Mind with permission from Little Brown

Learning point 2

- Can your client accept compassion from others?
- Can your client be self-compassionate, particularly when things go wrong?
- Is your client motivated to work on their eating difficulty using compassion for their suffering, or by fear?

Key questions to ask clients:

- When other people are upset, do you want to care for them and help them?
- When you are upset, do you find it difficult to allow other people to care for you?
- When you are upset, do you find it difficult to care for yourself like you would a friend?

Compassion Focused Therapy

CFT was developed by Professor Paul Gilbert. (For an overview of this approach see Gilbert, 2010.) It focuses on three motivational systems that help us to survive and thrive (often called 'The Three Circles model'). CFT proposes that mental health problems develop when these three systems are unregulated and/or unable to adapt to current circumstances. These systems are:

- The Threat system: This system is associated with rapidly activated emotions (such as anxiety, anger and disgust) and defensive behaviours (such as avoidance, aggression and submissiveness).
- The Drive system: This is a positive emotional system linked to feelings of achievement, joy and celebration.
- The Soothing system: This is our rest and digest system, which links to feelings of contentment, wellbeing and safeness, and is activated by giving and receiving affection, care, nurturance, and affiliation

Key questions to ask clients:

- Which system do you spend most time in currently?
- Which system do you find it hardest to access?

Figure 28.2 shows a typical pattern for some people with an eating difficulty. If your client reports high levels of shame and self-criticism, struggles with regulating these three systems and/or giving or receiving compassion, you might want to consider CFT-E2.

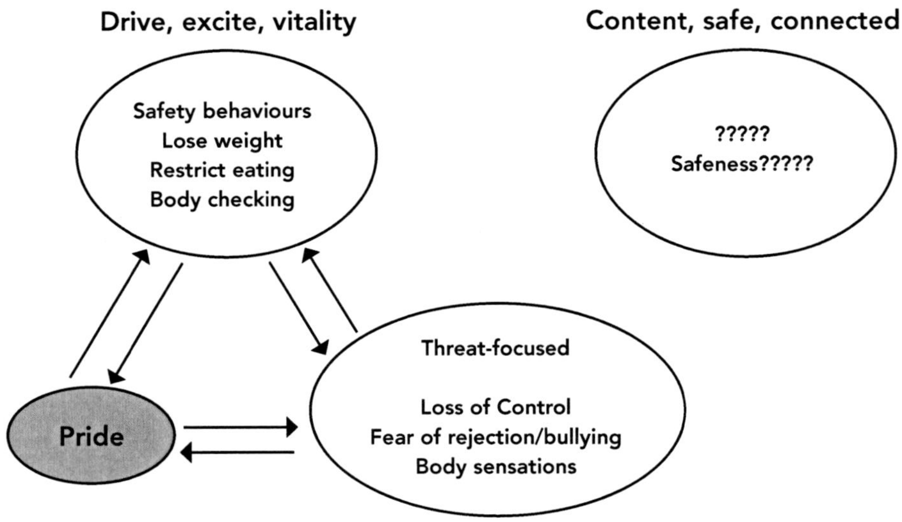

Figure 28.2: Types of affect regulator systems in eating disorders

The principles of CFT-E2

CFT-E2 is based on several key principles. These can be summArised as:

1. Eating enough food regularly is important but not sufficient for recovery.
2. Regular planned eating makes eating more predictable and allows a graded approach to changing calorie intake and food variety.
3. Planned eating may be required for at least 3-6 months before the client's hunger-satiety system is working and clients can move towards intuitive eating.
4. Mindful eating early in recovery is counter-productive, as clients initially experience more intrusive thoughts and feelings of anxiety about eating. This can reduce compliance with eating change and lead to treatment dropout.
5. There needs to be a gradual shift from planned and mindless eating (e.g. following a meal plan while paying attention to other things during eating) to mindful eating. Mindful eating can help clients become aware of feelings of hunger and satiety. It can also help them focus on the sensory experiences of eating including enjoyment of different tastes and textures. (For more information, see Chapter 30.)
6. A hierarchy of harm, developed with the client, clarifies the order of therapeutic work. This usually begins with eating regularly and sufficiently, followed by work on health damaging behaviours (e.g. laxative abuse, vomiting) and moving towards life interfering issues later (e.g. feared foods, social eating).

7. Body image work focuses initially on developing a compassionate motivation to care for the body and being compassionate with the body as it changes through therapy. This progresses to learning to live compassionately at one's set point (Harris, 1990) later in treatment.
8. Therapy needs to address the social challenges of recovery (e.g. comments/criticism from others about size and shape, living in a dieting culture).
9. Therapy is not perfect; lapses and therapeutic misunderstandings are normal. They are opportunities to learn and grow. It is important to be alert to the impacts of self-criticism and to validate and encourage compassionate self-correction in both clients and clinicians.

The flow of CFT-E2

In CFT-E2 we aim to help clients develop and use compassionate competencies to recover from their eating difficulty. Compassion involves three flows: compassion towards others (which many people with an eating difficulty are very good at); compassion from others; and self-compassion. People with an eating difficulty often struggle with self-compassion and are fearful of compassion from others. On a positive note, reductions in shame and improvements in the flows of compassion are linked to better treatment outcomes.

CFT-E2 follows a specific flow, however clinicians can and will move between the different aspects of therapy based on client need. The basic flow of treatment is as follows:

1. Psychoeducation

Psychoeducation is key to engaging clients with an eating difficulty. It helps clients to understand why their brains are tricky, the common human processes involved in eating, and the side effects of interrupting the regular intake of food that all humans need.

Some of the most important messages are:

- Infant feeding takes place while the child is being held and soothed. Infants fail to thrive/feed if they don't receive positive social contact when eating.
- Food can therefore become a very important source of comfort, particularly when we feel lonely or disconnected from others.
- Throughout life, feeding behaviour can take on many different functions, including pleasure and punishment.

- Human bodies have evolved to reproduce and function within a wide body fat percentage. This has helped us breed successfully even at times of food shortage.
- As outlined in setpoint theory, our bodies will work very hard to keep us in a specific range for body fat. If we are below this range, our bodies will drive us to eat and our physical and psychological wellbeing will be significantly compromised. This system also ensures that weight loss is difficult to achieve without extreme calorie deficits and makes sustained weight loss nearly impossible.
- If cultures name and shame particular body shapes/sizes, people will try to change their body to avoid stigmatisation, discrimination, internal shame and self-criticism.
- The side effects of restricted food intake (e.g. preoccupation with food, delayed gastric emptying leading to bloating, urges to binge) can lead to further psychological suffering. However, sometimes the effects of restriction (e.g. emotional numbness, preoccupation with food diverting attention from other painful thoughts and feelings) can help people to manage distress.
- We need carbohydrates as they can create a soothed state in the brain.
- Humans have a low tolerance for hunger but a slow and relatively unreliable system for knowing when we are full. This makes us prone to overeating and weight gain when food is plentiful, and our food industry produces high-calorie, easy-to-eat foods at a relatively low cost.
- Humans can override their hunger-satiety system, for example by comfort eating. If they do so, they can exceed their biologically healthy set point and this can also have health consequences.
- Weight fluctuations are normal during recovery and it will take time and courage for clients to reach their 'set point'.
- Therapy cannot help clients reach their 'ideal' weight and shape, but it can help them learn to find their set point, live more compassionately with their body, and find other ways to manage life's tragedies and challenges.
- The food industry spends billions encouraging us to eat more, while the diet, fitness and fashion industries spend billions encouraging us to eat less to meet thin/muscled ideals. These two opposing social pressures cause conflict and can lead to shame and self-criticism for overeating and/or failing to lose weight, or to become more toned.

Learning point 3

- How does this information change how you would work with someone with an eating difficulty?
- How do you think your client would respond to these key messages?

2. Formulation

We have two ways of working with formulation: looking at how clients' 'Three Circles' (systems) are functioning in the present, or exploring a historical understanding of the development and maintenance of their eating difficulty. The Three Circles model can be particularly helpful if clients find it difficult to recall or tolerate thinking about their past.

3. Developing and using soothing and grounding capacities

CFT-E2 helps clients to find ways to access and develop their soothing system early in treatment. It is important to discuss how the soothing system is used in CFT, which is to help stabilize or ground the mind and body before doing things that require wisdom and courage. It is not about being totally calm in the face of high levels of threat, soothing fear away, or becoming fearless.

We use a range of exercises including sensory soothing, soothing breathing rhythm and soothing imagery at this stage. We ensure clients can access their soothing system before we move on to working on eating related thoughts, feelings or behaviours, and we always ask them to activate their soothing system before working on these themes inside and outside of sessions. We also use this system as a gateway to engaging the compassionate mind (see Goss, 2011, for further details).

It is important to work with any fears, blocks and resistances (FBRs) to soothing at this stage. We have found that giving clients time to practice in the session, and to validate and work through FBRs, pays dividends further into treatment.

4. Enhancing and using the compassionate motivation system

We use Gilbert's (2010) Compassionate Mind Training Model. We begin with developing a shared understanding of the CFT model for compassion and any FBRs to compassion. We then explore ways for the client to work on allowing compassion to be helpful to them and others.

We use several key exercises to help people develop their compassionate capacities. These include:

- memories of being compassionate to others
- memories of receiving compassion from others
- memories of caring for the self
- Compassionate Companion imagery
- Me at My Best compassionate imagery

(Goss, 2011)

All these exercises have the potential to activate painful emotional experiences, including feelings of emptiness, vulnerability, unworthiness and grief, and need to be managed sensitively by clinicians at a pace the client can tolerate. Group work can be particularly helpful, as it gives clients the opportunity to practice expressing compassion for others and receiving compassion in a safe space, and FBRs can be worked through as they Arise.

5. Developing alternative foci for drive and pride

Many clients find it difficult to access the drive system, and it is important to help them explore and engage in fun and pleasurable activities as part of their recovery. Many clients find it difficult to recognize or express emotions (including positive ones) and/or can have a fear of positive feelings. If clients do not have other ways to feel positive about themselves apart from their size, shape or eating/exercise behaviours, they will continue to rely on these. We work on developing a sense of joy and pride in other activities early in therapy. We do not criticise pride in eating behaviours. Instead, we help clients explore alternative ways of accessing this feeling.

6. Enhancing social connections and managing the competitive mentality

Clients may have experienced or observed abusive behaviours from others, leading them to protect themselves from social contact. They may also struggle with issues of social comparison and often feel relieved and de-shamed when we explore these themes. Group work can be a good way for clients to build social connections and experience a secure base/safe haven. Clinicians may need to explore these issues more explicitly if they are working individually.

7. Enlisting the compassionate mind to help with eating behaviour change

It is important to develop a compassionate motivation for recovery and encourage compassionate responses to relapse. Without this, clients often motivate themselves via their threat system, and the changes they make in eating behaviours are unlikely to be sustained. In CFT-E2 we always ask the client to engage their compassionate mind to:

- Help them understand the functions their eating difficulty serves.
- Develop alternative ways to address these functions.
- Motivate them to engage in behaviour change.
- Use their courage to change eating behaviours.
- Tolerate giving up previously important goals (for example weight loss).

- Address lapses with compassion rather than self-criticism.
- Work with the emotions that arise when they commit to living life without their eating difficulty (including grief and regret).

Conclusion

CFT-E2 is a promising approach to helping people recover from an eating difficulty. If you feel this approach would be helpful for your clients, we suggest reading the references included in this chapter. You can also explore the Compassionate Mind Foundation's website (www.compassionatemind.co.uk) for further information (including measures of shame, self-criticism, compassion and fears of compassion) and training opportunities.

References

Gilbert P (2010) *Compassion focused therapy: Distinctive features*. London Routledge.

Goss K (2011) *The compassionate mind approach to beating overeating: Using Compassion Focused Therapy*. London, UK: Robinson.

Goss K & Allan S (2014) The development and application of compassion-focused therapy for eating disorders (CFT-E). *British Journal of Clinical Psychology* **53** (1) 62-77. doi: 10.1111/bjc.12039.

Harris RB (1990) Role of set-point theory in regulation of body weight. *The FASEB Journal* **4** (15) 3310-3318.

29. Finding the middle ground: Building a live worth living with Dialectical Behaviour Therapy

By James Downs

Summary

Written from the perspective of lived experience, this chapter aims to illustrate the ways in which eating difficulties often sit alongside experiences of overwhelming feelings, intolerable levels of distress and difficulties in maintaining stable and balanced relationships. The core components of Dialectical Behaviour Therapy (DBT) consist of skills-based training in the areas of:

1. Interpersonal effectiveness
2. Emotion regulation
3. Distress tolerance
4. Mindfulness

As such, DBT in its full intensive form, or adapted for use in other contexts, can potentially be of great use to those experiencing eating difficulties.

Drawing on real-life examples, this chapter seeks to offer relevant and practical insights into managing some of the underlying drivers of eating difficulties, acknowledging both the difficulty and the possibility of finding alternative ways of coping. Ultimately, the goal of DBT can be described as 'building a life worth living'. This chapter offers a hopeful story of how in the right context – with support, patience, perseverance and practice – change is possible.

Introducing DBT

Dialectical Behaviour Therapy (DBT) was originally developed by Marsha Linehan (1993) as an intensive treatment programme for those experiencing chronic suicidal behaviours. Taking a 'multi-modal' approach, DBT draws together strategies ranging from methodical analysis of unhelpful behaviours and psychoeducation, to exposure-based techniques and skill-building challenges. Over time, DBT has been modified for specific subgroups, such as for people experiencing substance misuse, and more recently those with eating difficulties (Palmer *et al*, 2003). This came out of a recognition that existing treatments for eating difficulties were only moderately effective, and that many people experiencing eating difficulties share struggles addressed by DBT such as difficulty regulating emotions, ambivalence about change, and suicidal thoughts and feelings (Linehan & Chen, 2005).

Many people find the word 'dialectical' a curious one. It refers to the overall epistemological framework within which DBT is situated and conducted, which says that the knowledge we have about the world is obtained through the discourse or dialogue between contradictory figures, ideas or truths. For example, teachers in ancient Greece used the dialectical method of back-and-forth debate to help students refine their ideas (Maybee, 2020), and the 19th century German philosopher Hegel systematized a dialectical approach to thinking and knowing based on acknowledging the 'opposing sides' that can exist not just between people but between ideas, ways of thinking and consciousness (Hegel, 2018).

Hegel's description of the three 'moments' of the dialectical process says that at first, we rationally understand a concept, which is a moment of fixity and stability. The second moment, the 'dialectical' or 'negatively rational' moment, is when the restrictedness of our first understanding comes to the fore and we are aware of its opposite, bringing a moment of instability. The third moment is the 'speculative' one, where we realise that there is some kind of unity in the opposition between two ideas or truths, where both can be held and preserved without negating the other. Hegel describes this moment as 'positively rational', and perhaps being able to comprehend nuance, hold competing tensions or integrate opposing ideas is what it is to have a more flexible, dialectical stance toward life (Hegel, 2018).

The central dialectic recognized by DBT is the one between acceptance and change, and it is perhaps for this reason that, despite being a therapy aimed at behavioural change, DBT draws extensively on mindfulness practices in order to develop a greater acceptance of self, others and life in general (Welch, 2006). DBT suggests mindfulness can be enhanced by practicing 'observing', 'describing' and 'participating' with phenomena experienced in the present moment – the 'what' –

and remaining 'non-judgemental', 'one-mindful' (i.e. doing one thing at a time) and 'effective' (doing what works) – the 'how' (Gratz *et al*, 2005). While mindfulness is one of the four areas of 'skills training' in DBT, it is viewed as underpinning all the other skills as well as the therapy as a whole and helps in recognising which other skills to use and when.

How, though, is this seemingly obscure philosophical stance relevant to helping those experiencing eating difficulties?

My journey to DBT

Like many people experiencing eating difficulties, my route to accessing help and support was not straightforward. I was diagnosed with anorexia when I was in my mid-teens. Already in treatment for obsessive compulsive disorder (OCD) and depression, I struggled to feel seen or understood. My family and school teachers couldn't see how devastatingly bored I was and left me to my own devices because I would get A*s. The psychiatrists didn't see the distress that was driving my OCD and the feelings of being unsafe and unacceptable to others that pervaded my life – they only saw a clever person who would supposedly recover simply because they could grasp the ideas of cognitive behavioural therapy (CBT).

My need to be stimulated, to feel like I belonged, for someone to 'get me' and see what I needed – all of these were overlooked, including by the people who were supposed to help me. This was deeply frightening; if the professionals couldn't understand me and meet me in my suffering, then who would? Because I was bright, came from a respectable family and appeared competent, it seemed like nobody thought I needed very much. But however we may appear, whatever our backgrounds or life experiences or prospects, we all have needs.

DBT draws on literature from emotion-focused therapy which provides a really helpful way of understanding needs, and the core painful feelings that can Arise when those needs are unmet (Timulak, 2015). The need for safety is an existential one, and without it we feel insecurity, invasion, terror. The need for love and connection also provides us with security – we only survive in communities. Without this, we feel alone, isolated and unloved. When the need for validation and a sense of value and agency is lost, we can feel ashamed, worthless and rejected. None of us can sustain having our needs violated or unmet – either in key moments or over time – without it leaving its mark. The emotional pain we feel from this isn't some abstract thing that is all in our heads. Emotions are called 'feelings' for a reason – we feel them in our bodies, and the body experiences and keeps a record of our emotional pain in the same way it remembers physical pain, illness and injury (Van der Kolk, 2014).

I understand my own experience of developing eating difficulties as emerging from a complex mosaic of factors, where many pieces of different sizes and shapes slotted together to reinforce feelings that I was not safe, loved or worth loving. Linehan's model describes how difficulties in regulating emotions, establishing internal safety and forming a stable self-concept often emerge in an 'invalidating environment', which isn't necessarily a singular physical place such as the home. This is a concept that really rung true for my experience of the world, which at worst didn't provide me with a framework for understanding what was even real. This is perhaps the 'borderline' between psychosis and neurosis referred to by the contested diagnostic label of 'borderline personality disorder' (for which DBT was originally developed) – an idea I could relate to profoundly.

Instead of focusing on the needs I was meeting through destructive eating behaviours, clinicians repeatedly told me that I simply needed to stop my behaviours and everything would be fine. Only the reality was that weight restoration, supervised eating and enforced cold-turkey from exercise didn't make me feel better at all. I felt like I had been sold a lie. I felt so much worse after I gained weight because all the emotional pain I didn't have to feel when starving came back, and worse. More dysregulated, more intense for being squashed down so long, and more frightening. All the security I gained from restriction, gone.

Unable to tolerate distress, I would jump out of my feelings into other eating difficulties – this time binge eating and purging. There was no middle ground. I ended up in and out of hospital with low potassium, suicide attempts and para-suicidal overdoses. I didn't know how to ask for help when it had been so painfully refused before. I poured myself into helping others and into abusive relationships as a way of not having to be with myself – to focus on the other or reinforce that I was worthless. I was able to get a place on any university course I wanted, but was unable to sustain anything except my eating difficulties. They became a way of being through which I experienced and dealt with the world.

I wish that professionals could have seen that, for me, my eating problems were the best way I knew to meet my needs. For all the times I was told 'you are going to kill yourself', 'you're putting your health at risk', and, ' you should stop your anorexic behaviours', I wish someone had said, 'I see you are in pain', 'your experience is valid', and, 'well done for coping in the only way that you could – how resourceful you are to have survived'. I also craved for someone to see beyond my eating problems and see a person that had so much more to offer and enjoy in life, but who couldn't recover without acceptance, validation and support.

Learning point 1

Before reading further, take a moment to reflect on any eating difficulties you may have encountered, be that relating to your work, your own experiences or those of someone who are supporting.

- Think of the reasons why those eating difficulties may have developed, worsened or been maintained. Can you view these often complex factors with compassion?
- What functions might eating difficulties perform in someone's life?
- What feelings might there be about change which could make it difficult to replace eating difficulties with other, more adaptive behaviours?

The DBT view of eating difficulties

The model of emotion regulation was explained to me when I finally had to pause my studies as a medical student following multiple suicide attempts. It was a massive relief to understand the role of my eating behaviours through this lens, which proposes that eating difficulties serve to regulate intolerable feelings, especially where less harmful or 'adaptive' emotion regulation skills are present, or eating difficulties have been 'over-learned' and reinforced as an 'escape behaviour' over a long period of time. For instance, DBT views binge eating and purging behaviours as an attempt to escape or block distressing physiological responses and feelings which can be triggered by thoughts relating to food, eating, body image, interpersonal situations and more. The escape response becomes increasingly automatic, more difficult to intervene in, and more likely to elicit distress if not enacted. This makes the idea of changing such behaviour inherently challenging and requiring a whole set of skills to tolerate the initial distress that can be caused by not using your 'target behaviour'.

In the case of restrictive eating difficulties, the drive to lose weight and weight loss itself can both be seen as an attempt to block emotions and physiologically reduce feeling. DBT also notes how eating difficulties in themselves can be emotionally painful, physically damaging and interpersonally traumatic – all of which can result in secondary emotional distress, including shame.

In a dialectical sense, distress sits at one end of the spectrum, and not feeling at the other. When feelings are so overwhelming, who wouldn't want to escape them? But continually opting out of feeling only serves to reinforce emotions as intolerable and difficult eating behaviours as the solution. As Hegel suggests, the sublation of one truth or state to another isn't an easy fix – it is a moment of tension (Hegel, 2018). Over time, DBT aims to recognize that both intense feelings and a desire to escape them are valid, real and acceptable experiences. Only through acceptance can we respond from where we are at, and so both acceptance and change are necessary for increasing psychological flexibility, growing in skillfulness and, ultimately, recovery.

While being in DBT can feel like you are between a rock and a hard place, the choice being presented isn't actually between the two difficult situations of feeling or not feeling. The challenge is between recognising your automatic and unhelpful ways of dealing with emotions and choosing *new ways of coping*. The key is in being 'willing' to try something new, rather than remaining 'willfully' committed to what you know. For this, you need intensive support, a therapeutic stance which radically accepts your experiences but challenges you to grow, and a whole lot of courage.

Learning point 2

- Thinking of the central dialectic of acceptance and change, can you identify where you or someone you might be supporting are on this scale?
- When considering change, what might be some of the barriers to changing eating difficulties?
- Why might acceptance be difficult for someone experiencing eating difficulties?
- What might help with holding this tension between the pain and grief of acceptance and fear and ambivalence about change? What support might be needed?

DBT: the key components

DBT takes a particular structure:

- Weekly group sessions (generally around 2-3 hours in length) focusing on teaching, learning and practicing behavioural skills.
- Weekly individual therapy sessions where the therapist teaches and reinforces adaptive behaviours.
- Telephone coaching which is extensively available to support the use of skillful responses to emotional difficulties and distress. Telephone coaching can help bridge the gap between practicing DBT skills in a therapeutic setting and being able to normalise their use in day-to-day life.
- Weekly DBT consultation group for therapists who tend to work in teams, to support each other and their work with people who often have severe and complex difficulties.

The therapeutic stance of DBT involves the therapist validating and accepting the client, while challenging them to step into more skillful ways of responding to their emotional pain, rather than rescuing them or taking them out of crises (Linehan, 2014).

The learning content of DBT falls into four modules[1]:

1) Distress tolerance

While many approaches to emotional distress aim at removing or modifying sources of distress, few radically accept the presence of distress in the way that DBT does. DBT teaches mindful awareness of distressed states, their triggers and the ways they are felt in the body. Accepting distress does not have to mean liking it – it is to non-judgementally notice it and then think about how to bear this pain skillfully.

DBT suggests skills such as appropriate distraction from peak distress, so as to deploy other tactics once the peak has passed, such as self-soothing or 'improving the moment' with techniques such as using imagery and meaning-making activities. Thinking of the pros and cons of the different responses we can take to pain. To balance our 'emotional mind' and 'reason mind', the dialectical stance helps to develop a 'wise mind' which validates that tolerating distress and taking skillful action is all emotionally hard, but will be helpful in the long run.

2) Emotion regulation

In DBT, understanding emotional distress is situated in understanding emotions more broadly – how they are perceived, our responses to them and how they are a product of our experiences in the world. As such, DBT skills include increasing our mindfulness/awareness of emotions, reducing vulnerability to 'emotion mind' and challenging our automatic responses to emotional states (such as shame creating the desire to disappear, fear to either freeze or escape). All emotions are seen as valid in DBT, but the intensity of an emotion or the nature of our response can sometimes be seen as 'unwarranted'. While this module has some focus on more enhanced distress tolerance techniques, it also looks at increasing the emotional states we experience as positive, and even at radical ways of challenging impulsive responses to emotions such as taking the 'opposite action' to avoidant responses.

3) Interpersonal effectiveness

I've always been known for having excellent communication skills and a high degree of empathy, but having interpersonal skills is not the same as being interpersonally *effective*. This is about making sure relationships and the ways you interact with people around you are helpful, balanced and not damaging. For

---

1 For a more detailed overview of DBT skills see www.dbtselfhelp.com

example, I was always excellent at being able to give help, but I learnt that asking for help was risky and potentially hurtful. DBT taught me effective strategies for asking for what I need, how to assertively say 'no' and set boundaries, and how to manage situations of interpersonal conflict.

4) Mindfulness

DBT describes the 'what' of mindfulness as to 'observe', 'describe' and 'participate' with the present moment. The 'how' of practicing mindfulness is to do so 'non-judgementally', 'one-mindfully' and 'effectively' – doing what works without judgement, and with our fullest attention. Mindfulness skills aren't simply one of the four skills modules taught in DBT groups, they are viewed as underpinning all dimensions of skillful behaviour and decision-making.

Learning point 3

- Having read about the different domains in which DBT aims to develop skillful behaviour, and some examples of these, can you see why these skills might be useful in relation to eating difficulties?
- Are there any skill areas which you recognise as difficult for yourself or someone you might support with eating difficulties? Are there any areas of strength?
- How might someone incorporate mindfulness skills into daily life when trying to make decisions about how to cope with difficult thoughts and feelings? Are there any particular exercises that might resonate with yourself/the person you are supporting?

People who struggle with eating are not deficient, but they may have over-rehearsed ways of coping with emotional pain that cause harm. Replacing eating difficulties with more 'skillful' behaviours requires a whole raft of techniques which can be acquired over time through group learning, intensive support and real-life practice.

DBT uses a hierarchy of 'treatment targets' – first of all, targeting 'life-threatening' behaviours; then 'therapy-interfering' factors; then other 'quality of life' limiting behaviours; and finally 'skill acquisition'. Similarly, the overall model of DBT proposes progressive stages of treatment. In stage one, the aim is to move out of a state of being dominated by uncontrolled and damaging behaviours. In stage 2, the patient is said to be in a state of 'quiet desperation', a phrase made famous by Henry Thoreau's 1854 assertion that 'the mass of men lead lives of quiet desperation' (Thoreau, 1993). Here the target behaviours are viewed as under control, but emotional experience inhibited. Freud may have been happy to end here – his aim in psychoanalysis being to help the patient transform 'hysterical misery into common unhappiness' (Kaye, 2014).

In Stage 3, the challenge is to cultivate more peace and happiness and to work towards self-determined goals. For some people, Linehan proposed a fourth stage of treatment that is centred around finding deeper meaning, purpose and fulfilment beyond 'recovery'.

Who might DBT help?

There has been an increasing popularity for using the skills outlined in DBT in psychoeducation groups, without the full structures of a formal DBT programme. There is emerging evidence that DBT might help in modified forms such as this – for instance in the form of guided self-help (Kenny *et al*, 2020) or through the use of DBT 'diary cards' which are a methodical way or recording emotional states and target behaviours with those who experience binge eating difficulties (Klein *et al*, 2013)[2]. Outcomes of DBT can be predicted by a number of factors, including the duration and age of onset of eating difficulties (Safer *et al*, 2002), and it won't be suitable for everyone. DBT reminds us, though, that being effective and 'doing what works' is more important than sticking to convention.

DBT may help a variety of people who struggle with emotional difficulties and harmful ways of responding to them. Whether or not someone undertakes DBT, key principles such as acceptance, skill-building and awareness of emotional experiences can be of benefit to many.

Conclusion

My years of experience living with eating difficulties have taught me that they exist for a reason. They are dysfunctional, but that's still a kind of functional. They provide a false sense of security, which is better than no security at all. They provide something to connect with when you might feel dislocated from the world around you. They are powerful tools for regulating emotions, even if you wished your emotions were not so dysregulated in the first place.

I've learnt from DBT that the support, skills and effort you need to come anywhere near to matching the automaticity and effectiveness of eating difficulties are really hard to come by. I've also realised that it's not my fault that I have the problems that I do. But it is my responsibility to be willing to try something new, however painful my experiences have been before. With DBT, I was finally given the framework and the support I needed to make steps towards a life worth living. I hope many others benefit from this support, too.

2 For examples of DBT diary cards, see www.dbtselfhelp.com/html/diary_cards1.html

References

Brown TA, Wisniewski L & Anderson LK (2020) Dialectical Behavior Therapy for Eating Disorders: State of the Research and New Directions, *Eating Disorders* **28** (2) 97-100, DOI: 10.1080/10640266.2020.1728204

Downs J (2019) *Choosing a life without an eating disorder meant confronting why I needed it in the first place* [online]. ORRI Guest Bloggers. Available at: www.orri-uk.com/choosing-a-life-without-an-eating-disorder/ (accessed August 2021).

Gratz KL, Tull MT & Wagner AW (2005) Applying DBT mindfulness skills to the treatment of clients with anxiety disorders. In: *Acceptance and mindfulness-based approaches to anxiety* (pp147-161). Springer, Boston, MA.

Hegel G (2018) *Georg Wilhelm Friedrich Hegel: The Phenomenology of Spirit* (Cambridge Hegel Translations) (T. Pinkard & M. Baur, Eds.). Cambridge: Cambridge University Press. doi:10.1017/9781139050494

Kaye HL (2014) *After Freud Left: A Century of Psychoanalysis in America*. Burnham J (ed).

Kenny TE, Carter JC & Safer DL (2020) Dialectical behavior therapy guided self-help for binge-eating disorder. *Eating Disorders* **28** (2) 202-211. DOI: 10.1080/10640266.2019.1678982

Klein AS, Skinner JB & Hawley KM (2013) Targeting binge eating through components of dialectical behavior therapy: Preliminary outcomes for individually supported diary card self-monitoring versus group-based DBT. *Psychotherapy* **50** (4) 543–552. https://doi.org/10.1037/a0033130

Linehan MM (1993) Dialectical behavior therapy for treatment of borderline personality disorder: implications for the treatment of substance abuse. *NIDA research monograph* **137** 201-201.

Linehan MM & Chen EY (2005) Dialectical behavior therapy for eating disorders. In: *Encyclopedia of cognitive behavior therapy* (pp168-171). Springer, Boston, MA.

Linehan MM (2014) *DBT skills training handouts and worksheets*. Guilford Press.

Maybee JE (2020) *Hegel's Dialectics* [online]. The Stanford Encyclopedia of Philosophy. Available at: https://plato.stanford.edu/archives/win2020/entries/hegel-dialectics/ (accessed August 2021).

Palmer RL, Birchall H, Damani S, Gatward N, McGrain L & Parker L (2003) A dialectical behavior therapy program for people with an eating disorder and borderline personality disorder description and outcome. *International Journal of Eating Disorders* **33** 281–286.

Robins CJ, Rosenthal MZ & Cuper PF (2010) Dialectical behavior therapy. In: JJ Magnavita (Ed.), *Evidence-based treatment of personality dysfunction: Principles, methods, and processes (p49–78). American Psychological Association*. https://doi.org/10.1037/12130-003

Safer DL, Lively TJ, Telch CF & Agras WS (2002) Predictors of relapse following successful dialectical behavior therapy for binge eating disorder. *International Journal of Eating Disorders* **32** 155-163. https://doi.org/10.1002/eat.10080

Thoreau HD (1993) *Civil disobedience, and other essays*. Courier Corporation.

Timulak L (2015) *Transforming emotional pain in psychotherapy: An emotion-focused approach*. Routledge.

Van der Kolk B (2014) *The body keeps the score: Mind, brain and body in the transformation of trauma*. Penguin: UK.

Welch SS, Rizvi S & Dimidjian S (2006) Mindfulness in dialectical behavior therapy (DBT) for borderline personality disorder. *Mindfulness-based treatment approaches: Clinician's guide to evidence base and applications* 117-139.

30. Mindful eating: A new behavioural approach for improving our relationship with food and treating eating difficulties

By Dr. Ifigeneia Giannopoulou

Summary

Mindful eating is a new behavioural approach focusing on eating behaviours and our relationship with food. Through mindfulness practices, the approach aims to bring balance to and minimise any struggles and difficulties with eating.

Mindful eating promotes a new way of eating. It is about being aware of our relationship with food, how we feel and think about food, and how much we enjoy eating. It is about being in the present moment and aware of our eating practices and choices. Once we have established this awareness, we have already taken the first step towards a healthier relationship with food.

This chapter will introduce the basic principles of mindful eating to support a better understanding of eating and its effects on mood. I will then provide some reflective exercises that will allow you to become more mindful in your eating practice.

What is mindful eating?

As with mindfulness, mindful eating applies practices of Buddhist origins to your eating behaviours. Specifically, it focuses on the observation of your eating practices, choices and habits, with the goal of bringing awareness and understanding to your relationship with food and your body. The main parameters of mindful eating are:

The present moment: Through the use of meditative practices and 'slowing down', mindful eating allows you to stay in the present moment and make you the focus of your life. Mindful eating creates the time and space to observe oneself and one's eating behaviours. In this way, self-care becomes an intuitive practice.

Awareness: Mindful eating brings awareness to your eating. It focuses on the observation and understanding of the following aspects that drive your eating behaviour: *how*, *where*, *when*, *what*, *why* and *how much you eat*.

Examples:
How: "Do you eat fast or slow?"
Where: "Do you eat in front of your computer?"
When: "Do you eat when you are hungry or stressed?"
What: "Do you choose what you eat without thinking or based on your likes and dislikes?"
Why: "Do you eat to comfort yourself emotionally?"
How much: "Do you listen to your body and eat until you are full, or do you eat too much or too little?"

Lack of judgement

Mindfulness in eating advocates the use of gentle and kind language when referring to our eating behaviours and our bodies. Thinking mindfully and compassionately about your eating and your needs allows you to let go of any judgemental inner voices and thoughts that create struggles and generate difficult emotions in your eating.

Learning point 1

Being in the present moment, observing non-judgmentally and gaining awareness about your eating practices and their effects on your emotional state, can bring balance and ownership to your eating.

Reflective practice

You might like to use a notebook to write down your answers and reflections during your practice.

1. How, when, where, why, what, and how much do you eat?
2. Do the above answers change depending on how you feel? I.e. when you are feeling stressed versus when you are feeling lonely or bored?

The science behind mindful eating and its effects on eating difficulties

In the last decade, mindfulness has emerged as a new behavioural approach with important health effects and benefits in clinical conditions such as obesity, diabetes and cardiovascular disease as well as depression and anxiety (Godsey, 2013; O-Reilly *et al*, 2014). Mindfulness is based on Zen and Tebetah meditation techniques and can be described as the practice of purposefully being in the present moment while attentive of how one feels, without judgement. Recently, mindfulness in eating was developed based on the application of mindfulness theories and techniques specifically to issues related to struggles with eating and difficulties with food (Wanden-Berghe *et al*, 2010). The cultivation of mindfulness in eating can result in transformative changes in eating behaviours and improve wellbeing and quality of life, for example reductions in the frequency of bingeing and the amount of food eaten (Katterman *et al*, 2014; Kristeller *et al*, 2010); increased self-regulation through an enhanced connection with the physical cues of hunger and fullness (Mantzios & Wilson, 2015); and reduced influence of emotional triggers to overeating (Kristeller & Wolever, 2013).

Such changes in eating behaviour have been shown to reduce calorie consumption for those over-consuming calories, facilitate weight regulation and improve body image and related anxiety and depression in individuals with eating difficulties (Carrière *et al*, 2017; Kristeller *et al*, 2014). Moreover, the introduction of just a few brief mindfulness instructions immediately before eating high calorie snacks has been shown to reduce portion sizes and lead to a healthier selection of snacks (Arch *et al*, 2016).

Mindful connection with our needs and body cues of hunger and satiety

Have you ever eaten out of habit? Or simply because the food smelt or looked good and not because you were hungry? Have you ever eaten in front of your computer without even realising what you are eating? Have you ever cleared your plate despite being full? These are eating behaviours and choices that are very common and we should not feel bad about them. They do not necessarily denote that there is a 'problem' with our eating behaviour and we should not feel guilty or ashamed about them. However, these behaviours are potential signs that you may have been eating mindlessly or automatically without paying attention to what your body was telling you.

Mindless eating is very common in Western societies, where the fast pace of life dictates, for the most part, our food habits and choices. As a result, we may not listen to our bodies and can learn to disconnect from our needs. We may forget to eat or fail to recognize how hungry or how full we are. As a result, we may neglect our nutritional and physical needs.

Observing and listening to your hunger and satiety/fullness cues is a central component of mindful eating and can radically transform your relationship with food, your body and your basic needs. When our body is lacking energy, physical cues of hunger such as a rumbling empty stomach, headache, lack of concentration and sleepiness due to low blood sugar levels, can inform us of the need for feeding. On the other side, when we are full, our bodies will send physical signals of satiety (i.e. fullness) as experienced by sensations of stomach fullness/bloating and pressure, no longer enjoying food and possibly sluggishness. It is important that we listen and respond to these physical cues in order to retain the homeostasis (energy balance) in our body. When we ignore these cues we can observe disturbances in energy levels, cravings, binge episodes etc. that can lead to struggles with food and related emotional experiences such as guilt, stress, anger and self-blame. Mindfulness in eating trains you to observe these physical cues and respond to them intuitively.

Types of hunger

Different types of hunger are very commonly experienced. The definition of hunger can become very complex due to several factors that 'trick' us into thinking we are hungry when we are not, such as our emotional state (e.g. loneliness or stress), social events and parties, or just the irresistible smell of freshly baked goods. Specifically, there are four main types of hunger that can drive our eating practices and the amount of food we consume:

- Physical, 'true' hunger: the physiological need for energy for our body to function.
- Psychological hunger: eating due to emotional states.
- Taste hunger: desire/cravings due to seeing or smelling a food that appeals to you.
- Practical hunger: a drive to eat due to routine or scheduling.

By not listening to our hunger cues, it is challenging to stop eating when we are full. Many people start eating their meals already feeling overly hungry; hence, they end up eating too fast and too much, continuing beyond their fullness levels. This can have negative consequences on weight regulation and, most importantly, can lead to potential difficult emotions towards ourselves such as self-blame, self-anger, guilt and feelings of failure. Mindful eating practices involve re-training so we can listen to our body cues with the aim of bringing significant improvements in our food intake and eating behaviours.

Learning point 2

Developing self-awareness of hunger and fullness cues can offer a sense of ownership of your eating behaviours. Through a better understanding of what your body needs and wants, you can be free to eat as you like, without disregarding your biological needs.

Reflective practice

1. What types of hunger do you experience and when?
2. How hungry and full are you now? Use the Hunger Scale below (Figure 30.1) (Forde, 2017) to assess your hunger and satiety levels. Repeat before, halfway through, and at the end of one of the main meals of the day.
3. Complete the sentence: "Noticing when I'm physically hungry is helpful because..."
4. Complete the sentence: "Noticing when I'm physically full is helpful because..."

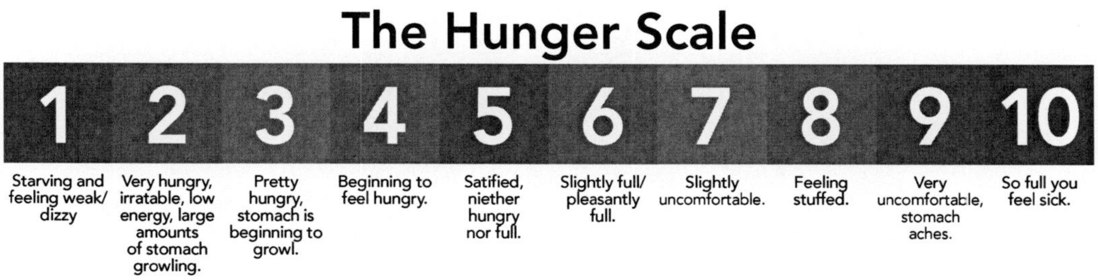

Figure 30.1: A visual analogue scale (VAS) to assess hunger levels, prior to, during and after the consumption of a meal (Forde, 2017).

Mindful exploration of the triggers for overeating or undereating

The environment and its triggers frequently alter the way we eat, either leading to overeating or binge eating or driving chronic, yo-yo dieting behaviours and undereating. Identifying and being aware of these triggers can help you to understand under what situations you face eating difficulties. Particularly, external environmental triggers can disconnect us from our needs and wants and lead to eating difficulties. Some very frequent triggers of overeating or undereating are:

- Emotional: such as stress, boredom or loneliness.
- Social/cultural: such as eating with friends, being at a restaurant/party, dealing with family culture and traditions/pressure etc.
- Social media influences: such as advertisements portraying what your body 'should' look like, or promoting new diet fashions and weight loss regimes.

Emotional eating, in particular, is one of the most prevalent triggers for over or undereating which, over time, can create new routines wherein food is used for comfort and the numbing of difficult emotions. Once this routine is established, we may learn to deal with difficult emotions in a mindless way without really resolving them; rather masking them, thus further exacerbating the problem. Mindful eating trains us to build emotional connections and deal with difficulties through awareness, acceptance and self-love.

Reflective practice

1. Identify one or two triggers that led you to overeat or undereat this last week.
2. Explore further how these triggers led you to fail to listen to your body and what you *really* wanted to eat, and how they changed your eating behaviour in other ways.
3. Make a list of the ways you could have behaved in response to your identified triggers, e.g. calling a friend.
4. Identify what types of personal experiences trigger emotional eating for you.

Mindful re-enjoyment of food

Society's and social media's preoccupation with diets and strict food rules ('good' versus 'bad' foods), and the obsession with weight loss and the 'ideal body type' has disconnected us from the enjoyment of eating and brought guilt and shame into our relationship with food for many people. We may often forget that food is life and nurture and should be tasty and fun! One of the key skills one develops with mindful eating is the re-enjoyment of food through an exploration of taste, flavours and the awakening of the senses. Once you start re-engaging with the fun aspect of food and bring back the pleasure of eating, it can become easier to eat as much as you want and need, slowly and mindfully, with no strict rules, 'shoulds' or 'musts'. You may become happier with your food choices. Moreover, through specific mindful eating exercises you can learn to deal with any feelings of guilt and shame that might accompany eating certain foods or eating in a certain way, and reduce potential anxiety or fear of overeating and/or gaining weight. Such a change in your eating behaviours and experience is proven to have a significant positive impact on the treatment of eating difficulties and your overall physical and psychological wellbeing (Warren *et al*, 2017).

Reflective practice

1. Mindfully eat a raisin or some fruit. Follow the instructions below in the bullet points and reflect on how you felt and what the experience taught you.
2. Repeat the previous exercise with a food that you tend to avoid or binge on.
3. Complete the sentence: "I've been surprised by how the taste of food changes when I eat mindfully. For example..."

Mindful eating exercise instructions

Close your eyes and take two or three relaxed breaths. Slowly open your eyes and ***take one raisin*** *and look at it with curiosity as if you have never seen one before. Examine the folds, the colour, the shape etc.*

Now close your eyes and smell the raisin, feeling it against the outside of your lips. Slowly place it into your mouth, but do not chew it yet. Move the raisin around your mouth and notice the sensations. Begin to chew it slowly and notice how the taste changes. Resist the urge to swallow.

Notice any thoughts or feelings about eating this raisin. Notice the experience of the impulse to swallow. Swallow the raisin when you are ready. Are there still any tastes or sensations now?

Open your eyes, pick up the ***second*** *raisin and follow the same process. Has anything changed? Repeat with the* ***third*** *raisin. Now look at the* ***fourth*** *raisin. Decide whether you want to eat this raisin or not. Be aware of* ***how*** *you are making this choice. If you choose to eat this raisin, lead yourself through the practice. If not, simply be aware for a few moments of your breath, thoughts, feelings and sensations in your mouth. Gently open your eyes.*

Mindful acceptance, self-love and letting go

The way we eat and the food choices we make are often governed by strong, critical automatic thoughts and self-talk. Negative thoughts such as: "I failed again", "I ruined my diet", "I will never achieve my goal" and "I am not good enough" can adversely affect our eating behaviours and emotional state. An absence of awareness of such automatic thoughts can lead us to overeat or undereat, and can cause binge eating or severe hunger and chronic dieting, with negative impacts on our eating behaviours. It can also result in difficult emotions such as guilt, regret and self-critical thinking, negative self-talk, distorted body image and anxiety.

Mindful eating teaches us to *let go* of negative, critical thinking, and to accept ourselves non-judgmentally for who we are, embracing our choices and our needs. Respect and self-care are central components of mindfulness that ground our behaviour and our relationship with ourselves.

At the core of mindful eating is *self-love*: the capacity to love yourself unconditionally for who you are, what you need and what you like. Once we start practicing self-love, acceptance and self-care, we put ourselves at the centre of our own lives. We become free to be authentic in our eating and respectful of our needs.

Reflective practice

1. Remember a time when you 'used' food for reasons other than being hungry. Reflect on what happened: Did food provide a solution and real comfort? Was there a *lasting* effect? Did it resolve the problem?
2. How do you usually deal with feeling lonely or uncomforted? What are some ways to find emotional fulfilment and comfort and self-love *besides* eating?
3. Make a list of self-love practices e.g. a luxurious bath or a relaxing walk. Reflect on which difficult situations they can be used to bring you comfort. Practice one of them today!

Conclusions

Mindful eating is a new behavioural eating approach and practice that has been shown to improve the health and wellbeing of some individuals with eating difficulties (Warren *et al*, 2017). This approach is based on the principles of non-judgmental awareness, being in the present moment, accepting and letting go of any critical thinking and listening and respecting bodily needs.

With mindful eating we can shift our experience with food to a positive one and can start reconnecting with our needs and ourselves while inviting back the joy of eating and self-love. Training yourself and developing an awareness of what drives your eating behaviours and habits through a mindful eating practice will allow you to become the 'carer' and 'decision-maker' of your eating.

Please see below for some resources and reading material about mindful eating which could further your understanding and practice of mindful eating.

Resources

Mindless Eating: Why we eat more than we think, by Brian Wansink, 2006, Bantam Books, New York, NY.

The Joy of Half a Cookie: Using mindfulness to lose weight and end the struggle with food, by Jean Kristeller and Alisa Bowman, 2015, Perigee, New York, NY

The Mindful Eating Center by Jean Kristeller. https://www.mb-eat.com/

The Center For Mindful Eating: Mindful Eating Position Statements. www.thecenterformindfuleating.org/Position-Statements

The Center for Mindful Eating: Resources: www.thecenterformindfuleating.org/Mindful-Eating-Resources

References

Arch JJ, Brown KW, Goodman RJ, Della Porta MD, Kiken LG & Tillman S (2016) Enjoying food without caloric cost: The impact of brief mindfulness on laboratory eating outcomes. *Behav Res Ther* **79** 23-34. doi: 101016/jbrat201602002

Carrière K, Khoury B, Günak M & Knäuper B (2018) Mindfulness-based interventions for weight loss: a systematic review and meta-analysis *Obes Rev* **19** (2)164-177.

Forde C (2017) Measuring Satiation and Satiety Chapter 101016/B978-0-08-101743-200007-8.

Godsey J (2013) The role of mindfulness based interventions in the treatment of obesity and eating disorders: An integrative review. *Complementary Ther Med* **21** 430-439. doi: 101016/jctim201306003

Katterman S, Kleinman B, Hood M, Nackers L & Corsica J (2014) Mindfulness meditation as an intervention for binge eating emotional eating and weight loss: A systematic review. *Eating Behaviors* **15** (2) pp197-204.

Kristeller J & Wolever R (2010) Mindfulness-Based Eating Awareness Training for Treating Binge Eating Disorder: The Conceptual Foundation. *Eat Disord* **19** (1) 49-61.

Kristeller J, Wolever R & Sheets V (2013) Mindfulness-Based Eating Awareness Training (MB-EAT) for Binge Eating: A Randomized Clinical Trial. *Mindfulness* **5** (3) pp282-297.

Kristeller J & Wolever R (2014) Sheets V Mindfulness-Based Eating Awareness Training (MB-EAT) for Binge Eating: .Randomized Clinical Trial *Mindfulness* **5** (3) 282-29.

Mantzios M & Wilson J (2015) Mindfulness Eating Behaviours and Obesity: A Review and Reflection on Current Findings *Curr Obes Rep* **4** (1) 141-146.

O'Reilly G, Cook L, Spruijt-Metz D & Black D (2014) Mindfulness-based interventions for obesity-related eating behaviours: a literature review. *Obes Rev* **15** (6) 453-461.

Wanden-Berghe R, Sanz-Valero J & Wanden-Berghe C (2010) The Application of Mindfulness to Eating Disorders Treatment: A Systematic Review. *Eating Disorders* **19** (1) pp34-48.

Warren J, Smith N & Ashwell M (2017) A structured literature review on the role of mindfulness mindful eating and intuitive eating in changing eating behaviours: Effectiveness and associated potential mechanisms. *Nutrition Research Reviews* **30** (2) 272-283 doi:101017/S0954422417000154.

31. How may cognitive behavioural therapy help individuals with eating difficulties?

By Yngvild Danielsen and Guro Rekkedal

Summary

Cognitive behavioural therapy (CBT) models hold a transdiagnostic view of eating difficulties, indicating that many of the underlying maintaining mechanisms are similar in all eating difficulties. CBT systematically aims at weakening and breaking factors maintaining the eating difficulty. These factors might be cognitive, behavioural, emotional and/or interpersonal. CBT treatment helps with understanding the eating difficulty as being a self-maintaining system, that is separate from personal identity. It offers tools to address unhelpful behaviours, thoughts and feelings, and provides support for clients in tolerating ambivalence and anxiety that Arises when starting to challenge the eating difficulty. Furthermore, it aims at establishing healthy self-perception, relationships and emotion regulation. For the treatment of eating difficulties, CBT (eating disorders versions) is currently recommended as best evidence in treatment guidelines (NICE, 2017). This chapter will provide insights into how CBT treatment might help people with eating difficulties.

Eating difficulties as being a vicious maintaining circle

Eating difficulties may start developing in the teens, with the individual using restrictive eating or binge eating as a means of handling and communicating their emotional pain, loss of control or self-esteem. For others it starts as a weight-loss endeavour or fitness program, with an underlying desire to change appearance.

At some point, however, the eating difficulty starts living its own life, demanding stricter and stricter rules and obeyance of these. More or less consciously, an increasing number of rules regarding food, eating and other weight control behaviours are developed. Examples include eating only at particular times, avoiding certain food items, consuming very few calories each day, cutting the food into small pieces or going to the gym twice a day. The system becomes so rigid, extensive and strict, that it is impossible to adhere to these rules, while at the same time staying healthy. The circle is closed into a downward spiral, that leads to either low weight (and negative somatic consequences), or being caught by the body's biological drive for energy. This causes rule breaking and episodes of loss of control over one's eating.

At this point the eating difficulty affects both relations with other people, thoughts and emotions. It has become a self-maintaining vicious circle that is extremely anxiety provoking to break. Cognitive behavioural models of eating difficulties describe the maintaining factors of eating difficulties and their interaction (Fairburn *et al*, 2003; Waller *et al*, 2007).

At the core of this cycle is a dysfunctional scheme for self-evaluation and self-worth. Most people evaluate themselves in several aspects of their life, such as relationships, friends, values and beliefs, work achievements, different abilities and hobbies. When a person has an eating difficulty, their self-evaluation has become mainly based on their appearance, shape and weight, and the ability to control these. Consequently, it becomes extremely important to succeed in this one project. This dominance results in a marginalization of other areas of life (Fairburn, 2008).

Learning point 1

- Please ask yourself: What is important in my personal self-evaluation? When you have created a list, think about the relative importance of each point.
- Take a minute to reflect upon the following question – How would failure in one of these areas affect me?

Breaking a dietary rule or losing control over food intake may cause very difficult feelings when someone has an eating difficulty, creating a drive to compensate or forming stricter rules. Vomiting is the most common way of compensating for a loss of control over food intake (binge eating), and it gives an immediate sensation of relief. For some, this circle of bingeing and vomiting becomes established and maintains itself. The possibility of vomiting makes the bingeing more likely to happen. The stress relief following bingeing and purging provides a sense of a reward that makes it an effective short-term reaction to interpersonal conflicts and difficult emotions. In that way both restrictive eating, breaking dietary rules and interpersonal problems may trigger binges.

Many people associate eating difficulties with being underweight. Before we mention starvation symptoms, we would like to highlight that most people with eating difficulties are a normal weight. However, when an individual is underweight, starvation symptoms evolve and enforce the rigidity and compulsiveness of the eating difficulty. The symptoms resulting from starvation become a major driving force for the eating difficulty. This is why it is impossible for an individual to get well from an eating difficulty without re-establishing their personally healthy weight.

Learning point 2

- Did you know that common starvation symptoms involves a reduction of cognitive flexibility, and includes experiencing intruding thoughts about food and eating, having a need for routines, social withdrawal, low mood and slow gastric emptying that promotes the sensation of fullness?

All the maintaining cognitive, physiological, emotional and behavioural changes discussed take place within a life (in a family, a relationship, a work, or school context) that also influence the individual. Some individuals with eating difficulties, for instance, react to stress or difficult situations by restricting eating or exercising excessively. CBT treatment of eating difficulties aims at weakening and breaking this maintaining circle and developing healthy strategies to deal with life-stress.

Ambivalence: making the decision to break the circle

Even though it is possible to recover from an eating difficulty through treatment (Linardon *et al*, 2017), the decision to start treatment or saying goodbye to the eating difficulty often takes time. Drop-out from treatment and several attempts to get well are rather the rule than the exception (Fassino *et al*, 2009; Gregertsen *et al*, 2019). Ambivalence is also present during treatment. Why is it so hard to make this choice to break the circle, act on it and endure the battle? And how does a CBT model address this ambivalence?

The mode of CBT stresses the agency and responsibility of the individual. Before starting treatment, an active choice has to be made and obstacles for treatment cleared away. This could involve e.g. ensuring that the individual is able to attend sessions, or moving away from an invalidating environment. For individuals with binge eating disorder, it would include coming to terms with the necessity to give up weight reduction until the eating difficulty is stabilized.

Furthermore, it is highlighted that no one, other than the client, should decide whether to start CBT treatment or not. On the other hand, the therapist stresses that ambivalence is expected to be a part of the process throughout treatment. Completing all treatment sessions is highlighted from the beginning as being crucial for there to be a successful outcome.

When starting to explore pros and cons of choosing treatment, the therapist starts with examining the patient's reasons for maintaining their eating difficulty. It is important to acknowledge and validate the protective, regulating function the eating difficulty may have provided before exploring the reasons for leaving it behind.

- Think about a time in your life when you needed to make a decision about changing behaviors or perceptions about something. Make a list of what helped you decide (i.e. past history, thoughts about the future, values, negative consequences, support from others).
- What characterised the people you experienced as supportive in this process?

Letting go of the eating difficulty, challenging the rules and gaining weight (when underweight) is scary and anxiety provoking, and might make the person feel very vulnerable and lonely. Preparing for these feelings by talking about them in advance and discussing how the therapist could be of support is helpful. Establishing a safe alliance with the therapist is crucial. Before starting treatment, it is important to ensure that patients are medically safe. Furthermore, a broader assessment of mental health through clinical interview is necessary in order to tailor treatment and address barriers for CBT.

Treatment: breaking the circle

As we have discussed, an eating problem develops into a self-maintaining system, that is, a vicious circle. CBT-Enhanced (CBT-E) is one of the most widely used versions of CBT treatments for eating difficulties (Fairburn, 2008). In the following we will describe CBT-E tools that are designed to help break this circle.

In order to help clients to step back from their eating problem, observe and understand it, we jointly create a personalized formulation. A formulation is a hand-drawn visual representation of the processes that are maintaining the client's eating problem (see Figure 31.1 for an example). The process of creating this formulation together with the client serves many functions. First of all, it gives the client the opportunity to realise how toxic and self-sustaining the eating problem is. Secondly, the realization is made that the eating difficulty is not part of their personality, but quite similar to the eating problems of others. This may offer a possibility to start distancing from the problem. Furthermore, the personalized formulation guides treatment and serves as a map for intervention.

The first behavioural strategy in CBT-E is to start real-time self-monitoring. The clients are asked to record everything they eat or drink and whatever else is going on at that specific time, each day between sessions. The purpose of the self-monitoring is two-fold. First of all, it reveals the exact nature of the eating problem. Secondly, it helps the client to change behaviours that prior to this point have seemed automatic and out of control. Through real time self-monitoring, the client will be able to observe behaviours from the outside.

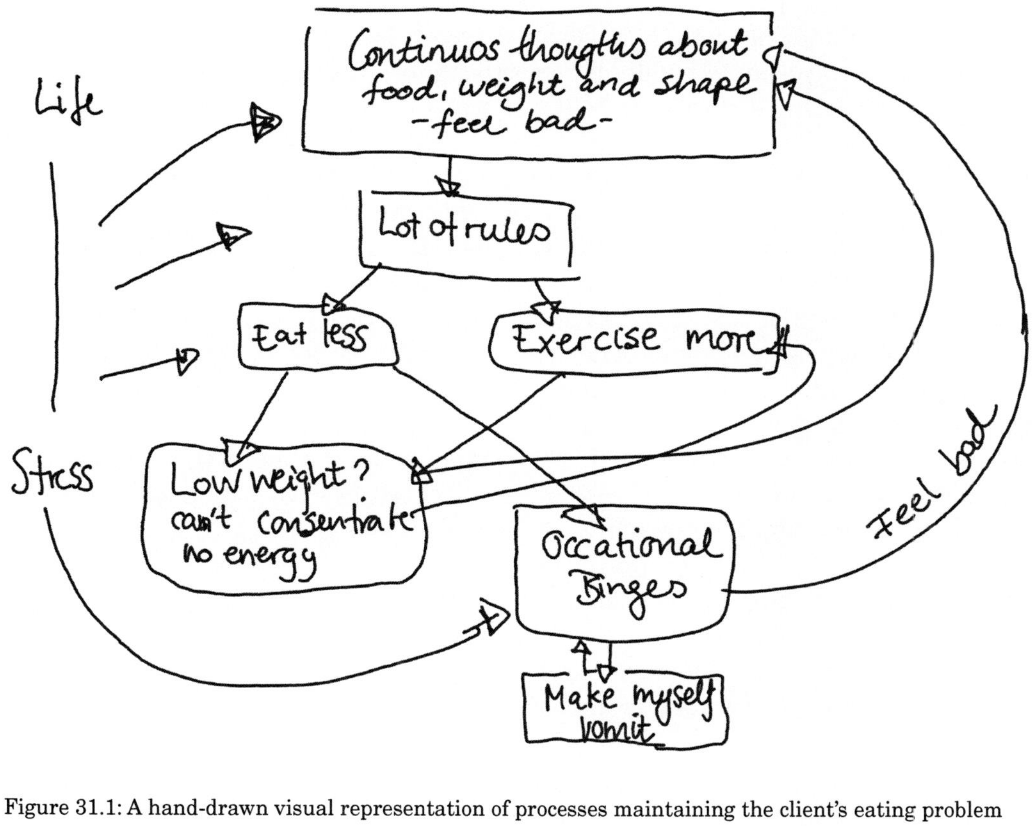

Figure 31.1: A hand-drawn visual representation of processes maintaining the client's eating problem

The two next steps in CBT-E are to establish in-session collaborative weighing and a pattern of regular eating. During this first phase of treatment, information about eating difficulties and how it might affect an individual is of the utmost importance. Every client needs research-based knowledge about the eating problem, about weight and weight change, and information concerning how irregular meals affect both body and brain and how this in turn maintains the eating problem.

Learning point 3

- Did you know that weight fluctuates during the day and that a stable weight might fluctuate with +/- 3 kg?
- Knowing this, how often would you consider it necessary to weigh yourself in order to be sure that you have a stable weight?

Clients with eating difficulties often weigh themselves too frequently, or not at all. Collaborative in-session weighing once a week (and no weighing outside the therapy session) is important, since frequent weighing often maintains dieting, and no weighing (avoidance) increases fear of weight gain. Collaborative weighing and the plotting of weight graphs help individuals to have a more realistic interpretation of their weight changes, and provides an objective alternative to the easily triggered feeling of loss of control of weight.

After clients have started self-monitoring, we introduce a pattern of regular eating. This intervention is the basis upon which all other changes in CBT-E are made. The client plans meals following specific criteria. First of all, meals must be planned ahead (often the day before). There should not be more than four hours between meals. It is important to complete all planned meals, and not eat between the planned meals. The type or amount of food is not important at this stage. Note that this intervention addresses one form of dieting (postponing meals). It also displaces binge eating in cases when the binge is a result of postponed meals. Once regular eating is established, planning will also involve eating the amount of food necessary for gaining weight (0.5- 1 kg a week if underweight) or stabilising weight.

Up until this point in treatment, the focus has been on creating an alliance with a therapist, understanding the nature of the eating problem, creating a personalized formulation and starting the process of behavioural change. An eating problem, however, is so much more than an individual's behaviour.

Decomposing the eating disordered self-evaluation

A self-perception mainly based on ability to control weight and shape is at the core of eating difficulties (referred to as overvaluation). In the third stage of CBT-E, this overvaluation is decomposed and addressed. Normally, a client with an eating difficulty will have to challenge strict dieting, concerns about shape, weight and eating, feeling fat and the marginalization of other important areas of life (see Fairburn, 2008).

The client's scheme for self-evaluation is assessed and made explicit in the sessions, and change is initiated through two processes. That is, individuals are encouraged to diminish their focus on weight and shape in self-evaluation, while also magnifying other aspects of their life. Body checking is one of the behaviours that enforces the weight and shape-based self-evaluation. Several techniques are used to reduce body checking. Examples include removing mirrors, or using bracelets that make a sound when you move the hands to check the collar bone or to reduce the use of triggering social media sites. Furthermore, behavioural activation is sought through planning more activities and engage in a social life that is experienced as rewarding and in accordance with personal values.

Learning point 4

Think about how scrutinising the body parts that you are most dissatisfied with ten times a day would influence your mood or self-evaluation?

When working with dietary restraint, it is important to keep reminding the client, using their personalized formulation, that dietary restraint is a problem, not a solution. Through regular eating of appropriate amounts of food, delayed eating and restriction are already addressed. Clients will further learn to challenge their avoidance of certain types of food and unhelpful dietary rules through systematic behavioural exposure.

'Feeling fat' is a common phenomenon both in people with anorexia nervosa, people who diet and non-dieters (Cooper *et al*, 2007). Thus, this somatic sensation is not exclusively an eating difficulty phenomenon. However, people with eating problems tend to equate this sensation of 'feeling fat' as 'being fat', independent of the individual's weight and shape. In CBT-E, feeling fat is considered a result of mislabelling certain physical or emotional states. This misinterpretation seems linked to the overvaluation of shape and weight in people with eating difficulties. Feeling fat increases concerns about shape and weight, which in turn prompts dieting. In order to observe this phenomenon from a distance, clients are encouraged to use the self-monitoring sheet to identify the triggers of (intense) feelings of fatness and how the sensation fluctuates. The goal is to help the client to ask: "What else am I feeling right now?" whenever they feel fat, and further to use problem solving to cope with the triggering events or feelings. A similar approach is used to identify and address emotional and interpersonal triggers of binge eating.

Towards the end of treatment, the emphasis shifts to the future. There is a focus on dealing with setbacks and maintaining the changes that have been obtained.

Conclusion

Treatment guidelines for eating difficulties recommend CBT as first-line treatment for adults (NICE, 2017), as this is the treatment with biggest documentation of helping adults with eating difficulties. CBT focuses primarily on the processes maintaining the eating difficulty. Different cognitive and behavioural techniques are used to build healthy eating patterns, weight, self-evaluations and emotion regulation strategies. It is important to note that CBT demands hard work and dedication from the client, as well as from the therapist. Therefore, obstacles to treatment, such as severe depression, substance abuse, or major life crises might need to be addressed before starting CBT treatment.

References

Cooper MJ, Deepak K, Grocutt E & Bailey E (2007) The experience of 'feeling fat' in women with anorexia nervosa, dieting and non-dieting women: an exploratory study. *The European Eating Disorder Reviews* **15** (5) 366-72.

Fairburn CG (2008) *Cognitive Behavior Therapy and Eating Disorders*. New York: The Guilford Press.

Fairburn CG, Cooper Z & Shafran R (2003) Cognitive behaviour therapy for eating disorders: a "transdiagnostic" theory and treatment. *Behaviour Research and Therapy* **41** (5) 509-528.

Fassino S, Pierò A, Tomba E & Abbate-Daga G (2009) Factors associated with dropout from treatment for eating disorders: a comprehensive literature review. *BMC Psychiatry* **9** (67). Available at: https://bmcpsychiatry.biomedcentral.com/articles/10.1186/1471-244X-9-67 (accessed August 2021).

Gregertsen EC, Mandy W, Kanakam N, Armstrong S & Serpell L (2019) Pre-treatment patient characteristics as predictors of drop-out and treatment outcome in individual and family therapy for adolescents and adults with anorexia nervosa: A systematic review and meta-analysis. *Psychiatry Research* **271** 484-501.

Linardon J, Wade TD, de la Piedad Garcia X & Brennan L (2017) The efficacy of cognitive-behavioral therapy for eating disorders: A systematic review and meta-analysis. *Journal of Consulting and Clinical Psychology* **85** (11), 1080–1094.

Lock J & Le Grange D (2013) Treatment Manual for Anorexia Nervosa: A family-based approach. New York: Guilford Press.

NICE (2017) *Eating disorders: recognition and treatment [NG69]* [online]. Available at: www.nice.org.uk/guidance/ng69 (accessed August 2021).

Waller G, Corder H, Corstorphine E, Hinrichsen H, Lawson R & Mountford V (2007) *Cognitive-Behavioral Therapy for Eating Disorders: A comprehensive treatment guide*. Cambridge, UK: Cambridge University Press.

32. Mentalization-based treatments for eating difficulties: A new treatment model for severe eating disorders

By Finn Skårderud & Bente Sommerfeldt

Summary

The aim of this chapter is to forward the understanding of how mentalization-based treatments (MBT), which originate from treatments for 'borderline personality disorder', are tailored and expanded to support those with eating difficulties. MBT-ED has been developed as a structured treatment model for severe diagnosed eating disorders. The traditional MBT model is always a combination treatment, i.e. a combination of psychoeducation, individual therapy and group therapy (Bateman & Fonagy, 2016). For children and adolescents, this may also be in conjunction with family therapy. This chapter presents the theoretical background, clinical stances and interventions, and therapeutic structures for 'mentalization-based treatment for eating disorders' – MBT-ED. The chapter also presents some practical recommendations and guidelines in work with severe and enduring eating difficulties.

We will describe 'mentalizing' as a concept, and our understanding of the nature of severe eating difficulties. We hope to enrich the understanding of eating difficulties by presenting an updated theoretical perspective. Within this framework, there is solid evidence to describe eating difficulties as *severe forms of impaired mentalizing*. To make therapy indeed therapeutic, we are convinced that an understanding of underlying psychological processes will inform treatment innovation, which in turn can be the subject of empirical investigation. MBT-ED is based on severe and enduring cases, and many of our patients will have been in other treatments without the wanted and necessary benefits.

MBT-ED as a clinical and therapeutic model is developed by the authors in collaboration with the British psychiatrist Paul Robinson. The theories behind it, implementation of treatment, therapeutic stances and practical guidelines are extensively developed in the manual *Hunger: Mentalization-based Treatments for Eating Disorders* (Robinson *et al*, 2019), and for further understanding we refer to this book.

Why MBT-ED?

A therapeutic treatment of eating difficulties will be effective to the extent that it is able to enhance the patient's psychological, physiological and social capacities without generating too many iatrogenic effects, i.e. negative effects of treatment. Work still needs to be done to move beyond the efficacy of today's evidence-based therapeutic models for eating difficulties, which requires an openness to innovation. Severe eating difficulties may last for decades, cause patients to retreat from normal social and family activity, destroy and break up families, and lead to severe physical harm and death, with anorexia nervosa being the psychiatric disorder with the highest mortality. Hence, the clinical challenges are obvious, and are as much to do with therapists and treatment systems as they are the significant difficulties someone with an eating difficulty might experience.

Establishing good working alliances is a major requirement for any treatment to be effective. Many people experiencing eating difficulties do not seek treatment themselves, may struggle with motivation to change, and research data demonstrates a high number drop out of therapy (Campbell, 2009). Mentalization-based treatments (MBT) have a specific focus on establishing healthy working alliances and preventing dropout.

Paradigms for treatments can vary widely. For example, a *medical model of psychotherapy* may involve the patient, based on assessment and diagnosis, being served a 'dose' of sessions with specific techniques and interventions, as though being prescribed a drug. Public services often work within such an ideological and administrative framework. MBT is not independent from such a model, but proper mentalization-based therapy is, as stated, far more based in *the relational model of psychotherapy*. A relational model of psychotherapy is a more person-centred than a disorder-centred approach.

This is highly relevant for eating difficulties, since establishing sound working alliances is often a problem. In MBT there is explicit focus on the quality of the clinical encounter. People with severe eating difficulties can often be perceived as 'hard to reach' in various clinical settings, and hence, an ethos in the mentalizing tradition is *how to reach those who are hard to reach*. As such, relational competences are important qualifications for the therapist (Robinson *et al*, 2019; Bateman & Fonagy, 2016).

Learning point 1

Before you continue reading, think about some of your own experiences, be that of living with or supporting someone with an eating difficulty, or working professionally with people experiencing long-term, significant eating difficulties.

- What kind of challenges and obstacles have you experienced?
- What has been the focus of any treatment?
- If you are a professional involved in treatment of eating difficulties, what is your focus? What do you value in treatment?
- What are your treatment goals? What do you value and prioritise as an outcome of treatment?

What is mentalizing?

Mentalizing can be described as a form of emotional knowing. All of our processes of perception are suffused with emotions. As we grow and mature, our experiences of brain and body (or brain within body) produce our *mind*. A central part of this is our interactions with others, which are essential to mental growth. Our physical encounters and relational experiences develop into internal representations, creating a world of assumptions, and as such, the *physical becomes mental*.

This understanding unlocks the unique possibility to use our minds to reflect upon our own minds, and others' minds. Instead of acting on strong emotions and impulses, we may use our minds for reflection and, hopefully, the establishment of realistic, healthy and friendly ways of behaving (Allen & Fonagy, 2006).

Mentalizing is the normal ability to ascribe intentions and meaning to human behaviour – to understand 'unwritten rules'. It involves both self-reflective and interpersonal components which provide the individual with a well-developed capacity to distinguish inner from outer reality, physical experience from mind, and intrapersonal mental and emotional processes from interpersonal communications. Mentalizing can be described as being able to see oneself from the outside, and other people from the inside. It is a major social competence, central to human communication and relationships.

It is of great clinical relevance that mentalizing fosters *emotional regulation*. But mentalizing is also important for *identity*, for knowing oneself, and experiencing *sense of agency*. Mentalizing is also important for real *intersubjectivity* and healthy relationships with others. Impaired mentalizing often leads to loneliness, or may cause social confusion and misunderstandings from acting on false assumptions. Being or feeling misunderstood is also highly aversive, and may generate powerful emotions that result in coercion, withdrawal, hostility, over-protectiveness or rejection. To mentalize means to be able to understand one's misunderstandings.

The relevance of mentalizing in eating difficulties

Mentalizing represents a new paradigm by integrating knowledge from different realms – including evolutionary theory, developmental psychology, attachment theory, theory of mind and neurosciences. Mentalizing is a model to understand human behaviour in general and psychopathology in particular, and it is used to inform the application of psychotherapy.

A person with an eating difficulty with impaired mentalizing will often experience a vicious circle in which impaired mentalizing creates misunderstandings and ruptures in relationships, and an already-insecure world becomes even more insecure. Such stress, fear and emotional arousal can further impair the mentalizing capacity. This can result in someone with an eating difficulty being perceived as an island of control and predictability (Skårderud & Fonagy, 2012). Hence, *eating difficulties are as much social and emotional difficulties as they are about eating* (Robinson *et al*, 2019).

Mentalization is operationalized for research as a *reflective function* (RF). In a study from the Cassel Hospital in the UK, 82 patients with diagnosed eating disorders scored lowest on reflective function along with patients diagnosed with 'borderline personality disorder'. Persons with anorexia nervosa scored lower than persons with bulimia nervosa and borderline personality disorder (Fonagy *et al*, 1996). The RF-scale is also used in a study (Rothschild-Yakar *et al*, 2010), showing that low mentalization is a risk factor for eating difficulties, with high mentalization being a protective factor.

Clinical examples

Diagnostic manuals characterize the set of symptoms experienced by those with eating difficulties into distinct disorders. These presentations are central in the clinical phenomenology of these disorders. We also focus on symptoms as manifestations of underlying psychopathology. In the language of mentalizing, eating difficulties are understood as manifestations of underlying deficits in self- and emotional regulation. The psychiatrist and psychoanalyst Hilde Bruch described the person with eating difficulties as suffering from *interoceptive confusion*, with perceptual and conceptual disturbances in the sense of *not knowing oneself*, both in matters of identity and also sensorimotor experiences of one's own body (Bruch, 1962; Skårderud, 2013).

There are numerous forms of impaired mentalizing. One of the most prominent forms in eating difficulties is how bodily traits can often be a focus for attention and preoccupation. When psychic reality is poorly integrated, the body may take on an excessively central role for maintaining a sense of self, *literally being a body of evidence* (Skårderud & Fonagy, 2012). Body serves as mind. We call this *concretism*, and the *concretistic* symptoms essentially serve the function of maintaining the cohesion and stability of a tenuous sense of self.

Let us link the conceptual model of mentalizing to the clinical phenomenology of eating difficulties with some examples.

Case study 1: When the solution becomes the problem

Eating difficulties represent a special case in the realm of mental health problems, in the sense that many actively use body modification to improve their sense of self. The individuals want to change themselves, in self-esteem and social acceptance, and such changes are sought to be fulfilled physically. *The individual's experience may be that the mind can be controlled by making the body work.*

> *Elsa was very unhappy and felt that she didn't fit in anywhere. She started to focus on her eating and exercise, and felt more mastery and self-control. She got more attention from friends and family. It worked for a while. After some months with restrictive eating and frequent workouts, she experienced a loss of control over thoughts and emotions related to food and body. It turned into a kind of obsession. This made her days more challenging, having problems with concentrating on school, and not at least being together with friends.*

Case study 2: Concretism and its contagions

Corporeality in eating difficulties may mean experiencing one's body as *too real* and *too unreal*. At the same time there may be an unduly negative focus on exterior, combined with incapacity to distance oneself from this dissatisfaction. The body is experienced more via weighing scales, in the mirror, measuring circumferences of limbs, and via fantasies about being looked at by others, than by *feeling* one's own *lived body* (Merleau-Ponty, 1962).

This is also important for treatment, because we as clinicians can also have a tendency to overemphasize weight, numbers and physical traits. Hannah illustrates this. Hannah has a severe eating difficulty with low weight over a long time. Because of no progression in weight gain, there has been an agreement between the team and Hannah that a three-week stay in an inpatient unit could be useful. In a therapeutic session she is frustrated and tells her therapist:

> *I am nothing but a number. I am the diagnosis. They don't ask me how I am anymore, they are just telling me numbers, weight and what I need to eat.*

Case study 3: Outer-directedness

Where self-regulation is difficult, someone may turn to others for response and confirmation of their self-esteem and wellbeing. This can be described as being *outer-directed*, where inner life is to a great extent an external affair. But an increased awareness of others as potential validators or invalidators of the self should not be confused with mentalizing capacities to understand others' minds; rather the opposite. Bodily preoccupation will often impede appreciation of others' bodies, which can impair social communication. This process is described by Frank:

> *I completely lost sight of the world. The self-centredness of it was remarkable. I did not care. Today I feel ashamed about it. I also felt shame at that time, but was thrown back on my own embodied preoccupations. I was preoccupied with my own body and trying to control it. So rather than thinking of others I thought about whether my stomach was flat or not.*

Another person, Lisa, described how she had challenged therapists and clinicians by questioning and checking again and again. Inner distrust may also be expressed as distrust towards other people, including healthcare professionals and carers, and fear of not being in psychological control can lead to controlling behaviour towards others.

> *If I am going to eat this, you need to eat the same.*

Learning point 2

Good mentalizing is expressed by a flexible mind, playfulness, and the capacity to see different perspectives and change perspective.

Think of your own personal or professional experiences in relation to eating difficulties.

- Do you recognise how the symptoms, mental functioning and behaviour related to eating difficulties can be understood and described as impaired mentalizing?
- Are there some parts you relate to, or reject, more than others?

Mentalization-based therapies for eating difficulties

Most forms of psychotherapy foster mentalizing, as long as it is not strict behaviourism, but mentalization-based therapy is the *systematic focus on the enhancement of these competences*. In MBT there is an explicit model of humans as relational beings. The mentalizing approach has roots in psychodynamic psychotherapy and more specifically a relational or intersubjective tradition developed in the second half of last century (Bateman & Fonagy, 2016). In practical terms, this implies a belief that mentalizing, symptom reduction and clinical improvement is best forwarded through therapeutic relationships over time (Allen & Fonagy, 2006; Robinson *et al*, 2019). There is specific emphasis on the therapeutic encounter itself – that the cooperation works, and that meetings are experienced as safe enough settings in which beliefs about oneself, others and behaviour can be challenged. Again, mentalization-based therapy has a *systematic and explicit focus on how to work with the therapeutic relationship.*

Psychotherapy provides an excellent opportunity to experience and learn from 'failures' in mentalizing, and examples of such can be worked with in therapeutic encounters. We advocate a mentalization-based approach for severe eating difficulties because it is structured, manualised and based in a comprehensive theoretical model. Mentalizing as an intellectual framework can be helpful in organising the confusing and challenging phenomenology presented by experiences of eating difficulties, which can also help carers and professionals to comprehend difficult situations (Robinson *et al*, 2019).

Structure of treatment

In the case of severe eating difficulties, mentalization-based treatment is to be considered a long-term treatment. The mentalization-based treatment program is structured as a combination of psychoeducational work in groups, individual therapy, dynamic group therapy, the active use of written case formulations and crisis plans. Treatment is structured with the explicit intention to stimulate mentalizing through a combination of treatment formats. There is also a focus on strengthening therapeutic alliances and preventing dropout.

MBT-ED is a double-minded therapy, with focus both on minds and on symptom reduction (Robinson *et al*, 2019). Specifically, because of the possible severe somatic consequences of eating difficulties, there is a need to also have a specific focus on symptom reduction. The MBT-ED therapist also will have a weighing scale. We have been met with strange beliefs from therapists, that we in psychotherapy should not be working with the normalization of eating, weight and exercising when working with people with eating difficulties. We believe that we should. The explicit ambition of MBT-ED is the double focus: to be able to work constructively with symptoms, while at the same time fostering curiosity about the meeting of minds. People experiencing eating difficulties are often stuck in their view of psychological and corporeal reality, and through a curious therapeutic activity, one aims to enrich reflective functioning. Paraphrasing Donald Winnicott (1971), we provide a structure to play with embodied realities.

Therapists' minds

The model of mentalizing is not only about the person *in therapy*, but also about *us as therapists*. In the contexts of great therapeutic challenges, the therapists' reflective function may collapse. Well-known examples from everyday clinical work are how, for example, fear, frustration or anger among therapists can create a tunnel vision with a one-sided focus on somatic and bodily traits such as weight and blood tests. In this way, severe eating difficulties can be seen as 'contagious', with both patients and clinicians overemphasising bodily traits, and focusing less on what is going on in the mind. Or the opposite: clinicians might ignore somatic traits and threats, and instead have a one-sided focus on inner life and relationships. There is a practical but also an ethical aspect to all of this – too often people experience getting worse through treatment.

In MBT we focus not only on characteristics of 'patients' and 'disorders', but also on our own emotional reactions as therapists. Emotions are contagious, and so are mentalizing capacities and impaired mentalizing. Few symptoms create stronger reactions in therapists than those that often present with eating difficulties – particularly anorexia nervosa – and few conditions require more forbearance and self-questioning. Trying to support people with severe eating difficulties can compromise the therapist's reflective mode and mentalizing, with the risk of enactments and over-reactions due to intense emotional reactions. A lack of understanding can lead to a lack of commitment and patience, or worse, to aggression and rejection. Eating difficulties are challenging for mental health practitioners in both clinical and intellectual terms.

Learning point 3

Think of different feelings you may have had when working with or meeting people experiencing eating difficulties, either as a carer, professional or individual.

- Can these feelings tell you anything about your own mind?
- How might this awareness help you in supporting someone with eating difficulties?

Practical MBT-ED guidelines

Here we present what we see as useful competencies required of MBT-therapists.

Competency areas for an MBT-therapist
(Bateman & Fonagy, 2016)
1. The not-knowing, genuine and inquisitive therapist stance.
2. Support and empathy.
3. Clarification.
4. Exploration.
5. Challenge.
6. Affect focus.
7. Focus on relationships, not at least the patient-therapist relationship.

We propose the additional treatment competencies for an MBT-ED therapist (Robinson *et al*, 2019)

The dual track
An ability to simultaneously promote mentalizing in the dialogue and systematically work to reduce symptoms.

Minding the therapist's mind
An ability to maintain one's own mentalizing in the midst of the specific challenges these patients may present.

Nutrition and somatic health
Substantial knowledge about nutrition and the somatic manifestations of eating difficulties, including the psychology and physiology of hunger and malnutrition, and of chaotic eating.

The concretised mind
An ability to assess and share with the patient the specific impairments of mentalizing in eating difficulties, such as substantial bodily concretisation of emotions and relationships.

Minding the body
An ability to stimulate the patient to be more aware of their bodily feelings and sensorimotor experiences.

Minding the symptoms: pros and cons of eating difficulties
An ability to help the patient develop curiosity about the many functions that their behaviours and symptoms may have, both positive and negative, e.g. eating behaviours as self-regulation.

Ambivalence
An ability to understand and deal with the ambivalence about change and recovery often presented by these patients.

Negotiate non-negotiables
An ability to negotiate non-negotiables in a mentalizing dialogue. For example, in anorexia nervosa this means negotiating around sufficient nutrition and weight gain, or having regular blood tests in patients who purge.

Meeting alexithymia
An ability to regulate one's own activity when dealing with alexithymic traits. For example, assisting the patient to develop a language for his or her own experiences, but not being 'too helpful' by labelling experiences for the patient.

Covert feelings
An ability to recognise and deal with pseudo-cooperation, pseudo-compliance and pseudo-mentalizing.

The silent patient
An ability to stimulate mentalizing with 'the silent patient'.

Learning point 4

Among the competencies listed above, reflect a little more on the idea of 'ambivalence'.

- Do you recognise ambivalence in your experience of eating difficulties, or supporting others?
- Do you understand this ambivalence? What function might it serve? What is it about? Where might any uncertainty come from?
- How might appreciating and exploring ambivalence help you to better support someone experiencing eating difficulties, be that yourself or someone you care for?

Conclusion

Eating difficulties come in different forms for different people – from restrictive eating to bingeing and purging, to name just a few. They are also experienced in highly varying degrees of severity, with some being enduring and highly serious. The risk to life – with anorexia nervosa having the highest mortality of all psychiatric conditions – cannot be understated. Hopes, futures and families are ruined for too many people. Hence, there is always a need for innovation, both in the ways in which we understand eating difficulties and also the ways in which we respond to them across healthcare and statutory services.

If we are honest, existing therapeutic models are not efficient enough in helping a range of people experiencing a range of different psychological problems. Mentalizing, however, is an updated theoretical model that aims describe and understand mental life, offering new insights for many different experiences and diagnoses. In this chapter, we have applied models of mentalizing to clinical cases of eating difficulties, trying to demonstrate clinical encounters that use mentalization-focused approaches to increase mentalizing and thereby reduce eating difficulties.

Impaired mentalizing, could be described as 'contagious' – in the sense that the mentalizing capacities of carers and therapists may be challenged in the course of their work. Hence, it is important to identify the presence of concretism, impaired emotional regulation and black-and-white thinking in encounters with people experiencing severe eating difficulties, and seek always to retain a central understanding that good mentalizing requires flexibility of minds and flexibility between minds.

References

Allen JG & Fonagy P (2006) *Handbook of Mentalization-Based Treatment*. Chichester, W Sussex: John Wiley.

Bateman A & Fonagy P (2016) *Mentalization Based Treatment for Personality Disorders: A Practical Guide*. Oxford: Oxford University Press.

Bruch H (1962). Perceptual and conceptual disturbances in anorexia nervosa. *Psychosom Med* **24** 187-194.

Campbell M (2009) Drop-out from treatment for the eating disorders: A problem for clinicians and researchers. *Eur Eat Disord Rev* **17** 239.

Fonagy P, Leigh T, Steele M, Steele H, Kennedy R, Mattoon G, Target M & Gerber A (1996) 64 22-31. The relation of attachment status, psychiatric classification and response to psychotherapy. *J Consult Clin Psychol*, 64, 22-31.

Merleau-Ponty M (1962) *The Phenomenology of Perception*. London: Routledge and Kegan Paul.

Robinson P, Skårderud F & Sommerfeldt B (2019) *Hunger. Mentalization-based treatments of eating disorders*. London: Springer.

Rothschild-Yakar L, Levy-Shiff R, Fridman-Balaban R, Gur E & Stein D (2010) Mentalization and relationships with parents as predictors of eating disordered behavior. *J Nerv Ment Dis* **198** (7) 501-507.

Skårderud F (2013) Hilde Bruch (1904–1984) – the constructive use of ignorance. *Adv Eat Disord* **1** (2) 174-181.

Skårderud F & Fonagy P (2012) Eating disorders. In: A Bateman & P Fonagy (Eds.), *Handbook of Mentalizing in Mental Health Practice*. Washington DC: American Psychiatric Publishers.

Winnicott DW (1971) Playing and Reality. London: Tavistock.

33. The role of exercise in recovery from eating difficulties

By Brian Cook

Summary

The role of exercise in recovery from eating difficulties is not clearly defined, with competing views about its importance and safety existing among clinicians working in this area. Recent research and clinical work have discerned important nuances that can indicate if or when individuals may safely include exercise in recovery. This chapter will provide a brief review of the current state of understanding of how exercise may be a beneficial aspect of recovery from a range of eating difficulties.

The primary focus of this chapter is on understanding the functional relationship of exercise in recovery. Specific content includes an overview of factors that can help identify readiness to exercise during recovery, specific motivations to exercise among those experiencing eating difficulties, and information on how to successfully maintain a safe exercise routine during recovery. Several activities and practical examples are included throughout to help illustrate specific functions of exercise during recovery.

Background

Experiences of eating difficulties and recovery can often involve complex relationships with movement and exercise. Many people find exercise a fulfilling part of their journey that helps create and nurture social connections, respects the physical self, and calms the mind. Others find that they must avoid exercise altogether, as it can bring up many unpleasant emotions and sensations that lead to relapse. These extremes describe two ends of a continuum of the relationship that one may have with exercise. Neither end can be, nor should be, the sole focus when approaching exercise. Rather, everyone's journey during recovery is unique. Deciding if, when, or how exercise will be a part of recovery is a deeply personal decision. Not everyone experiencing eating difficulties can or should exercise, especially during the initial phases of recovery (Cook *et al*, 2016). This chapter will briefly review some of the key aspects of what to consider when determining how exercise may fit into recovery.

Research, clinical work, and personal stories from individuals with eating difficulties overwhelmingly shows there is no 'one-size-fits-all' exercise routine in recovery. A rapidly growing body of research and clinical evidence has shown that identifying the functional relationship between exercise and eating difficulties is key to reaping the benefits of exercise while avoiding the potential for harm (Cook *et al*, 2016; Dobinson *et al*, 2019; Hay *et al*, 2018; Mathisen *et al*, 2020). The main challenge around exercise during recovery is developing a mindful approach that honestly respects the body and recognizes the underlying motivations for exercise.

Learning point 1

Considering the psychological factors underlying the function of exercise for any individual experiencing eating difficulties (such as their beliefs and motivations) can help assess if exercise can be a part of their recovery (Cook *et al*, 2011; Lipsey *et al*, 2006). When considering someone you may be supporting, or your own experiences in relation to exercise, you might like to think about the following questions:

- What might be the function of exercise for you or the person you are supporting?
- What are the motivations, what purpose does exercise serve?
- Are there any clear benefits or drawbacks in this relationship with exercise?
- Are there any elements of these exercise behaviours that help maintain difficulties with eating?

Readiness for exercise in recovery

There are many things to consider when deciding whether exercise can be included in recovery. Here are a few factors to keep in mind.

Accepting that exercise is not mandatory

Exercise during recovery from eating difficulties is a process. Building intuition around when to, and when not to, exercise can be an important step in this process. Exercise during recovery requires full awareness, mindfulness, and an honest appreciation of the mind-body connection. It's essential to listen to the body in order to recognize the need for rest and properly fuel and hydrate. Being flexible enough to skip an exercise session, take consecutive days off or exercise with less intensity or for a shorter duration can be challenging. Having good social support that understands that the relationship with exercise can be very different for those experiencing eating difficulties is important too.

Remember, there will be times when exercise is desired, but the body might not be feeling up to it. A key to distinguishing when exercise is possible is to listen to bodily signals like being tired, sore, or feeling the effects of stress. The mind may say exercise can help, but often these sensations are ways that the body indicates a need for rest.

Challenging beliefs about exercise and expected outcomes

Eating difficulties can sometimes change beliefs about the function of exercise (Lipsey *et al*, 2006). To exercise during recovery, it can help to understand what the function of exercise is at the current moment. Are exercise beliefs and expectations rational? Where did they come from? Remember that exercise is not the cure-all that many people believe it is. This can be especially challenging given the barrage of 'fitspiration' on social media and misleading marketing from the fitness industry. Exercise beliefs can lead to a perception that exercise-related outcomes are a carrot dangling just out of reach. In fact, these outcomes, while highly desirable, are often unattainable.

Recognising progress

Recovery from eating difficulties can often involve a lot of hard work, honest reflection, and struggle through adversity. Skills and strategies developed along this journey can also be used to stay on track during recovery. A great way to build upon previous successes is to gradually progress with an exercise routine (Cook *et al*, 2016). Going slow allows time to process emotions, connect with the body, and reflect on how to keep exercise as a safe part of recovery. The saying 'sometimes less is more' definitely fits here!

Finding alternatives

Many people exercise to 'clear their head' or deal with a bad day. Remember that exercise is not the only way to cope with negative emotions, bad days, or stress in general. Think of different enjoyable activities that can help boost mood which could be used instead of fulfilling the desire to exercise. For example, meditation, writing in a journal, or playing with a pet are examples of alternatives people may find useful. It may help to fill in the blank of this sentence (Johnson & Cook, 2013): 'Instead of exercise, I will ______________.' For instance, 'Instead of doing a high intensity workout after a stressful day, I will call my best friends so we can meet up.'

Finding functional motives of exercise

Exercise alongside eating difficulties has been linked to several detrimental outcomes, such as increased depression and anxiety, earlier onset of symptoms, poorer treatment response, and higher risk of relapse (Cook *et al*, 2014). These association suggest that exercise should be avoided during recovery. However, these associations fall short of specifying when or for whom exercise may become problematic during recovery (Meyer *et al*, 2011). Moreover, such associations fail to provide theoretical or empirically testable guidance on how to intervene and change the functional relationship of exercise from problematic to supportive of overall health and sustained recovery.

Fortunately, research and clinical work over the past decade has identified potential targets for interventions that may allow for exercise during recovery to not increase risk for relapse (Cook *et al*, 2011; 2014; 2016; Meyer *et al*, 2011). Specifically, a compulsive drive to exercise can be a predictor of eating difficulties. Compulsions are defined as urges to perform a behaviour in order to relieve negative emotions arising from the perceived negative consequences if the behaviour is not performed (Meyer *et al*, 2011). Thus, the function of compulsive exercise is to reduce negative emotions or prevent troublesome things happening. Identifying when exercise is related to compulsions is important for those experiencing eating difficulties and can help to formulate ways of replacing exercise with other coping skills such as emotion regulation and stress management techniques. This may help limit any harm that may be caused by compulsive exercise in conjunction with eating difficulties.

Learning point 2

Before you continue reading, think about your experiences of when you exercise, or those of someone you might be supporting. Have any of the following motives influenced exercise behaviours?

Exercise to manage negative emotions

Many people struggling with eating difficulties may use exercise to deal with unpleasant feelings like shame, or anxiety or guilt, and may feel disappointed with themselves when missing an exercise session.

- Honestly reflect on whether exercise may be part of avoiding something else that is bothering you.
- Why are you really upset that you missed an exercise session?
- What are some non-exercise activities that may fit more holistically into recovery?
- Try journaling about how your emotions relate to exercise, why you hold exercise in such high regard (if you do), and think of identifying any alternatives to exercise that may help you cope with unpleasant feelings.

Exercise to boost positive emotions

Exercising to boost mood is certainly a benefit! However, this can become problematic when exercise is the primary or only thing that is turned to for mood improvement.

- Can you think of any other activities that you can find joy in?
- Has exercise ever distracted you or taken you away from other opportunities?

Exercise to control weight or shape

Exercising to lose weight can be a part of someone's experience of eating difficulties. Try to identify the source of why you believe you need to control your body weight or shape and why exercise is an option for this.

- Where do your beliefs about weight and shape come from?
- Are there any ways in which your motivation for exercise interferes with recovery?
- If the source of your beliefs is external (e.g., social media, friends), are these sources valid?
- How can exercise be a truly joyful experience, rather than something that is done for weight control? What might that look like for you?

Lack of enjoyment when exercising

Exercising despite not enjoying it can indicate a disconnection between mind and body and could suggest that exercise may be detracting from other areas of life.

- Reflect on whether you are using exercise as a self-punishment.
- How is doing something you don't enjoy related to other areas of who you are?
- What other things can you do, or have you been putting off, instead of exercising?

Exercise rigidity

Following strict patterns or rules about exercise behaviour can lead to problems.

- Are there any ways in which you can be flexible when something conflicts with your exercise schedule?
- Come up with a list of things you could do instead of exercise. Perhaps you could plan to try one new non-exercise activity every week, or something manageable for you?
- Reflect on your experience of trying new things and breaking old patterns.
- Can you be ok with not exercising?

Maintaining recovery

Maintaining an exercise routine during recovery requires self-efficacy and an honest appraisal of why you are exercising and the usefulness of it for you. Self-efficacy may seem like confidence, and in some ways it is. In fact, confidence can help us to be more effective in our choices. Self-efficacy is a deeper understanding of exactly how to do a task and the role it plays for us. This includes recognising barriers, anticipating limitations, and maintaining rational expectations for success. Self-efficacy has been shown to be an important factor in maintaining recovery (Haskins *et al*, 2018; Johnson & Cook, 2013).

Learning point 3

The following activities may help increase self-efficacy and could be useful for someone experiencing eating difficulties to try.

Learning from previous experiences

Think about positive experiences of exercise when they weren't associated with eating difficulties.

- Describe in detail how you exercised, included rest, and listened to your body.
- What can you learn from your previous experiences?
- How are these experiences different from exercising with eating difficulties?

Imagine your future

Close your eyes and picture yourself in the future while thinking about the following questions:

- What does your relationship with exercise look like?
- Describe how you feel using exercise for recovery rather than as part of your experiences of eating difficulties.

Turning to others

It is helpful to have someone that understands the risks and nuances of exercise during recovery (e.g. a therapist, close friend or family member). Who can you turn to for support?

Listen to your body

Our minds have a way of making our body do things that we probably shouldn't.

- How can you improve the way you listen to your body when it is telling you to exercise to manage emotions, despite needing more rest, or when you are running on empty?

Thinking about your emotions

Exercise is often used as an emotional coping mechanism. Ensure exercise is not masking emotions or used as a sole method to feel better.

- Keep a journal of your emotions immediately before, during, and after exercise.
- Describe emotions on rest days, when life gets in the way of exercise routines, or when you are sick or injured and cannot exercise.

Plan for barriers

- Setbacks happen. List coping skills you have or can develop to deal with triggers, negative emotions, and/or when exercise is overtaking your recovery.

Conclusion

Exercise is a dynamic and deeply personal behaviour that can be a helpful part of recovery for many people. However, solely focusing on the behaviour of exercise overlooks key considerations that can differentiate whether exercise can be beneficial in recovery or lead to difficulties during recovery. Current evidence suggests that understanding the function of exercise can help with the recovery process. Honestly examining motives, beliefs and expectations about exercise is necessary to identify the underlying function of exercise. Therefore, determining if, when, and how to exercise requires a mindful approach that respects the body and recognizes often overlooked factors that can help support recovery. Safely maintaining an exercise routine during recovery is possible by learning from previous experiences, keeping supportive relationships with people who understand how exercise can present unique challenges, and recognising how emotions can motivate exercise behaviour.

References

Cook B, Hausenblas H & Freimuth M (2014) Exercise addiction and compulsive exercising: Relationship to eating disorders, substance use disorders and addictions. In T Brewerton & A Dennis Baker (Eds). *Eating Disorders, Addiction and Substance use Disorders: Research, Clinical and treatment Perspectives*. (pp. 127-144). Springer.

Cook B, Wonderlich S, Mitchell J, Thompson R, Sherman R & McCallum K (2016) Exercise in eating disorders treatment: Systematic review and proposal of guidelines. *Medicine & Science in Sport & Exercise* **48** (7) 1408-1414.

Cook B, Hausenblas H, Tuccitto D & Giacobbi P (2011) Eating disorders and exercise: A structural equation modeling analysis of a conceptual model. *European Eating Disorders Review* **19** (3) 216-225.

Dobinson A, Cooper M & Quesnel D (2019) The Safe Exercise at Every Stage (SEES) guideline – A clinical tool for treating and managing dysfunctional exercise in eating disorders. See www.safeexerciseateverystage.com/ (accessed August 2021).

Hasking P, Boyes M & Greves S (2018) Self-efficacy and emotionally dysregulated behaviour: An exploratory test of the role of emotion regulatory and behaviour-specific beliefs. *Psychiatry research* **270** 335–340.

Hay P, Touyz S, Arcelus J, Pike K, Attia E, Crosby RD, Madden S, Wales J, La Puma M, Heriseanu AI, Young S & Meyer C (2018) A randomized controlled trial of the compuLsive Exercise Activity TheraPy (LEAP): A new approach to compulsive exercise in anorexia nervosa. *The International journal of eating disorders* **51** (8) 999–1004.

Johnson S & Cook B (2013) Building Motivation: How Ready Are You? In: C. Nigg (Eds) *ACSM's Behavioral Aspects of Exercise*. (pp. 103-128). Lippincott Williams & Wilkins.

Lipsey Z, Barton S, Hulley A & Hill A (2006) "After a workout …" Beliefs about exercise, eating and appearance in female exercisers with and without eating disorder features. *Psychology of Sport and Exercise* **7** (5) 425-436.

Mathisen TF, Rosenvinge JH, Friborg O, Vrabel K, Bratland-Sanda S, Pettersen G & Sundgot-Borgen J (2020) Is physical exercise and dietary therapy a feasible alternative to cognitive behavior therapy in treatment of eating disorders? A randomized controlled trial of two group therapies. *International Journal of Eating Disorders* **53** (4) 574-585. doi: 10.1002/eat.23228.

Meyer C, Taranis L, Goodwin H & Haycraft E (2011) Compulsive Exercise and Eating Disorders. *European Eating Disorders Review* **19** 174–189.

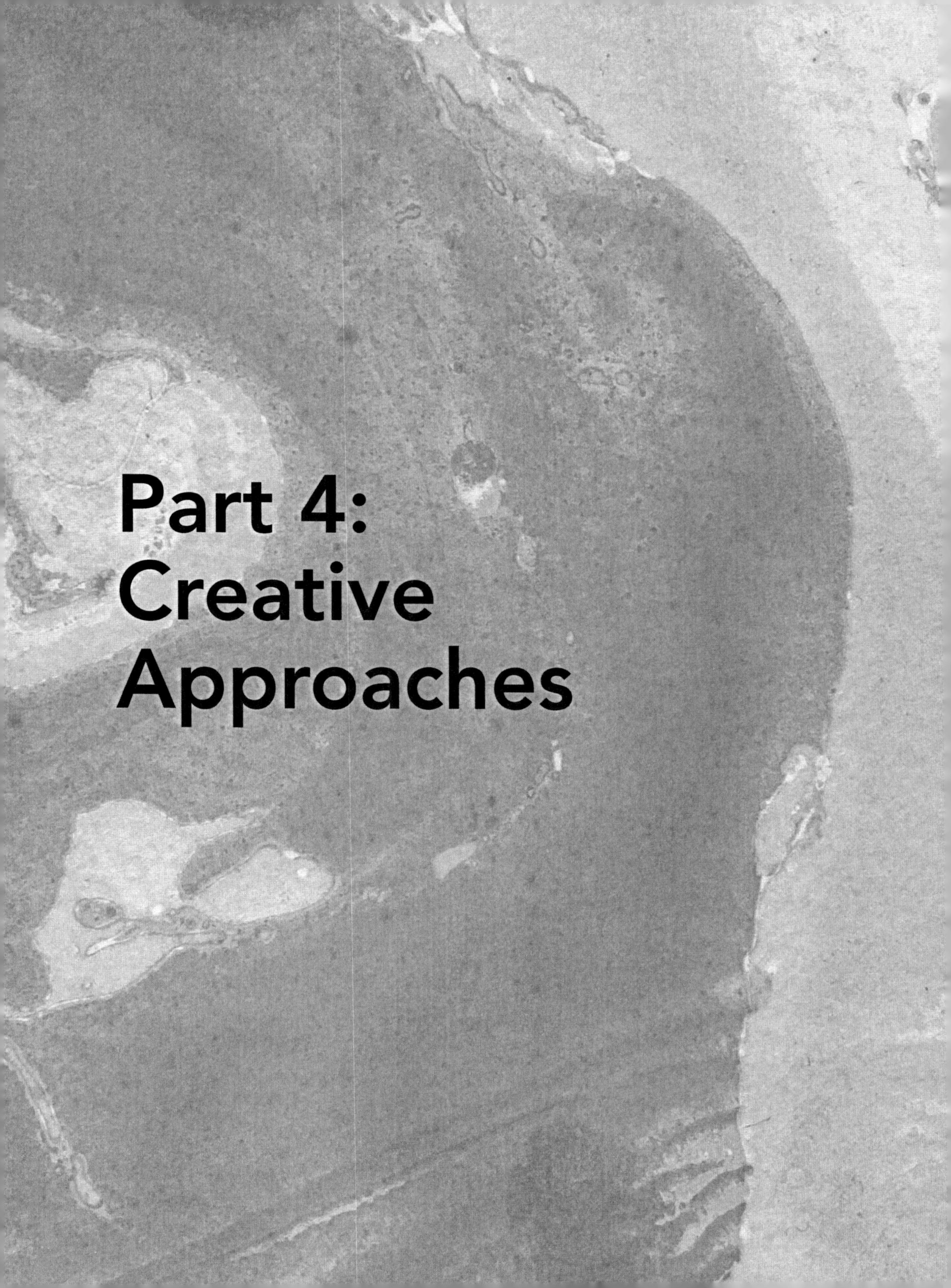

Part 4: Creative Approaches

34. An embodied approach in the prevention and treatment of eating difficulties

By Estey EEE, Pollack SR & Cook-Cottone CP

Summary

Recently, eating difficulty (ED) researchers have been examining protective mechanisms that promote 'positive embodiment' – the experience of inhabiting and befriending one's body with nonjudgmental acceptance and appreciation for its function, rather than appearance. One of these mechanisms is mindful self-care (MSC), a set of formal and informal practices that exemplify caring for the body with awareness, loving kindness, and compassion. The six domains of MSC outlined in this chapter address both inner and outer aspects of the self, providing a basis for working towards a life-long, harmonious balance between attending to one's inner needs and meeting external demands with self-regulation and efficacy. Integrating research findings, best practices and practical suggestions, this chapter takes a salutogenic approach to EDs by offering treatment providers and consumers alike a framework for cultivating and maintaining a positive, embodied self-connection that supports flourishing in and from the body. This chapter also details the Embodiment of Self Model within the context of embodiment theory, providing a model for assessing the body's needs and the development of a mindful self-care plan.

Introduction: prevention, treatment, and the shift

"You can't hurt others without hurting yourself; you can't love others without loving yourself."
Debasish Mridha

Embodiment refers to an ongoing, moment-by-moment experience of the self in the body as one grapples with the domains of life, both internal (e.g. thoughts, emotions) and external (e.g. social, cultural) (Cook-Cottone, 2015a). Positive embodiment is the unfolding of being in the world characterized by the ability to attend and meet one's needs, self-agency, purpose and meaning, and appreciation for the body (Cook-Cottone, 2015a). It is the experience of *living in and from* the body (Cook-Cottone, 2020a), a fluid existence that allows us to "taste the joy of being fully present, alive and connected with all of life" (Brach, 2003, p. 97).

Disparities in embodiment are prevalent; there are those who experience their body as part of a whole and a resource to rely on, while others view their body as an object, an enemy, or are not even aware of their body (Cook-Cottone, 2020; Emerson & Hopper, 2011). For those with EDs, the relationship with one's body is often rife with complications. At the core of EDs is a profound disconnection between the mind, heart and body (Sands, 2016). This disconnection is often caused or influenced by factors such as societal pressures to attain an ideal body (Cook-Cottone, 2015b; 2020; Fredrickson & Roberts, 1997; Tylka & Agustus-Horvath, 2011), family or cultural factors (Cook-Cottone, 2020), and/or traumatic stress (Brach, 2003; Emerson & Hopper, 2011).

Considering the high rates of EDs and their outcomes (Joint Commissioning Panel for Mental Health, 2013; Le Grange *et al*, 2012), researchers and clinicians alike have sought to address individuals' complex, adverse relationship with their body (Cook-Cottone, 2020). Early approaches aimed to measure and reduce the dysfunctional aspects of perceiving and relating to the body (e.g., negative body image, dissatisfaction with the body; Webb *et al*, 2015). In recent years, contemporary approaches have shifted away from symptom reduction and towards examination as well as cultivation of the protective qualities (e.g., self-regulation, body appreciation; attuned self-care; Cook-Cottone, 2015b; 2016; Mahlo & Tiggemann, 2016; Piran, 2015; 2016; Webb *et al*, 2015) and practices (e.g., yoga, mindfulness; Cook-Cottone *et al*. 2017; Neumark-Sztainer, 2014; Piran, 2015, 2016) integral to positive embodiment. One of these approaches, *the embodied approach to eating disorders* (Cook-Cottone, 2020), is proposed in this chapter as one process for helping individuals build positive embodiment from within.

Learning point 1

- What experiences have prompted me to leave, disconnect from, or hate my body?
- What effect did these experiences have on my relationship to food/eating, physical activity, my sense of self, and other people?
- Currently, how present am I in my body on a daily basis?

If you are a clinician, after reflecting on your experiences, reflect on those of your clients.

Positive embodiment, attunement, and mindful self-care

Abra Fortune Chernik, an American feminist and essayist wrote, "We must claim our bodies as our own to love and honor their infinite shapes and sizes. Fat, thin, soft, hard, puckered, smooth, our bodies are our homes" (Weekes, 2007, p51). Chernik's words propose two important notions: (1) embodiment is a basic human right (Cook-Cottone, 2020), and (2) the process or journey to enact this right on an ongoing basis, while challenging and difficult, can lead us back to body – back to home. This path to recovery consists of attending to one's internal and external world with balanced awareness, defined here as *attunement*, as well as involvement in *mindful self-care* (Cook-Cottone, 2015a; 2020).

Case study

Throughout the course of her childhood, Mattie was sexually abused by her alcoholic and physically violent father. Growing up, Mattie attempted to cope in any way she could: drinking, eating, and she was eventually caught in a cycle of bingeing and purging almost every night. Each post-binge morning, she'd wake feeling shame and self-hatred, deciding yet again to starve herself as punishment. Each new diet, exercise program, and weight-loss strategy offered some hope to Mattie, until she soon found herself again disillusioned, loathing the figure that stared back at her in the mirror. Her dating partners usually made negative comments about her weight or cheated on her; as a result, she further stifled her own needs and became even more disconnected from her emotions. Mattie felt trapped in an addictive loop of behaviours that never satisfied her need to be safe, to be connected to others, to experience and express her emotions without being overwhelmed by them, or to feel at home in her body. To restore her connection to her body and find ways to meet its needs, she would need to learn and practice the principles of positive embodiment outlined in the following sections.

Positive embodiment

In the 20th century, the idea that the body is an integral part of self and that embodiment is a central aspect of the existence of all beings emerged as new ways of perceiving the body – replacing antiquated notions that the body is separate from, and inferior to, the mind (Cook-Cottone, 2020; Smith, 2017). From the perspective of the body as a unified whole, being embodied represents a continual experience of living *from within* the body, as opposed to having a body, thinking about the body, or judging the body from the stance of an observer (Cook-Cottone, 2020). For a practice on experiencing the body from within, see Appendix A: The Journey Inward Exercise on page 327.

From the basis of the aforementioned philosophical origins, efforts to define, measure and quantify embodiment have yielded a multifaceted construct backed by models that take into consideration the various dimensions of self (i.e., internal, external), the interpersonal as well as existential factors, and larger constructs that affect embodiment (i.e., social, cultural, political systems (Cook-Cottone, 2020; Estey, 2020; Piran, 2016)). While it is difficult to define and measure embodiment due to its association with a wide-range of constructs, its unique manifestation in individuals, and changing, fluid nature (Cook-Cottone, 2020; Estey, 2020), one current definition of 'positive embodiment' is as follows:

> *"... a way of being (non-dualistic conceptualization self) in which being is understood as residing in and manifesting from the body as one experiences the internal (i.e., physiological, emotional, cognitive), external (i.e., interpersonal, social, and cultural), and existential dimensions of life."* (Cook-Cottone, 2020, p22).

In the *Embodiment of Self Model* by Cook-Cottone (2020), embodiment is thought to be a developing experience of the self that is expressed through attunement to inner and external experiences of the self. Positive embodiment is facilitated and maintained by continual utilization of strategies that allow individuals to be aware, responsive, and active in meeting bodily needs and desires through mindful self-care practices (Cook-Cottone, 2020; Estey, 2020). Consequently, the body is listened to, felt, and attended to instead of silenced and ignored (Cook-Cottone, 2020). In Cook-Cottone's (2020) model, attending to the body includes intentional engagement in embodying practices (e.g., yoga, mindfulness, mindful eating), maintaining a balance between one's needs and external demands, involvement in supportive relationships, and the developing the wisdom to discern between factors that pose a risk to one's wellbeing, and those that contribute to flourishing in and from the body.

From theoretical and conceptual models of embodiment, prevention and treatment interventions have been developed to support individuals in learning to sense, feel and care for the body (Ariel-Donges *et al*, 2019; Cook-Cottone *et al*, 2017; Cook-Cottone *et al*, 2020; Cox *et al*, 2017; Halliwell *et al*, 2018). These approaches hold that the ongoing act of turning towards the body through self-care behaviours, rather than away, is the path home (Cook-Cottone, 2020; Cook-Cottone & Guyker, 2018; Estey, 2020). For Mattie, she will need to practice listening to and paying attention to her body, lovingly tending to the neglected parts of herself.

Learning point 2

- What aspects or parts of myself have I neglected or abandoned?
- How do I sense this neglect or abandonment in my body?
- What unmet need is showing up through this felt-sense?
- In what way might I care for this part of myself in the next few minutes or hours? See Appendix A for a felt-sense exercise that expands upon these questions (page 326).

Attunement

Central to embodiment is attunement (Cook-Cottone, 2020). Attunement is a process which an individual balances, coordinates and integrates the internal and external experiences of self in a manner that maintains positive embodiment, health and wellbeing in regard to one's self as an individual, as well as results in a sense of effectiveness, voice and self-determination within the context of one's self in the world (Cook-Cottone, 2020). It can be thought of as a process that maintains our sense of personal integrity and requires skills in both self-regulation and working with others.

The process of attunement is a two-part process. First, it is an ongoing process of cultivating mindful awareness and presence of your inner experience of self (physiology, emotions and cognitions) as well as the external experience of self (i.e., family, close friends, community, culture; Cook-Cottone, 2020). This aspect of attunement can be referred to as Being-With and the skills that help you cultivate mindful awareness and presence in both the inner and outer experiences of self, can be referred to as *Being-With Skills* (Cook-Cottone, 2020). These skills include mindfulness techniques and practices, distress tolerance skills, and somatic experiencing techniques (see Dialectic Behavioural Therapy, see also Cook-Cottone, 2015b and 2020). In this step of attunement, the goal is to be aware of what is present in one's experience via development of the meta-awareness skill of noticing. I am aware and I am aware that I am aware. More, I can regulate that awareness.

Some mindfulness texts refer to this as developing the *witness* aspects of self, the part of self that can notice what is happening inside and out, with acceptance, equanimity, and perhaps compassion and living-kindness (Cook-Cottone, 2015b; 2020). Effective mindfulness-based prevention and intervention programs integrate instruction and practice in being with skills (e.g., Borden & Cook-Cottone, 2020; Cook-Cottone *et al*, 2017).

The next step in attunement involves *Working-With Skills*. Interestingly, many prevention and treatment programs overemphasize this aspect of attunement, moving directly to working with emotions, cognitions, and interpersonal difficulties without first supporting the development of being with skills. Many experiences, issues, emotions and/or stressors do not necessarily need to be fixed, changed or worked with. Much can be accomplished by being with what is, acknowledging it, and allowing (Cook-Cottone, 2015b; 2020). The first step, then, for *working-with* is *being with*. In the case that being with appears insufficient, then working-with skills can be implemented. It can be very helpful to teach and practice these skills before they are needed, so that when distress, craving or compulsion occur, the *working with* skills are readily at hand. These skills follow a basic problem-solving model (e.g., identify the problem, generate solutions, choose a solution, engage in the behaviours, and evaluation effectiveness) and include distress tolerance, emotion regulation, somatic experiencing, interpersonal effectiveness, response prevention, and therapeutic yoga practices (Cook-Cottone, 2020). The goal of *working-with* skills is to manage either the internal or external stressors, changes or demands in a manner that supports a positively embodied internal experience of self and an effectiveness in the external experience of self. Both the *be-with* and *work-with* skills are meant to functionally prevent the formation of, or replace, the role of symptoms in an individual's coping repertoire.

Learning point 3

- What types of internal and external experiences might a person with an ED have that might trigger ED symptoms?
- How might learning to notice and be-with these experiences support recovery?
- What working-with skills might support an individual with an ED rely less on their ED symptoms to cope?

Mindful self-care

Mindful self-care can be a powerful proactive tool in preventing and treating eating difficulties, as it is positively associated with body esteem and negatively associated with ED behaviour (Cottone & Guyker, 2018; Cook-Cottone, 2020).

In order to manage eating difficulties, we can use mindful self-care to shift our attention and behaviours to our relationship with ourselves and the body (Cook-Cottone, 2016; Cook-Cottone & Guyker, 2018). Mindful self-care involves a set of informal and formal practices that care for the body with loving-kindness and compassion. These practices can influence a shift to occur from judgmental and critical concern with the body to a loving appreciation and care for the mind-body connection. As demonstrated in the Mindful Self-Care Scale (MSCS), we will discuss the six domains of mindful self-care that address both inner and outer aspects of the self.

Physical care

Physical self-care includes nutrition, hydration, and exercise practices (Brown & Gerbarg, 2015; Cook-Cottone, 2015b). Items on the MSCS consist of exercising 30-60 minutes a day, planning daily exercise, engaging in a mind/body practice such as yoga, adequately hydrating, eating nutritional foods, and planning meals and snacks (Cook-Cottone & Guyker, 2018). When practicing self-care, it is helpful to focus on the nutritional value of food, variety, planning regular meals without skipping, and paying attention to our body's hunger, thirst, and satiety cues (Cook-Cottone & Guyker, 2018). Engaging in recommended exercise can also cultivate a positive body image and prevent and treat EDs (Cook-Cottone, 2020). Exercise reduces stress by releasing endorphins into the bloodstream and improves psychological wellbeing (Cook-Cottone, 2015b). There should be a shift to focus on moving the body in healthy ways as opposed to a focus on weight, size, and shape as a path to physical health (Dollar *et al*, 2017). By focusing on physical care in our self-care plan, we can self-regulate and better manage eating difficulties.

Supportive relationships & supportive structure

To assess supportive relationships, items on the MSCS ask if an individual is spending time with individuals who are good to him/her, if he/she feels supported and has someone who will listen, schedules time with supportive people, and has people in his/her life that respect his/her choices (Cook-Cottone & Guyker, 2018). Interpersonal problems are associated with EDs which is why building relationship awareness with ourselves or with our clients can help develop the support system necessary to recover (Cook-Cottone, 2020). Supportive structure consists of having a healthy living/work environment and a schedule with sufficient rest and restoration. Items include keeping work areas organized, maintaining a comfortable and pleasing living environment, creating a balance between demands of others and our own internal needs, and maintaining a manageable work schedule (Cook-Cottone & Guyker, 2018). Self-care involves planning breaks from our current activities such as taking days off, week-long vacations, or short 5-10-minute breaks away from work, the computer, or interpersonal interactions (Cook-Cottone, 2020).

Mindful relaxation and mindful awareness

Mindful relaxation includes mindfulness practices and self-soothing to enhance self-care. It is important to participate in creative activities or engage the senses to relax (Cook-Cottone & Guyker, 2018). Self-soothing skills like progressive muscle relaxation, deep breathing, reading and writing can help calm the self when physically and emotionally stressed (Cook-Cottone, 2020). Mindful awareness involves having a calm awareness of thoughts, feelings, and the physical body, as well as an intentional choice of which thoughts and feelings we use to guide our actions (Cook-Cottone & Guyker, 2018). Specific practices such as engaging in meditation, yoga, mindful eating and gratitude can enhance our mindful awareness and self-care.

Self-compassion and purpose

Self-compassion means "treating oneself with kindness, recognizing one's shared humanity, and being mindful when considering negative aspects of the self" (Neff, 2011, p1). By practicing self-compassion, we can grow and flourish when facing struggles and protect ourselves against negative body image and eating pathology (Cook-Cottone, 2015b; Braun, Park, & Gorin, 2016). Items include engaging in supportive and comforting self-talk, permission to feel feelings, and acknowledging that failure and challenges are part of the human experience (Cook-Cottone & Guyker, 2018). Combined with self-compassion, purpose can be a source of strength and may even function like a spiritual, long-term goal allowing individuals to pick themselves up and persevere (Cook-Cottone, 2015b).

By taking the MSCS, we become mindfully aware of our current strengths and areas of improvement in our self-care behaviours. It is important to continually reassess our self-care plan based on our changing needs and external demands. MSC is a foundational self-regulating practice that cultivates overall mental health and integrates embodiment practices to prevent and manage eating difficulties (Cook-Cottone, 2020). Many people say that they will take better care of themselves and engage in healthier behaviours once they feel better, but MSC is the fundamental practice for feeling better (Cook-Cottone, 2015b; Cook-Cottone *et al*, 2013). MSC is the practical pathway towards embodiment, attunement, and improving our quality of life.

Learning point 4

- What consistent behaviors and activities (if any) are you consistently engaging in?
- Which self-care domains are your strengths? Which can you focus on more?
- What specific activities can you engage in to better take care of yourself?

Resolution with case study

Healing into positive embodiment requires a journey inward to connect to those aspects of ourselves that need to be seen, acknowledged and attended to (Brach, 2017; Cook-Cottone, 2020). For Mattie, the journey was a difficult one, but well worth-it. She took the Mindful Self-Care Scale (Cook-Cottone & Guyer, 2018) and formed a self-care plan with her therapist. She has started gardening, enjoying the sensation of dirt in her hands and the sun on her face. She and her therapist helped Mattie develop be-with and work-with skills. When feeling overwhelmed at work, she pauses to feel her feet supported by the floor and the warmth of her hand over her heart as she whispers to herself, "You are okay, I'm here for you". At night, as urges to binge or purge Arise, she practices identifying and labeling her emotions and sensations; she uses the feeling of her hands on her belly and her breath as an anchor until the urge passes. She loves to bake and uses an embodiment practice (mindful eating) to enjoy a cookie without spiraling into shame and self-loathing. Her day ends with a gentle yoga practice and a soothing meditation. In her personal and social life, she makes decisions based on her embodied knowledge – the north star of her inherent worth and value.

Conclusion

As you start on the path to positive embodiment, know that the body can be a guide that leads you back to your capacity to live from the very center of yourself. Bringing mindful attunement to your body's needs and external demands with an awareness of your inner resources can support you in showing up to life with a sense of agency. This *being-with* and *working with* what unfolds moment-to-moment (Cook-Cottone, 2020; Treleaven, 2018) using the skills as well as the practices discussed here, can reveal your body's resilience and wisdom.

References

American Psychiatric Association (2013) *Diagnostic and statistical manual of mental disorders: DSM-5 (5th ed.)* American Psychiatric Publishing.

Ariel-Donges AH Gordon EL Bauman V & Perri MG (2019) Does yoga help college-aged women with body-image dissatisfaction feel better about their bodies? *Sex Roles* **80** 41-51 https://doi.org/10.1007/s11199-018-0917-5

Blondin S (2020) *Heart minded: How to hold yourself and others in love* Sounds True.

Brach T (2003) *Radical acceptance: Embracing your life with the heart of a Buddha* Bantam.

Braun TD Park CL & Gorin A (2016) Self-compassion body image and disordered eating: A review of the literature *Body Image* **17** 117-131.

Brown RP & Gerbarg PL (2015) *Nutrients phytomedicines and mind-body treatments for substance abuse* In: N El-Guebaly G Carra & M Galanter (Eds.) *Textbook of addiction treatment: International perspectives* (pp747–772) New York: Springer.

Cook-Cottone CP (2013) Dosage as a critical variable in yoga research *International Journal of Yoga Therapy* **23** 11–12.

Cook-Cottone CP (2015a) Incorporating positive body image into the treatment of eating disorders: A model for attunement and mindful self-care *Body Image* **14** 158–167 http://dx.doi.org/10.1016/j.bodyim.2015.03.004

Cook-Cottone CP (2015b) *Mindfulness and yoga for self-regulation: A primer for mental health professionals* New York: Springer.

Cook-Cottone CP (2016) Embodied self-regulation and mindful self-care in the prevention of eating disorders Eating Disorders: *The Journal of Prevention and Intervention* http://dx.doi.org/10.1080/10640266.2015.1118954

Cook-Cottone CP (2020) *Embodiment and the treatment of eating disorders: The body as a resource in recovery* W W Norton & Company.

Cook-Cottone C, Beck M & Kane L (2008) Manualized-group treatment of eating disorders: Attunement in mind body and relationship (AMBR) *The Journal for Specialists in Group Work* **33** 61–83 http://dx.doi.org/10.1080/01933920701798570

Cook-Cottone C, Cox AE, Neumark-Sztainer D & Tylka TL (2020) Future directions for research on yoga and positive embodiment *Eating Disorders* **28** (4) 542-547 http://dx.doi.org/10.1080/10640266.2020.1763113

Cook-Cottone C P & Guyker W M (2018) The development and validation of the Mindful Self-Care Scale (MSCS): An assessment of practices that support positive embodiment *Mindfulness* **9** (1) 161-175 http://dx.doi.org/10.1007/s12671-017-0759-1

Cook-Cottone C Talebkhah K Guyker W & Keddie E (2017) A controlled trial of a yoga-based prevention program targeting eating disorder risk factors among middle school females *Eating Disorders* **25** (5) 392-405 https://doi.org/10.1080/10640266.2017.1365562

Cox A Ullrich-French S Howe SS & Cole AN (2017) A pilot yoga physical education curriculum to promote positive body image *Body Image* **23** 1-8 http://dx.doi.org/10.1016/j.bodyim.2017.07.007

Dollar E, Berman M & Adachi-Mejia AM (2017) Do no harm: Moving body weight loss to emphasize physical activity at every size *Preventing Chronic Disease* **14** 1-3.

Emerson D H & Hopper E (2017) *Overcoming trauma through yoga: Reclaiming your body* North Atlantic Books.

Estey E E (2020) Efficacy of Eat Breathe Thrive: A randomized controlled trial of a yoga-based program [Unpublished doctoral dissertation] University at Buffalo The State University of New York.

Fredrickson B L & Roberts T (1997) Objectification theory: Toward understanding women's lived experiences and mental health risks *Psychology of Women Quarterly* **21** (2) 173-206 http://dx.doi.org/10.1111/j.1471-6402.1997.tb00108.x

Halliwell E, Jarman H, Tylka T L & Slater A (2018) Evaluating the impact of a brief yoga intervention on preadolescents' body image and mood *Body Image* **27** 196-201 http://dx.doi.org/10.1016/j.bodyim.2018.10.003

Joint Commissioning Panel for Mental Health 2013 *Guidance for commissioners of eating disorder services* [online] Available: http://www.jcpmh.info/resource/guidance-commissioners-eating-disorder-services/

Le Grange D, Swanson S A, Crow C J & Merikangas K R (2012) Eating disorder not otherwise specified presentation in the US population *International Journal of Eating Disorders* **45** 711-718.

Neff K D (2011) Self-compassion self-esteem and well-being *Social and Personality Psychology Compass* **5** 1–12 http://dx.doi.org/10.1111/j.1751- 9004.2010.00330.x

Neumark-Sztainer D (2014) Yoga and eating disorders: Is there a place for yoga in the prevention and treatment of eating disorders and disordered eating behaviors? Advances in Eating Disorders: *Theory research and practice* **2** (2) 136-145 http://dx.doi.org/10.1080/21662630.2013.862369

Piran N (2015) New possibilities in the prevention of eating disorders: The introduction of positive body image measures *Body Image* **14** 146-157 http://dx.doi.org/10.1016/j.bodyim.2015.03.008

Piran N (2016) Embodied possibilities and disruptions: The emergence of the experience of embodiment construct from qualitative studies with girls and women *Body Image* **18** 43-60 http://dx.doi.org/10.1016/j.bodyim.2016.04.007

Treleaven D A (2018) *Trauma-sensitive mindfulness: practices for safe and transformative healing* New York NY: Norton.

Tylka T L & Augustus-Horvath C L (2011) Fighting self-objectification in prevention and intervention contexts In: R M Calogero S Tantleff-Dunn & J K Thompson (Eds.) *Self-objectification in women: Causes consequences and counteractions* (pp 187–214) Washington DC: American Psychological Association.

Sands S H (2015) Eating disorder treatment as a process of mind–body Integration: Special challenges for women *Clinical Social Work Journal* **44** (1) 27-37 http://dx.doi.org/10.1007/s10615-015-0540-7

Smith J E (2017) *Embodiment: A history* Oxford University Press.

Weekes K (2007) *Women know everything* Quirk Books.

Webb J Wood-Barcalow N L & Tylka T L (2015) Assessing positive body image: Contemporary approaches and future directions *Body Image* **14** 130-145 http://dx.doi.org/10.1016/j.bodyim.2015.03.010

Key references and websites

Books

Brach T (2003) *Radical acceptance: Embracing your life with the heart of a Buddha*. New York, NY: Bantam.

Cook-Cottone CP (2015) *Mindfulness and yoga for self-regulation: A primer for mental health professionals*. New York, NY: Springer

Cook-Cottone CP (2017) *Mindfulness and yoga in Schools: A guide for teachers and practitioners*. New York, NY: Springer.

Cook-Cottone CP (2020) *Embodiment and the treatment of eating disorders: The body as a resource in recovery*. New York, NY: W. W. Norton.

Neff K & Germer C (2018) *The mindful self-compassion workbook: A proven way to accept yourself, build inner strength, and thrive*. New York, NY: Guilford Press.

Websites

Mindful Self-Care

- Mindful Self-Care Scale Assessment: http://ed.buffalo.edu/mindful-assessment/scale/assessment.html
- Mindful Wellness Assessment: http://ed.buffalo.edu/mindful-assessment.html
- Catherine Cook-Cottone, PhD: https://www.catherinecookcottone.com/
- Mindful Self-Care Scale- 3 versions:
- https://www.catherinecookcottone.com/research-and-teaching/mindful-self-care-scale/
- Mindful Self-Care Scale: An Open Access Resource: https://www.catherinecookcottone.com/research-and-teaching/mindful-self-care-scale/

Self-Compassion:

- Center for Mindful Self-Compassion: www.centerformsc.org
- Self-Compassion: https://www.self-compassion.org/
- Christopher Germer, PhD: https://chrisgermer.com/
- Center for Mindful Self-Compassion: https://centerformsc.org/
- Kristen Neff, PhD: www.self-compassion.org

Appendix A: Felt-sense exercise

The following felt-sense exercise is drawn from the work of Peter Levine and Eugene Gendlin (Levine, 1997; Sandmaier, 2017) and adapted to support participants in moving from the perception of the body from an observer's stance (viewing it as an object), to experiencing it subjectively, with attunement to its needs. This exercise and other somatic mindfulness practices can be facilitated in session to help clients move towards a deeper sense of their bodies and attunement to their inner needs. As a clinician, you may need to set up the conditions for the needs of the client's body to be heard and listened to with compassion and understanding. This might entail providing brief psychoeducation on self-compassion (Germer & Neff, 2020) before facilitating the exercise, orienting the client to the difficult emotions or reactions that might Arise during the practice, and discussion of the ways in which they can meet internal stimuli using mindfulness. If the client is triggered or flooded, they may need to be prompted to use grounding tools (e.g. orientation to the environment, the sound of your voice, the breath, or a stabilizing part of the body). After a need has been identified, you can help them consider options for a small action step they might take to fulfill the need in a practical way (e.g. drinking tea, going to sleep early, calling a supportive friend).

Set the stage: Find a quiet, comfortable space. Give yourself time to settle into a chair, cushion, or yoga mat, feeling into the support. Lowering your gaze or softly closing your eyes, take a few deep breaths, noticing the breath on the inhale, letting go of any tension on the exhale.

Move from perception to experience: In your mind's eye, visualize your body, its size, weight, shape, and outline. Then, turning inward, scanning your body from your scalp, face, chest, hips, legs, down to your feet, toes – noticing any bodily sensations that call for your attention.

Notice the felt-sense and describe it: Allowing any words, images, or phrases to Arise that capture this information from your body. You might notice feelings or sensations (e.g. emotions [worry, joy, sadness, hunger], pain, pressure, air, tingling), environment or quality (e.g. temperature, size, weight, shape, movement, speed, texture, color), inner sounds (e.g. buzzing, ringing), tastes (e.g. bitterness, sweetness, no taste), smells (e.g. floral, minty, pungent), or emptiness (e.g. numb, space).

Label the felt-sense: As a felt-sense emerges, try labeling it non-judgementally. You might say to yourself "tight chest," "racing heart," "knot in stomach." Noticing that your felt-sense is not the whole of who you are, only a part of your overall experience.

Acknowledge the felt-sense: As it feels right, send a gentle acknowledgement or greeting to the felt-sense. It might be a kind nod, a tip of the hat – any way you can recognize its presence in your being.

Explore unmet needs: As you acknowledge the felt-sense of your body, you may inquire, "What does this felt-sense need from me?" Deeply listen from the place of your inner wisdom and insight. There may be a response that shows up in the form of a behaviour you can do in the next few moments to hours in response to the need, or perhaps an image, or a phrase emerges, or there may be a shift that occurs physically. Or there may be no response, and that's okay too – sometimes the body needs time to find its voice.

Receive the experience and thank your body: In your own time, sending a simple "thank you" to your body for its wisdom. Reminding yourself that you can return to this place of body-listening at any time, gently return to feeling the support of your cushion, chair, or mat and opening the eyes slowly, orienting to the space of the room you are in.

Journey Inward: A Meditation for Embodiment

Written by Esther Estey, LPC, Ph.D., RYT-200

This mindfulness practice supports individuals in cultivating the processes of Acceptance and Commitment Therapy (Harris, 2009) and self-compassion (Germer & Neff, 2020) for greater embodiment. If you are a therapist or other medical provider, you might introduce this exercise as an experiment of embodiment during a session, supporting the client in opening up to their experience of their body in the present moment. Facilitation of this exercise should be slow and gradual with sufficient pauses to allow time for individuals to identify internal stimuli as it Arises, and work with it using the concepts of ACT and self-compassion. Definitions of embodiment and self-compassion may be presented before the exercise is facilitated, tailored and adapted for patient comprehension (e.g. "embodiment is a way of experiencing your body as your home or developing a positive relationship with your body"). One clinical definition of positive embodiment is as follows:

> *"… a way of being (non-dualistic conceptualization self) in which being is understood as residing in and manifesting from the body as one experiences the internal (i.e., physiological, emotional, cognitive), external (i.e., interpersonal, social, and cultural), and existential dimensions of life."* (Cook-Cottone, 2020)

Introduction to practice and rationale

While positive embodiment, the capacity to live in and from the body, is something we are working towards, it is also a way of being already available to you now. The following is a brief practice to bring whole-hearted, kind presence to the experience of your body today.

I invite you to settle into a comfortable position, allowing the gaze to be lowered or the eyes to gently close. Taking a moment here, reflect on what your intentions are for cultivating an ability to live in and through your body. What do you value? Why is this meaningful for you? Recognize and honour your commitment to being with and working with all that Arises in your body with awareness, with presence, with compassion. Perhaps extending gratitude to yourself for all the ways in which you endeavored to show up here in your body today.

- Begin by taking a couple gentle inhales and exhales. Noticing where you feel the breath most prominently. Is it in the nose? The chest? The belly? Observe how the breath naturally knows how to breathe you.
- See what it's like to allow yourself to be gently rocked by the rhythmic flow of the breath. Each breath coming in, each breath going out.
- Now shifting your attention from the breath to the body. Inclining your awareness to the sensations of the body from the top of your head through each part of the body, and down to your feet.
- If there are difficult sensations, judgements, criticisms, or thoughts that arise, see if you can let them come and go, gently drawing your attention back to presence, back to your body.
- Now, choosing a part of the body to explore, the hands, feet, or belly, whatever area of the body will serve you to explore today. It is natural that certain parts of the body may have a certain charge or may hold intense emotions. Rather than getting caught in a tug-a-war with this part or the emotions arising, drop the rope. Bear witness to all that unfolds in your internal experience – letting it be exactly as it is. If it is not workable to stay with a certain part of the body, shift your attention to another, more neutral part of the body or focus on the breath as an anchor before returning to the part of the body you were attending to.
- Starting from the outside, noticing the outline, the form of this area of the body. Then sense into the feeling of the skin, the outer layer of the self.
- If any judgements, thoughts, or feelings come up about this part, as they will, send a gentle nod of acknowledgement and return to simply noticing the part with curiosity.

- If there's a sense of being an observer of your body, see if you can draw closer to the body, letting go as much as possible today, settling into being the body.
- In your own time, draw deeper inward, bringing awareness to the temperature (e.g. warmth or coolness), rhythms, and sensations (e.g. tingly, pulsating, firm) that are present in this area. Perhaps even feeling into the muscles, the tendons, the bones.
- Allowing this process to be one of kind curiosity, exploring and cultivating into an inner knowing of what it is like to inhabit, as much as you can today, this part of your body.
- Reflect on what this part of the body does for you every day, its function. Offering appreciation and gratitude for how it serves you. Or extending support and compassion if there is pain, an injury, or discomfort present in this part.
- If storylines about this part of the body begin to appear, as they will, know that this is what the brain does, it creates stories derived from our experience. Drop below the story into presence in this part of yourself. Meeting it as you would a dear friend, with warmth, and kindness.
- Let this journey be one of a slow, gradual process. Coming home to this body as much as you are able today. Perhaps arriving at the doorstep, opening the door, stepping into the entrance of this body. This is an experience of directly sensing, feeling, arriving into the home of your body – in essence, embodying your life.
- You can use gentle touch, placing a hand on this part of your body as a gesture of loving kindness and compassion, extending a warm greeting to yourself, or just rest here quietly in the body.
- Now opening and expanding out your awareness, sensing your body as a whole in the room that you are in, noting any changes in your experience of your body since you began this exercise.
- In your own time, gently flutter the eyes open, orienting to the support of your chair or cushion, the space you are in, and the ground beneath your feet.

35. Moving matters: living in the body after anorexia

By Grace Lucas, MA (Cantab), MSc, PhD

Summary

I used to live entirely inside my head. My body was an object that I appraised through mirrors and other people's opinions. During treatment for eating difficulties, psychiatrists asked me to focus on the dysfunctional thoughts in my head. I was not given any tools with which to enquire about my body and how it related to my sense of self. In the process of recovery from anorexia, it was this body-based self-inquiry that made the biggest positive impact on my healing.

In this chapter, I discuss how I was able to define what had happened to me through physical exploration in body-based practices including yoga, and by drawing on theoretical understandings of embodiment. I argue that mental health is not all in our heads and that how we live, feel and move in our bodies in the world is crucial to our wellbeing. This chapter advocates for a ground-up approach to eating difficulties and suggests emphasis should be put on the development of 'body sense' as much as mindfulness or talking as ways to work with distress – which does not need to be qualified as mental or physical.

Defining my eating difficulties

In medical definitions and psychiatric diagnostic criteria, personal experiences of eating difficulties become indexed and profiled. These definitions are important because they become the tools for people to represent and explain their experiences to others. Anorexia nervosa, for example, is defined as a mental disorder. The word 'mental' indicates that the problem is something to do with the mind or brain and its symptoms tell us that the 'physical' body suffers as a result. Cognitive-based, psychologically informed therapeutic approaches usually start to address the problem from the head down.

When I was diagnosed with anorexia, its categorization as a 'mental' disorder informed my understanding of what I was experiencing. I attended psychiatric appointments designed to address the dysfunctional thoughts in my head. Each word within my mental stream was analysed as a feature of the problem. I was so carried along in this rushing thought-stream that I lost all sense of contact with the rest of me. I repeated this 'troubled thinking' narrative to others, to explain what was happening to me.

After anorexia, many years later, I now begin with a different language, one that does not mimic medicine. Instead, I start the story of my eating difficulties with the feeling of being in my body in this world: I start with the cauldron of my guts; the weakness of my arms; the stiffness of my jaw; the thickness of my thighs; the insecurity in my feet and the shiver of my skin.

Learning point 1

Before reading further, reflect on how you understand mental illness and health and its relationship to physical health.

- How would you characterise this relationship?
- How might your understanding of eating difficulties or any experiences of treatment relate to the model described here?

Escape from the body

It's hard to identify when I left my body behind, but as a child I remember feeling a sense of unease with my physical self. I would reach to catch a ball and would miss it. I would run but my legs were jelly-like and shaky. As a teenager, I observed my body in the mirror and listened attentively to others' judgements of it, but I did not live in my body. Instead, I focused on my intellect and got on to an endless treadmill of academic achievement. In the shifting shape of puberty, when my body grew and changed, it felt more comfortable to slip out of my skin altogether and live almost entirely in my head. In the whirly, floaty head space that I inhabited, I vowed to get my growing form under control. Disconnection with my body transformed into fear of my body size and shape. It did not seem like a strange path to choose as I was simply complying with a 'mind over matter' culture where bodies were objects to manage and discipline.

Back to the body

The return back to my body happened unconsciously. In the process of trying yet another exercise regime to soothe my self-critical thoughts, I went to some yoga classes. I remember balancing in a tree pose – one foot pressing into the inner thigh of the other leg and finding a sense of ground and centre. Lying down, at the end of practice, energy spread over me – a tingling; a white light; the feeling of my belly breath surfaced and the noise in my head was strangely quiet. I had this sense of remembrance of my creative, intuitive, emotional self, rather than the rigid, overthinking person I had become through my eating difficulties.

Each time I came to the mat, I longed to re-find this feeling. Sometimes, I couldn't – my breath was strained and my energy tight and fixed. In those times, though, I observed how stress liked to occupy me and where it took root. This observation process was really important. Other days, the freeing feeling was there and I breathed and moved in such synchronicity and flow that the thought-torrent just dissipated.

I didn't have the words to explain the shift. I just knew I felt better. Eventually, through my academic research, I came across the term 'embodiment'. I became so interested in its meaning that I undertook a PhD to explore what it might mean for understanding and treating mental health problems (Lucas, 2017). Embodiment has been defined as the experience of living as a body engaging with the world (Piran & Teall, 2012). The sense of 'positive embodiment' I experienced stemmed from the bodily connection and comfort I was able to cultivate when I practised yoga and breathwork (Piran, 2016). The psychologist and yoga teacher Catherine Cook-Cottone explains how, when this happens, the body stops being your enemy – it is not separate from your sense of self, nor is it something that you manage and punish from the top down (Cook-Cottone, 2020).

Learning point 2

Before you continue reading, can you stop and think about what embodiment might mean for you?

- Is there a time that you recall that you felt a sense of flow in your body?
- How did this make you feel?

Learning to be whole

I began to ask myself – what if my mental health is in my whole body moving through the world, not only in the thoughts in my head or my brain? I reflected on where I felt physically uncomfortable. I noticed tiny patterns that were so rooted within me – in every breath and movement I made – they were barely perceptible. These habits told a story of my life's experiences and I needed to listen to them to heal.

When I was four years old I fell off a small chair and fractured my elbow. I screamed as the doctors manipulated my arm for the x-ray and bound it into a hard cast. I held my arm across my belly for six weeks in a beige, foamy sling. When the cast was removed, I was considered fixed. But I wasn't. My arm had been set in the wrong place. I could no longer easily touch my left hand to my left shoulder. When I was sad or stressed my left shoulder would slightly hunch up towards my ear. My elbow always felt weak, like it might collapse under me. I held myself differently and because of this, the connection to my shoulder, my chest and my heart all feel different. We are not a series of different parts – everything is connected.

Frederick Matthias Alexander, who established the Alexander Technique, came to bodywork as he attempted to deal with the voice hoarseness he developed practising lines in his work as an actor (Alexander, 1932). This technique focuses on inhibiting habits and, in doing so, improving movement and overall health. Alexander believed in working on the body as a whole and that it was not possible to separate mental and physical processes in human activity. Somatics practitioners also show us how to become more aware of our bodies by tuning into our sense of inner perception – often through movement – and this is underpinned by the understanding that 'everything we experience in our lives is a bodily experience' (Hanna, 2004, p.xii). When we tune into that idea, we may start to be able to interrogate the notion that our distress is all about perceptions and thoughts in our heads.

Learning point 3

Before reading on, can you reflect on any habits you have developed in your body that relate to how you feel? For example, if you feel stressed or anxious, can you locate how you react and where you feel that tension or stress?

The ground under your feet

I began to ask the question: what if my mental health is in my feet? What if the eating difficulties I had were linked to how I felt there? When I am stressed and out of control, I don't want to put my feet on the ground – I move fast as if I am trying to escape gravity. When I was unwell with anorexia, this was the feeling all of the time.

My yoga mat became a small, defined space of safety. Every time I planted my feet down, I began again. I practised being in my body. Each practice was entirely new. It didn't matter how I moved. I didn't plan to make certain shapes or achieve certain things. I found rootedness through this practice. I developed a sense of myself from the ground up. I learnt to feel into my weight and be calmed by it, rather than trying to escape it. Another useful expansion into my body came through walking in nature. Feeling my feet sink into the mud, crunch leaves underfoot and getting a sense of physical perspective of my body against the landscape cultivated further connection. Researchers have found that a connection with nature can accentuate calmness and sensory engagement for those recovering from eating disorders (Jepsen Trangsrud *et al*, 2020).

Embodied learning point 1: feeling through the feet

Send your attention to your feet. Feel the weight sink down into what you can sense beneath your soles. Staying still might feel challenging but try not to run, heave or resist. Feel the sensations that arise. Notice how there are tiny calibrations that keep you balanced and stable. Pay attention to the three corners of the foot – the back of the foot and just below the little and big toes. Root down. Lift your toes, spread them apart. Rock forward and back. Centre your weight. If you are standing, bend your knees and fold forward, put opposite hands in opposite elbows, let yourself hang and move as needed. Allow the ground to hold you up, sink down. When you are ready, roll up slowly. You are supported.

Gut in mind

The sense of satiation that comes with eating may bring with it fullness and, sometimes, bloating or discomfort. In the process of confronting the fear and feeling the belly expand, distress bubbles up. To feel this in the belly is to feel your embodied reaction. This may be more than just a stress response – another thing to manage from above – because evidence suggests that bodies once starved may experience alterations of the gut microbiome (Seitz *et al*, 2019). The gut and the brain interconnect and communicate and the signals go both ways – 'gut thinking' helps to collapse the idea of mind over body (Lucas, 2018).

Embodied learning point 2: breathing in the belly

Settling your hands against your belly may be too confronting at first, but eventually resting your hands there you might begin to feel the depth of your touch. Lying down in a comfortable position, perhaps try resting a small cushion there too, and feel the gentle calming compression as you begin to focus on the sense of the belly rising and expanding as you inhale and falling back as you exhale. Try slow and nourishing breaths, breathing in for a count of four and out for a count of four. What sensations come up for you? Does this help you feel more centred?

Worded resistance

Another way of exploring embodiment is to read how others have explained it and to think critically about the context for the development of eating difficulties. Involvement in activities such as political activism and community engagement have been shown to help in long-term recovery from eating disorders (Matusek & Knudson, 2009) and engagement with feminist texts has been trialled in treatment (Holmes *et al*, 2017). One useful reflection could be around how we perceive the capabilities of our bodies. We may think that our bodily capacities are due to our genes. I used to think I wasn't good at sport and wasn't physically strong because it was something inherent to me, but it is likely to be a lot more complex than this. Biosocial research helps to explain the mutual interaction of biology and the social world and how our environment can affect and shape our bodies.

The essay 'Throwing like a Girl' by feminist philosopher Iris Marion Young (1980), helped develop my thinking on this. Young argues that how we throw or learn to move more generally is a response to how bodies are taught by society that they are allowed to move or be. Bodies react to the way they are treated and begin to move differently as a result.

Eating distress is about relationships with the world that cannot be disentangled because the conditions of being in the world affect our bodies. The realization that power structures affect how bodies move and feel makes it possible to question the way you may have labelled or perceived your weakness, fears or failures. When you understand how you exist in relation to the space around you – how you have adapted to the world and how it has treated you – there is the chance to challenge the structures that define what bodies should be like. It may also help you resist ideas about controlling your health behaviour like you are a bounded individual. Embodiment can act as a challenge to the idea that the physical body is the object for the self in the head to sort out and manage.

Critical movement

Alongside developing a positive relationship with your embodied self, it may also help to think about the act of resistance you might make in returning to your body and in moving through your body with softness, care and compassion, without the agenda being about exercise and without tracking technologies counting steps or scales measuring weight. How might you stand up against raging diet culture that constantly reprimands us with a focus on endless self-improvement, that shouts at us through repeated mantras of: 'It's you versus you', 'mind over matter' or 'ignore the pain; talk over it'? What if we use a different language around movement – that movement is you *for* you and that connecting to each step or stretch is why we move – so that we can *feel*, not so that we can disconnect. What if it were possible to move for fun and to play, to find pleasure through moving your body and to find acceptance in relaxing and resting too?

The more the body is an object or an image in the mirror or a clothes hanger or a tracked and monitored machine, observed only through tiny social media squares, the more it becomes abstracted from the self. And when your body is not part of your sense of self, how easy is it to attack it; to use it to take back control from whatever is causing you anxiety, to respond to fear or pain and strike out at your flesh?

Learning point 4

Before you finish this chapter, can you identify the messages from society that may have taught you a particular way of being in your body? How might resisting cultural pressures be useful in creating change for yourself or others? Who has inspired you through their words or actions?

Moving on

We have an opportunity for an intervention to happen earlier than the moment someone's low self-esteem slides into self-damage and eating difficulties. We must begin to teach children and teenagers about their embodied selves and provide more opportunities for different forms of movement that help with establishing connections to their whole selves. While positive embodiment might be considered a state that we should naturally be able to access, given the dominance of mind over matter models of selfhood and body management, embodiment needs to be cultivated – it requires practice.

Author and yoga teacher Matthew Sanford talks about how anorexia is a way 'out' of a body and parallels this experience with his own paralysis following a car accident (Sanford, 2006, p69). Coming back to the body can be chest-tightening and stomach-knotting. There are many routes to connecting with your body. This is not a prescription but an invitation to practice and to make space for the idea that eating difficulties are not all in the head. I borrow from Toni Morrison's novel *Beloved* (1987): 'Anything dead coming back to life hurts'. But once life is full again, that pain subsides, the pleasures of being a body surface and the head can quieten down.

References

Alexander FM (2001; orig. 1932) *The Use of the Self*, London: Orion.

Cooke-Cottone C (2020) *Embodiment and the Treatment of Eating Disorders: The Body as a Resource in Recovery*. New York: WW Norton & Company.

Hanna T (2004) *Somatics: Reawakening the Mind's Control of Movement, Flexibility, and Health*. Cambridge, MA: De Capo Press.

Holmes S, Drake S, Odgers K & Wilson J (2017) Feminist approaches to Anorexia Nervosa: a qualitative study of a treatment group. *Journal of Eating Disorders* **5** (36).

Jepsen Trangsrud LK, Borg M, Bratland-Sanda S & Klevan T (2020) Embodying Experiences with Nature in Everyday Life Recovery for Persons with Eating Disorders. *International Journal of Environmental Research and Public Health* **17** (8) 2784.

Lucas G (2017) All 'in the mind'?: towards a new model of embodied mental health. Doctoral thesis, Birkbeck, University of London.

Lucas G (2018) Gut thinking: the gut microbiome and mental health beyond the head. *Microbial ecology in health and disease* **29** (2) 1548250.

Matusek JA & Knudson RM (2009) Rethinking recovery from eating disorders: spiritual and political dimensions. *Qualitative Health Research* **19** (5) 697-707.

Morrison T (2007; orig 1987) *Beloved.* London: Vintage.

Piran N & Teall T (2012) The developmental theory of embodiment. In: G McVey, H B Ferguson, M Levine, & N Piran (Eds) *Improving the prevention of eating disorders: Collaborative research, advocacy, and policy change* pp169-198. Waterloo, Ontario, Canada: Wilfred Laurier Press.

Piran N (2016) Embodied possibilities and disruptions: The emergence of the experience of embodiment construct from qualitative studies with girls and women. *Body Image* **18** 43-60.

Seitz J, Trinh S & Herpertz-Dahlmann B (2019) The Microbiome and Eating Disorders. *Psychiatric Clinics of North America* **42** (1) 93-103.

Young IM (1980) Throwing Like a Girl: A Phenomenology of Feminine Body Comportment, Motility and Spatiality. *Human Studies* **3** (2) 137-56.

36. Enacting change: the role of dramatherapy in the treatment of eating difficulties

By Mary Franklin-Smith & James Downs

Summary

This chapter aims to illustrate some of the ways in which the theoretical perspective and creative practices of dramatherapy can help in understanding and responding to eating difficulties. Starting with a specific focus on the Sesame Approach, the chapter will explore how dramatherapy might conceptualize eating difficulties and the theoretical basis of techniques that might be used. The following section offers a range of practical and imaginative ideas which, while sitting outside of traditional treatment models, have been shown to provide hope, meaning and change for people with eating difficulties.

What is dramatherapy?

Dramatherapy is a form of psychotherapy which makes use of a range of creative processes within the therapeutic relationship between the artist-therapist and the individual presenting with whatever difficulty they are grappling with in their lives. Dramatherapists often have backgrounds in theatre, dance and other creative arts, as well as healthcare or education, and undertake training at postgraduate level in the theory and reflective practice of dramatherapy.

The Sesame Approach, focused on here, is one such training route which emerged since the 1960s from Billy Lindkvist's dream of how the arts can contribute to the mental wellbeing both individually and culturally (Hougham & Jones, 2017). This reflects Karl Marx's proposition that sensory processes have the power to transform and actualize the potential of humans and society for the better (Rose, 1988). The interweaving of philosophy and action is central to dramatherapy, which makes use of predominantly 'oblique' or 'indirect' methods aimed at unlocking what Carl Jung sees as the innate and self-regulating tendency of our psyche towards balance, growth and awareness (Jung, 1960).

Using the example of eating difficulties, this might mean that, rather than imposing a medicalized model for 'treating' eating difficulties, the dramatherapist instead provides a structured, contained and non-judgemental environment in which creative methods are used to facilitate expression, uncovering healing and growth from within (Hougham & Jones, 2017). The dominant cognitive-behavioural model used in the treatment of eating difficulties in healthcare settings today (Cognitive Behaviour Therapy for Eating Disorders, or CBT-E) is concerned with stabilising eating patterns on the basis of challenging 'core psychopathology'. The focus on 'faulty' thoughts around food, weight and shape, and negative self-evaluation on the basis of these, is central and tackled via direct means (Fairburn, 2008). In contrast to this, dramatherapy suggests that attempts at 'making sense' of eating difficulties can be complemented by the use of *sensory* experiences, too.

This is essentially an embodied process, i.e. focused on 'the experience of living as a body engaging with the world' (Kiran & Teall, 2012), which appreciates the physicality of the relationship between the therapist and the client, the centrality of the body in the lived experience of eating difficulties, and how, for all of us, 'everything we experience in our lives is a bodily experience' (Hanna, 2004). Dramatherapy recognizes and seeks to avoid the trap of privileging the mind over the body; thought over feeling; brokenness over wholeness; and external knowledge over inner wisdom. The use of symbols, myth, movement and play are the central vehicles through which the dramatherapist and person experiencing eating difficulties create meaning, challenge identity, retell stories and ultimately enact change.

Learning point 1

Having read a little about dramatherapy, take a moment to reflect on any knowledge or experiences of therapy you may have already – be that personally, professionally, or both. If you have had little experience of psychological therapies, consider any ideas you have about what they might involve.

- How does the perspective of dramatherapy compare with your own experiences and ideas of what it is to be in therapy?
- Is there anything that stands out as different, or anything missing? Do you spot holes in the dramatherapy approach?
- What is your gut reaction to ideas such as embodiment, taking an indirect approach, or using play and storytelling in therapy?
- How do you feel ahead of reading the rest of the chapter?

How does dramatherapy explore and understand eating difficulties?

Dominant treatment models for understanding and responding to eating difficulties privilege 'top-down' cognitive processes over and above somatic or 'bottom-up' processes (Downs, 2021). For instance, emphasis is placed on executive functions such as inhibitory control – the ability to control one's thoughts, emotions and behaviours (Diamond, 2013), and language is the predominant vehicle for articulating and making sense of experiences.

Dramatherapy recognizes and actively seeks ways of knowing about ourselves and our experiences beyond the realm of language alone. When it comes to understanding, the range of eating difficulties that people can experience, the role of symbols, myth, movement and play are valued alongside language and verbal dialogue. Instead of thinking our way out of problems, dramatherapy suggests that we may be able to use other expressive tools to move our way through things, or – as Jung would suggest – allow our inherent wholeness to emerge from within (Pearson, 1996).

An indirect approach and working with embodied states may well be especially important where someone with eating difficulties has experienced trauma, as evidence shows that the executive functions relied upon so heavily in traditional therapies may be weakened amongst this group (Monteleone *et al*, 2019). Furthermore, emerging neurodevelopment and attachment research demonstrates the impact of traumatic experiences in embodied terms, and how developmental trauma can impact the five developmental gestures of yielding, grasping, pushing, reaching, and pulling (Loutsis *et al*, 2017). For the dramatherapist, enquiry into the quality of movement may be as relevant as assessing the quality or accuracy of thinking.

The entanglement of body and brain and the dependence of our cognitive functions on our baseline physiological state is clear. The use of role-based embodied techniques in dramatherapy with people experiencing eating difficulties has been shown to improve levels of emotional regulation, cognitive flexibility and self-attunement, with researchers suggesting that these measurable benefits are as a result of the capability for dramatherapy techniques to engage both cognitive and affective systems to promote optimal neural integration (Wood & Schneider, 2015).

While eating difficulties represent an array of experiences and behaviours which for any individual will be rooted in the context of their own lives, dramatherapy might approach the idea of 'clinical presentation' in terms of *representation* – asking questions about what eating difficulties might symbolise. 'Physical symptoms' might be viewed as signals, nudges or clues from a person's innate health, that signal a 'way forward' or a 'next step'. Embodied behaviours arising from eating difficulties might be viewed instead as symbols of distress; of roles people feel bound to fill; of things that are unspoken yet need to be communicated. The aetiology of someone's eating difficulty and its current 'formulation' might be as much about the cultural myths their social understandings have been informed by; the stories they've been told and tell themselves; an over-rehearsed pattern of movement; or the improvisation of some kind of equilibrium amidst chaos.

Jung described the psyche as a self-regulating system tending towards balance, growth, awareness, proposing that our psychological health depends upon the integration of unconscious material into consciousness (Jung, 1960). The 'language' of the unconscious does not take the form of words or cognition. Instead, the unconscious seeks expression via symbols, imagery, myth and movement. These Arise naturally in dreams, art, play, music, storytelling and dance. As a result, dramatherapy suggests that in order to work with blockage or imbalance in the psychic system, therapists and treatment providers are required to work with the media of the unconscious, too. In sessions, clients will be invited into the play space where creativity, inspiration and new ideas can be encountered and explored.

Learning point 2

Before reading further, take a moment to reflect on what you have read and your own responses to the ideas in this chapter.

- Have you encountered the privileging of mind over body? Do you think that there are any problems with mind and body being treated separately, especially in relation to eating difficulties?
- In what ways do you make sense of your experiences, come to understand what is true, and learn how to change in your life, besides through language?
- Besides language, how do you express your feelings, communicate what you need, or ask for help? Are some of these ways more helpful than others?
- Do you have any creative practices or art forms that you particularly like, or used to like? For example, perhaps you especially love comedy or music, or like to practice yoga or drawing, maybe you like to lose yourself in a film or book? How do you feel when you take part in these activities? What do they connect you with? Can you see how intentional use of the arts could be therapeutic and healing?

Examples of dramatherapy in action

So, what might dramatherapy with someone experiencing eating difficulties look like? This section illustrates some of the ways in which dramatherapists might work to incorporate some of the ideas in this chapter into practice.

Example 1: Using space and character to direct awareness

The dramatherapist can take many roles in the therapeutic relationship, ranging from actor or director, to explorer or witness. When working with someone with an eating difficulty, the director role could be used to encourage the creative use of space to examine roles, identities, stories and our own awareness.

The dramatherapist asks the client with experience of eating difficulties to use two chairs – one where the character of the 'eating difficulty' sits, the other where a more rational, oppositional character sits.

> *The therapist encourages the client to explore the relationship between these characters by using the space – getting down on the floor to see what the space is like between the characters; to look down from above and observe the opposition between the characters; to stand on one chair, either chair, or both chairs.*
>
> *Encouraging creativity, playfulness and curiosity, the dramatherapist might encourage the client to embody each of these characters – what would the eating difficulty say to the rational-minded character? Instead of just reflecting on this, the client is encouraged to embody each character.*
>
> *Lastly, the dramatherapist might ask the client, "Which character are you?" This might help the individual to see that they identify very much with one particular role today. Or perhaps, they see themselves as the witness of the drama playing out between these competing characters, rather than the characters themselves. As a result, they may bring to light a greater awareness of the different roles they inhabit, including that of their eating difficulty.*

Example 2: Evoking and expressing embodied experience

This exercise might be used in an established group setting where trusting relationships can allow for a little experimentation.

> *The dramatherapist introduces an activity for the session – something that will evoke discomfort and reluctance amongst the group. This might be to sing the first line of a song, or in the context of eating difficulties, to eat an unplanned snack together.*
>
> *Having introduced the activity, the dramatherapist acknowledges the discomfort people seem to have. In order to focus on the embodied nature of this, the therapist asks the group to close their eyes if they wish, and to feel where in the body any sensation has arisen. Group members might be encouraged to place their hands on the sensation – to identify what they are feeling and where in the body it is felt, as well as any action tendency that arises from it. For example,*

is the experience of fear felt as a clenched stomach accompanied with a desire to escape? The dramatherapist might ask, "Does the feeling have a sound? What would that sound be?", and may encourage people to make that sound, a movement, or express the feeling to the group in another suitable way.

It turns out that there is no singing activity or snack involved in this exercise. Instead, there are the stories and feelings that people may associate with the activity, which are reflected in the body and brought to light through this exploration. Perhaps these thoughts, feelings and stories were less about the food (or singing) than was previously thought.

Example 3: Golden moments

The Sesame Approach to Dramatherapy describes the phenomena of 'golden moments' – where something that might not be in the dramatherapist's plan may just Arise in the moment, its significance requiring full presence and witnessing. One example from Mary's practice:

A client was talking about how they felt like they had no worth, no use in life, and nothing useful to offer to the world. At that moment, a spider was spotted in the therapy room and having a phobia of spiders, the dramatherapist was immediately panicked. The client, however, was extremely calm and took control of the situation – seeing the spider out of the room and reassuring the therapist. This moment that had been shared showed the disparity between the client's story of feeling profoundly useless and the reality of their agency and helpfulness to another.

Learning point 3

Having read some of the examples of dramatherapy in practice, take some time to think about the following questions:

- Are there any examples here that you might use in your personal self-enquiry? For example, is there an activity you could do in your own time to creatively explore how you are feeling?
- If you work in a professional capacity with people experiencing eating difficulties, how do you feel about these examples? How might they contrast with your therapeutic approach? Are there any ways in which you could incorporate embodiment and more creative approaches in your work?
- Are there any further questions you have arising from this chapter? How might you continue to explore this subject? Perhaps you can look into the references below, engage with your own – perhaps forgotten – playful spirit, find a local creative activity group to join, or make time to be creative at home. You are also welcome to get in touch with Mary via her website at www.lightofmind.co.uk

Conclusion

Unfortunately, the dominant treatment models currently used in understanding and responding to eating difficulties are only moderately effective (Smink *et al*, 2013; Accurso *et al*, 2020). Enhancing the efficacy of these treatments will involve many things, including greater access to timely care and refining the ability of therapies to provide individualized treatments for diverse groups of people. Part of the picture of improving care for people with eating difficulties could also be about diversifying the range of options people have when it comes to therapy, and providing embodied, indirect approaches as well.

The creative arts are, by their nature, diverse. They allow for and celebrate freedom of expression and individual uniqueness. They can be an antidote for people with eating difficulties who may have been treated in settings which have disallowed freedom or reinforced a rigid identity of what it is to experience eating difficulties. Getting 'un-stuck' from eating difficulties may, for some people, involve removing old roles and functions through physical movement; telling a new story through symbolism, myth and play; and knowing what is true for them through felt experiences as well as intellectual ones. The role of dramatherapy in supporting those with eating difficulties can involve all of these things and more.

Martha Graham, a founding figure of contemporary dance, said, "There is a vitality, a life force, an energy, a quickening that is translated through you into action… and because there is only one of you in all time, this expression is unique. And if you block it, it will never exist through any other medium and will be lost" (as quoted in De Mille, 1992, p.264). Dramatherapy recognizes our nature as energy, movement and change in human form. By working with this nature – using the language and tools of our bodies and minds – dramatherapy aims to provide a structure and relationship within which people can connect with their inner wisdom, vitality and capacity for health. Our capacity for growth, wholeness and health is *already there*, we just need to find ways to bring it to light.

References

Accurso EC, Sim L, Muhlheim L & Lebow J (2020) Parents know best: Caregiver perspectives on eating disorder recovery. *International Journal of Eating Disorders* **53** (8) 1252-1260.

Badth.org.uk (2021) *BADth: What is Dramatherapy?* [online] Available at: www.badth.org.uk/dramatherapy/what-is-dramatherapy (accessed October 2021).

Brooke SL (Ed) (2008) *The Creative Therapies and Eating Disorders*. Charles C Thomas Publisher.

Butler C (2018) Billy's Drum: Feet and Rhythm in Sesame Therapeutic Practice. *Dramatherapy* **39** (2) 63-75.

De Mille A (1992) *Martha: The life and work of Martha Graham.* Vintage.

Diamond A (2013). Executive functions. *Annual review of psychology* **64** 135–168. https://doi.org/10.1146/annurev-psych-113011-143750.

Downs J (2021) Wellbeing in the body: yoga and movement in recovery from eating disorders. *Clinical Psychology Forum* **343** 22-26).

Fairburn CG (2008) *Cognitive behaviour therapy and eating disorders*. Guilford Press.

Hanna T (2004) Somatics: Reawakening the Mind's Control of Movement, Flexibility, and Health. Cambridge, MA: De Capo Press.

Hougham R & Jones B (2017) *Dramatherapy: Reflections and Praxis*. Macmillan International Higher Education.

Jung CG (1960) *The structure and dynamics of the psyche. Collected works: Vol. 8*. Trans. RFC Hull. Princeton: Princeton University Press.

Loutsis A, Hougham R & Jones B (2017) Body, movement and trauma. *Dramatherapy: Reflections and praxis* 145-168.

Monteleone AM, Monteleone P, Esposito F, Prinster A, Ruzzi V, Canna A & Maj M (2019) The effects of childhood maltreatment on brain structure in adults with eating disorders. *The World Journal of Biological Psychiatry* **20** (4) 301-309.

Pearson J (1996) *Discovering the self. Discovering the Self through Drama and Movement, The Sesame Approach*, London: Jessica Kingsley Publishers.

Piran N & Teall T (2012) The developmental theory of embodiment. In: G McVey, H B Ferguson, M Levine, & N Piran (Eds), Improving the prevention of eating disorders: Collaborative research, advocacy, and policy change pp169-198. Waterloo, Ontario, Canada: Wilfred Laurier Press.

Rose MA (1988) *Marx's lost aesthetic: Karl Marx and the visual arts*. Cambridge Univer-sity Press.

Royal Central School of Speech & Drama (2021). *Drama and Movement Therapy, MA* [online] Available at: www.cssd.ac.uk/courses/drama-and-movement-therapy-ma (accessed October 2021).

Smink FR, van Hoeken D & Hoek HW (2013) Epidemiology, course, and outcome of eating disorders. *Current Opinion in Psychiatry* **26** (6) 543-548.

Van der Kolk B (2014) *The body keeps the score: Mind, brain and body in the transformation of trauma.* Penguin UK.

Wood LL & Schneider C (2015) Setting the stage for self-attunement: Drama therapy as a guide for neural integration in the treatment of eating disorders. *Drama Therapy Review* **1** (1) 55-70.

37. Dance in the treatment of eating difficulties

By Lilian Prince

Summary

This chapter explores the relevance and possible therapeutic benefits of dance for people experiencing eating difficulties. The role of dance more generally as a way of experiencing the body, interacting socially and obtaining exercise, is explored, before focusing specifically on Dance and Movement Therapy (DMT) as a structured method of using dance to improve wellbeing. Alongside theoretical explanations of the mechanisms by which DMT might work to help people with eating difficulties, this chapter attempts to bring theory to life with examples of how this might work in practice. The learning points offer a chance to reflect on what you've learnt about the subject as well as suggesting some practical activities which you may like to try. The chapter aims to illustrate how the deep-rooted human experience of dance may offer an alternative way of working therapeutically with the body, and how this could offer hope and healing for people experiencing eating difficulties.

Introduction

Humans have used dance throughout history for several reasons, which include entertainment purposes, visual storytelling or as a means to keep healthy. Dance has roots in cultures all over the world: for example, the Chinese dragon dance, the Viennese waltz, and Brazilian Samba dancing (Starquest, 2021). The universal nature of dance means that it is bound to have benefits that exceed the traditional purposes of entertainment and storytelling. One of these supposed benefits is that dance can be used in a therapy setting to improve symptoms of mental health (Goodtherapy, 2018).

This therapeutic use of dance has been used to reduce symptoms of anxiety, improve mood in depression, and aid socialization in individuals with autism (Goodtherapy, 2018). Dance therapy, along with other creative therapies, have recently received interest since more traditional therapies continue to have ever growing waiting lists (Smith *et al*, 2018). Creative therapies could allow for patients to receive treatment while waiting for these traditional therapies.

What is dance therapy?

Dance therapy, otherwise known as Dance and Movement Therapy (DMT), was pioneered by Marian Chace, Mary Whitehouse and Trudy Schoop in the mid-20th century (ADMPUK, 2013). From there, several associations sprung up globally dedicated to the upkeep of professional standards within the dance therapy community. These associations include, but are not limited to, the Association of Dance and Movement Psychotherapy (ADMP)[1] in the UK, the Indian Association of Dance and Movement Therapy (IADMT)[2], and the American Dance Therapy Association (ADTA)[3]. There are thousands of licensed therapists and even more clients registered to these groups.

Dance therapy is described by the ADMP as an 'empathic creative process' that uses 'body movement and dance to assist the integration of emotional, cognitive, physical, social and spiritual aspects of life' (ADMPUK, 2013). In order to aid the participant/s, the therapist first needs to know whether they are working with an individual or a group. Secondly, the therapist needs to know of any specific difficulties the participant might be experiencing in order to determine how to target the therapy, so that it suits the individual needs of their client.

There are several ways that the therapist can tailor the therapy. First of all, the movement used in dance acts as a language between the participant and therapist, which the therapist will assess along with the participant's general body language, their non-verbal behaviours as well as their emotional expressions. Once these general assessments have been established, the therapist can use more specific dance therapy techniques, like mirroring or movement metaphors. Mirroring is when a therapist echoes or matches the participant's movements to imitate and portray empathy (Goodtherapy, 2018). Movement metaphors suggest that movement can be used to form a symbolic bridge between internal feelings and external experiences (Goodtherapy, 2018).

These activities, along with the fact that dance therapy works on improving the connection that an individual has with their body, seem to provide a good basis for dance therapy as a potential treatment for a range of eating difficulties.

---

1 www.admp.org.uk

2 https://iadmt.org/

3 www.adta.org

Learning point 1

Having read a little about the aims and methods of DMT, take a moment to consider your initial thoughts and responses. You might like to reflect on your experiences of movement and dance, and how that might relate to any personal or professional experiences of living with or supporting those with eating difficulties.

- Do you share the view that body movement and dance can 'assist the integration of emotional, cognitive, physical, social and spiritual aspects of life'?
- Have you had any positive or negative experiences of dance and movement yourself?
- In what ways do you think using dance and movement might be challenging for someone with an eating difficulty? What barriers might be encountered and what might that say about the relationship with the body?
- What might need to be considered when tailoring dance and movement therapies for someone with an eating difficulty?

If you wish, you could try this practical exercise to explore the relationship between movement, mirroring and empathy:

When you next see a trusted friend, try mirroring their movements. You can choose to tell them beforehand, or not!

- What happens when you reflect their patterns of movement?
- How does mirroring your friend change the interaction you have with them, what you notice about them, and how you feel?

How does dance therapy work?

There are a few theories as to why dance therapy could be beneficial to those experiencing eating difficulties. Key among these are the roles of embodiment, social interactions and exercise.

Embodiment

The psychological concept of embodiment is particularly important to consider when applying dance therapy to those with eating difficulties. However, we first need to establish exactly what embodiment is, and how it might be involved.

Embodiment can best be described as a combination of both the physical and mental processes which allow for an awareness of an individual's own body (Varga *et al*, 2018). However, there are variations in how embodiment is defined by researchers. Launeunu & Kwee (2018, as cited in Perey & Cook-Cottone, 2020) describe embodiment simply as the holistic experience of mind, body and spirit. These experiences can range from positive to negative and form the basis of our relationship with our embodied selves. On the other hand, Piran (2019, as cited by Perey & Cook-Cottone, 2020) suggests that amongst women and girls specifically, a healthy 'embodied experience' is composed of five elements. These include having agency over their body, as well as feeling comfortable in their connection to their body.

Though these descriptions differ, they agree that embodiment is the evolving experience of connection with one's own body. This explanation is particularly important when considering embodiment in the context of eating difficulties. A key diagnostic criterion for some diagnosable eating disorders is that the individual has a disturbance in the experience of their weight and/or body shape (APA, 2013). If dance therapy can improve an individual's embodiment, in theory it should be able to improve this aspect underpinning some eating difficulties.

Learning point 2

Before reading further, take a moment to reflect on the idea of embodiment, and consider the following questions:

- What does embodiment mean to you, if anything?
- Think about how experiences of being in a body might be shaped by experiences of eating difficulties, and vice versa. How might experiences of the body influence eating difficulties, and how might eating difficulties influence the way the body is experienced?

Try this practical exercise to explore the idea of embodied states a little more deeply. Be mindful not to push too deeply into any painful memories you may have, and feel free to leave this exercise if it feels too uncomfortable.

A "negative" embodied state

Bring to mind a simple example of a particular event when you felt 'bad' – this could be something very simple such as forgetting something and feeling embarrassed, or a time you felt annoyed or angry with someone. Think about the following questions:

- What is the feeling that is conjured in the body? Do you have a name for the emotion?
- How does this feeling manifest in the way that you move? Does it make you hold the body in a particular way? Where do you feel the feeling in your body?
- Is there any tension, impulse or direction to the feeling? Is it linked to movement? For example, does your feeling in the body bring about a desire to make yourself small, disappear, run away, lash out?
- What would a dance based on this feeling look like?
- Could you try making some simple movements – even with your hands or arms – that might represent or express this feeling?

Repeat this exercise for a 'positive' embodied state. Maybe you can remember a time when you felt at ease, held, or joyful. Think about the questions above in relation to this experience, too.

Social inclusion

Dance therapy can take place in a group setting, allowing a social component to be incorporated into the therapy. Socialization can be an important tool in any treatment, fostering a sense of reintegration with others, and belonging. Eating difficulties are often experienced as isolating, involving withdrawal from friends and family, especially in settings where food and eating have prominence. This can be as a result of specifically challenging eating behaviours as well as the presence of social stigma surrounding eating difficulties which can reinforce feelings of shame (Rotenberg *et al*, 2013). Humans need to have social interaction to function in a healthy way. The social aspect of dance therapy could help those with eating difficulties in this important dimension of life.

Exercise benefits

There is already a well-established link between exercise and mental wellbeing. Two popular theories behind this are the release of endorphins into the brain (the happy chemicals responsible for what is known as 'runner's high') and the 'thermodynamic hypothesis', which suggests that the increase in body temperature after exercise contributes to a decrease in levels of anxiety (Mikkelsen *et al*, 2007). However, a lot of research suggests that this improvement refers to the symptoms of depression and anxiety, and is not specific to experiences of eating difficulties.

Furthermore, eating difficulties may in part involve a dysfunctional relationship with exercise, where exercise becomes a means to lose weight rather than a route to improved health. This type of weight loss behaviour is seen in the general population to an extent, but becomes problematic when used as a compensatory behaviour for a normal or restrictive calorie intake. Where exercise is compulsive, significant distress may Arise when someone is unable to complete their exercise regime. Because of this, a lot of treatment plans for eating difficulties tend to steer clear of exercise all together.

However, recent studies have looked into whether exercise abstinence is actually the best course of action, and whether the supported reintroduction of exercise might be a more helpful approach for people recovering from eating difficulties (Quesnel *et al*, 2018). This is where dance therapy comes in. Dance therapy could be integrated into an exercise programme, as suggested by Quesnel *et al* (2018) to help establish or re-establish a positive relationship with movement.

Dance and movement therapy in practice

Obtaining these therapeutic benefits starts in the context of DMT with establishing an alliance between the therapist and the person experiencing eating difficulties. The therapeutic relationship would be established through the use of exercises such as 'mirroring'. In the first session, the therapist would first work with the individual to examine the role of exercise in maintaining their eating difficulty, and to consider how to individually tailor any treatment to meet their needs and preferences. During this session they may also assess the individual in terms of their body language and their emotional expressions. Further sessions may introduce more exercises, emotional and physical depending on the therapist's initial assessment of their client.

These dance therapy sessions could then form the basis of a re-introduction to gentle exercise. The therapist might organize their therapy sessions based on the similarities of eating behaviours or thought processes between the clients. This may ease the clients into the social side of the therapy, whilst also tackling their issues at the same time/with their peers. The dance therapist themselves provides a safe space for the individual to rediscover movement in a healthy and constructive way, and is able to assess whether the use of movement is helpful or where it might become problematic or an unsuitable activity for supporting recovery

This is a generalization of how dance therapy may work, and may not apply to all individuals taking part in DMT.

Conclusion

While researchers and dance therapy practitioners are optimistic about the benefits of using DMT with people experiencing eating difficulties, there is still some resistance to actively involving exercise in clinical settings. This is partly as a result of the distrust that can Arise around behaviours that may be involved in maintaining an eating difficulty, which may sometimes be used covertly (Quesnel *et al*, 2018).

However, the therapeutic benefits of dance as demonstrated in this chapter may be highly relevant in offering an alternative way of exploring some of these specific struggles. Exploring embodied experiences, creative movement and dance within structured context has been shown to help in addressing distortions of bodily experience and difficult relationships with exercise. Whilst research focussing on using dance for eating difficulties is lacking at present, it is clear that dance therapy offers a promising alternative to traditional therapies in this area and can support people as they move through recovery.

Learning point 3

Having read this chapter, contemplate the entirety of what you have learnt about the role of dance in the treatment of eating difficulties. Perhaps some parts seemed irrelevant to you, and others sparked your curiosity. Whatever perspective you are approaching this chapter from, you might want to consider the following questions in your reflection:

- What are your overall thoughts about the possible value of Dance and Movement Therapy?
- Do you recognise the components of eating difficulties discussed here that dance might be used to help with? These include tackling social isolation; improving awareness of embodied states; reformulating relationships with exercise, self-perception, and the body more generally?
- What might you do differently as a result of reading this chapter, be that in your personal life or professional practice? Is there anything you will try and keep in mind, or anything you might try in practice?

References

ADMPUK (2013) Home [Online] Available at: www.admp.org.uk (Accessed December 2020)

American Psychological Association (2013) Diagnostic and statistical manual of mental disorders (Fifth Edition) Arlington, VA

Good Therapy (2018) Dance/Movement therapy (DMT) [Online] Available at: www.goodtherapy.org (Accessed December 2020)

Mikkelsen K, Stojanovska L, Potenakovic M, Bosevski M & Apostolopoulos V (2017) Exercise and mental health, *Mauritas*, **106**, 48-56.

Perey I & Cook-Cottone C (2020) Eating disorders, embodiment, and yoga: a conceptual overview. *Eating disorders: The journal of treatment & prevention*, **28**(4), 315-329.

Quesnel DA, Libben M, Oelke ND, Clark MI, Willis-Stewart S & Caperchione CM (2018) Is abstinence really the best option? Exploring the role of exercise in the treatment and management of eating disorders. *Eating disorders: The journal of treatment & prevention*, **26**(3), 290-310.

Rotenberg KJ, Bharathi C, Davies H & Finch T (2013) Bulimic symptoms and the social withdrawal syndrome. *Eating behaviors*, **14**, 281-284.

Smith J, Kyle RG, Daniel B & Hubbard G (2018) Patterns of referral and waiting times for specialist child and adolescent mental health services. *Child and adolescent mental health*, **23**, 41-49.

Starquest (2021) Ten dances around the world [Online] Available at: www.starquestdance.com (Accessed January 2021)

Varga S (2018) Embodied concepts and mental health. *Journal of medicine & philosophy*, **43**, 241-260.

38. Equine facilitated psychotherapy and eating difficulties: An embodied, relational approach

By Dr Danielle Mills

Summary

This chapter will discuss what Equine Facilitated Psychotherapy (EFP) is and why we work therapeutically with horses, before discussing the theoretical rationale for this work with eating difficulties.

Research suggests that clinical practice may be improved by incorporating a focus on sensory experiences – this is where our four-legged companions come in. Embodied awareness through EFP supports an increase in the way clients experience and interpret their understanding of that they are doing, and how they are doing it (proprioception, neuroception and interoception – these terms will be defined later in the chapter). This helps us to explore and understand how these sensory experiences contribute to clients' experiences and is a way to provide novel interpretations for the motivations underlying frequently associated patterns in eating difficulties.

Practice examples will be provided in this chapter as a means of demonstrating ways in which theory can be applied to practice.

What is Equine Facilitated Psychotherapy?

EFP involves working alongside a horse or horses as a part of the therapeutic treatment team. Being with horses promotes different ways of thinking, being and relating. This helps clients to explore alternative ways of relating to their somatic (bodily) selves, others, and the world.

The principles that apply to building a relationship with horses can be translated into healthy human relationships. The non-judgemental response of the horse can make it easier for clients to identify and examine how they create those same patterns in relationship with themselves and with others, thus helping to support the client to take positive steps in how they relate to other people.

The three key principles of the HERD approach (Lac, 2017) within which I work are:

- **Here and Now:** our ability to remain in the moment in a fully embodied way. This includes both our internal (interoceptive) and external (exteroceptive) awareness. As practitioners, it is our job to support and explore the client's awareness of self, other and their environment. By supporting the client to stay in the here and now, we can support them to connect their cognitive and embodied awareness.
- **What and How:** is based on the philosophical concept of phenomenology. As practitioners, we seek to understand the client's experience without interpreting it. This allows the client to explore and make their own meaning from each experience.
- **I and Thou:** relates to Buber's (1965) concept of the moment of connection between self and other and the more objectified I-It relationship. The HERD approach focuses on the movement between these moments of connection and attending to the embodied nature of these encounters for all involved.

Learning point 1

- Working with horses and outside in nature allows for an embodied experience and exploration of the client's relationship with the self, other and environment.
- This allows for safe and contained experimentation of alternative ways of being.

It is important to note that there are differing approaches, belief systems, methods and acronyms that describe and define what, how, and why EFP is a valuable process for different populations (Hallberg, 2008). There is not scope in this chapter to address the different approaches and benefits of each of these; thus, the focus will be on the modality used by myself, the writer.

Reflection point 1

Before reading further you might like to consider the following questions:

- What might it be like working with more than one 'therapist' (with a horse as one such therapist) within a therapeutic relationship?
- What might be the barriers to working alongside horses in a therapeutic space?
- How might you address these barriers?

Why horses?

As animals who have evolved as prey, horses are highly attuned to their environment in order to sense potential sources of danger (Karol, 2007). They perceive the world very differently to humans. Horses possess a keen sense of smell, hearing, and sight, and have often been described as highly attuned to emotional cues of others in their environment (Brandt, 2004). A horse can detect a human's emotional state, intentions and needs immediately by reading a human's body language and 'energy' (Gehrke, 2010).

Working with horses involves a different type of communication and connection than humans may be typically used to (Sharpe & Strong, 2015). Just like humans, a horse demonstrates their emotions with changes in their body language; these changes are often more obvious in horses than humans, however, thanks to their large size.

Whilst their past experiences play a part in how horses interact with the world, they also appear to live in the moment more than humans who often find themselves telling stories about the past or future. This natural preference can potentially reduce the amount of bias and projection in the human-equine therapeutic relationship and create a non-judgmental space for the client to explore sensations, thoughts, and feelings (Ford, 2013).

Reflection point 2

- Before you continue reading, think about your own experience of spending time with non-human animals and the benefits you might have gained from this.
- How do you communicate with non-human animals and how difficult or easy is this?
- How could you increase your connection to non-human animals and nature in your life? What might the barriers be to this? And the benefits?

The theory behind working with eating difficulties through EFP

The model within which I work is an integrative one that takes a relational approach to the treatment of eating difficulties. The integration of Gestalt therapeutic theory can be applied to address two of the main processes that are involved in the development and maintenance of eating difficulties – the mind-body connection and relational processes (Lac *et al*, 2013). The relational element of the treatment is based on the theory that relationships are integral to the development and maintenance of body image, weight and eating concerns (Ambwani & Strauss, 2007; Jackson *et al*, 2005).

Clients with eating difficulties often experience a schism wherein the body is experienced as being separate from the mind, including a divide between thoughts and feelings (Lac *et al*, 2013). An awareness of this schism, and an attempt at integration, can support the client to increase their awareness of the process by which they make or break connection with themselves and others (Lac *et al*, 2013). This relates closely to the sensory elements of proprioception (perception of the position and movement of the body); neuroception (whether situations/people are safe, dangerous, or life threatening); and interoception (an understanding and feeling of what is going on inside one's body, as well as regulating this).

Interruptions within sensory processes may contribute to some of the pathology around eating difficulties through links to hunger and satiety, risk prediction errors, emotional awareness and body dysmorphia (Jacquemot & Park, 2020). Research has suggested that the pursuit of a low body weight and eating difficulties may be motivated, in part, by a desire to alter the experience of being in the body, rather than just by how it looks and is desired to look (Cserjesi *et al*, 2010; Sachdev *et al*, 2008; Zucker *et al*, 2013). The inclusion of sensory experiences in EFP supports the client to recontextualise sensation and how they respond to sensory information.

Learning point 2

- EFP with eating difficulties can support integration between body and mind, and support with related sensory issues.
- The exploration of sensory issues allows for an alternative conceptualisation of body image issues that may support the client to work a way that does not foreground cognitive issues.

Practice example one: proprioception activities

Activities exploring proprioception can support recovery from eating difficulties by providing a way into connecting cognitive and embodied processes through awareness of both internal and external experience and awareness. This can support the client in building awareness of where they externalize emotional difficulties by inscribing them on their bodies; this focus on body shape/size can provide a function of allowing a disconnection from cognitive processes. This supports a process of embracing the whole self through relating to another, in this case a horse. In addition, it provides a different way to consider the phenomenological experience of clients with eating difficulties.

Cally (pseudonym) was 14 years old and had experienced eating difficulties for a number of years. She had recently been in inpatient treatment for anorexia nervosa and was struggling to maintain recovery after discharge. She had tried talking therapies but had not found the cognitive focus to be helpful. Cally struggled with her awareness of her body. Breathing exercises had previously been too difficult for her and had increased rather than reduced her anxiety. Her focus on her 'fat stomach' meant that noticing her body while doing the breathing exercises was too distressing for her. While I was discussing this difficulty with her, Paddy, one of our horses, approached and placed himself in a position where his stomach was aligned with Cally's. I invited Cally to place her hands onto Paddy's abdominal region and notice the sensations. She verbalised noticing the fluffiness of Paddy's coat, the warmth beneath her hands, and the movement of his stomach. I invited Cally to notice the pattern of Paddy's breathing and to try to match her breathing with his.

This sensory experience allowed Cally to connect with the **Here and Now** in relationship with Paddy (**I and Thou**), giving her a break from some of the thoughts which plagued her general experience. The ability to incorporate appropriate touch in this way provided the opportunity for connection and healing (Chandler, 2012). This is related to the concept of co-regulation: the process mammals experience in attachment relationships whereby the presence of one enables the regulation of the other. Experiencing the felt sense of safety in relationship can set the conditions for co-regulation to occur with other humans, as well as supporting the development of self-regulation (Schlote, 2018).

After a number of sessions wherein this activity became a regular practice, I invited Cally to rest her stomach on Paddy's stomach and notice the relationship between the two. Cally was able to experience her body in relation to Paddy's. As she inhaled, Cally's stomach expanded into the space left by Paddy's stomach when he exhaled. Experiencing her stomach in relationship to this 'other' allowed Cally to feel her awareness of herself in a different way; in relation to the horse. Rather than solely focusing on the shape and size of her stomach, she could feel the horse's stomach filling up the space her exhalation left.

Practice example two: neuroception activities

Herd observation is a beneficial way for clients to watch the horses interact and practise noticing the body language they observe both in each horse and in the wider herd. It is important to remember that this is not a time to teach clients about equine behaviour and herd dynamics, but rather to facilitate an experience wherein they can explore how they make meaning from the world around them.

The size of the horses is significant here: the average horse weighs about 500kg, much bigger than a human. We need to consider safety in a wider sense, as well as the client's sense of safety around certain experiences. A simple activity to explore safety-specific neuroception can be focused around approaching a chosen horse or horses.

Steven (pseudonym) was 26 years old and had only recently realised that his thoughts, feelings and behaviour around food, weight and body image may be causing him some difficulties. Steven's relationship with the world felt unstable and he was questioning everything he knew. Steven was very aware of his internal experience but found it difficult to orientate to the external environment. When Steven felt ready, we entered the field with the horses and I invited him to notice what drew his attention, in the **Here-and-Now**, without judgment. The opportunity to be in an unfamiliar space allowed Steven to notice more of what was around him as he assessed how he felt in relation to the space that he was in, particularly around how safe he felt physically.

What I said	What Steven said	Theoretical Rationale
"I notice that all of the horses have looked up – what is that like for you?"	"My breathing has quickened, and my knees have locked – I'm scared they're going to come over."	I am exploring Steven's phenomenological experience of what I have noticed. Because Steven is more aware of his internal experience, I can draw his attention to what I might notice in the external world.
"What do you do when you're scared?"	"I don't like to feel scared – I get out of the situation. Who wants to feel scared?!"	Feeling into the body can trigger a feeling of danger for those with eating difficulties. This opportunity allows an embodied exploration of how the client experiences fear and experiment with ways to regulate around this.
"What would it be like to leave this situation now?"	"I would feel like I had failed, but it would be a bit of a relief. I prefer watching the horses from the other side of the fence."	We can learn to regulate the danger felt from body awareness through neuroception. In this case, Steven wanted to leave, and it was positive for Steven to acknowledge this need. His pattern was to ignore what his body was telling him and 'push through'. To acknowledge and address this need was significant.

To build on this, we might explore what activities would help Steven to regulate his fear (see Practice example one) and combine these activities to support him to practise this regulation in-vivo. We would plan to support Steven to try this activity in his daily life, for example with foods that made him feel scared. This would help translate the learning gained from EFP into exploring recovery behaviours.

Conclusion

In this chapter we have considered EFP in the context of eating difficulties. Working therapeutically alongside horses can provide safe opportunities for clients to explore sensory experiences in relation to themselves, others and their environment.

Working with a therapist to identify the **Here and Now**, **What and How**, and **I and Thou** can support clients to connect their cognitive and embodied awareness and to make their own meaning from each relational experience.

EFP provides an opportunity to engage clients affected by eating difficulties in a unique way. We have considered how holding the space for two simple activities can support clients to access their own embodied experience and to explore how to integrate these experiences into their recovery from eating difficulties. By facilitating these activities phenomenologically through EFP, the client can begin to make their own meanings and expand and deepen their relationship with the world beyond their eating struggles.

References

Ambwani S & Strauss J (2007) Love thyself before loving others? A qualitative and quantitative analysis of gender differences in body image and romantic love. *Sex Roles* **56** 13-21.

Brandt T (2004) A Language of Their Own: An Interactionist Approach to Human-Horse Communication. *Society & Animals* **12** (4) 299-316.

Buber M (1965) *Between man and man* (Trans Smith RG). New York, NY, USA: Routledge Classics

Chandler CK (2012) *Animal assisted therapy in counseling* (second edition). New York, NY, USA: Routledge Taylor and Francis.

Cserjesi R, Vermeulen N, Luminet O, Marechal C, Nef F, Simon Y & Lenard L (2010) Explicit vs. implicit body image evaluation in restrictive anorexia nervosa. *Psychiatry Research* **175** (1-2) 149-153.

Hallberg L (2008) *Walking the way of the horse: Exploring the power of the horse–human relationship.* Bloomington, IN, USA: iUniverse, Inc.

Jackson T, Weiss, KE, Lunquist JJ & Soderlind A (2005) Sociotropy and perceptions of interpersonal relationships as predictors of eating disturbances among college women: two prospective studies. *The Journal of Genetic Psychology* **166** 346-359.

Jacquemot AMMC & and Park R (2020) The role of interoception in the pathogenesis and treatment of anorexia nervosa: a narrative review. *Frontiers in Psychology* **11** (98) 281-289.

Karol J (2007) Applying a traditional individual psychotherapy model to equine-facilitated psychotherapy (EFP): Theory and method. *Clinical Child Psychology and Psychiatry* **12** (1) 77–90.

Lac V (2017) *Equine-Facilitated Psychotherapy and Learning: The Human-Equine Relational Development (HERD) Approach*. New York, NY, USA: Academic Press.

Lac V, Marble E & Boie I (2013) Equine-assisted Psychotherapy as a creative relational approach to treating clients with eating disorders. *Journal of Creativity in Mental Health* **8** 484-498.

Sachdev P, Mondraty N, Wen W & Gulliford W (2008) Brains of anorexia nervosa patients process self-images differently from non-self images: an fMRI study. *Neuropsychalgia* **30** (31) 2161-2168.

Schlote S (2018) Integrating Somatic Experiencing® and Attachment into Equine-Assisted Trauma Recovery. In K Trotter & J Baggerly (eds) *Equine-Assisted Mental Health for Healing Trauma* pp3-18. New York, NY, USA: Routledge.

Sharpe H & Strong T (2015). *Embodied relating and transformation: tales from equine-facilitated counselling*. Rotterdam, NL: Sense Publishers.

Zucker NL, Merwin RM, Bulik CM, Moskovich A, Wildes J & Groh J (2013) Subjective experience of sensation in Anorexia Nervosa. *Behaviour Research and Therapy* **51** (5) 256-265.

39. The role of music and music therapy in recovery from eating difficulties

By Dr Jennifer Bibb

Summary

Music is an integral part of people's lives and is regularly used to influence emotional states and facilitate healthy coping. This level of existing engagement with music and the accessibility of music in people's lives provides a platform for music therapists to connect with people experiencing eating difficulties. Music therapy is used internationally in clinical treatment settings for eating disorders, which is indicative of both the needs of patients and of professional advocacy for creative approaches to recovery.

Research provides evidence for the effectiveness of music therapy in significantly reducing anxiety after meals, and for managing distress for people experiencing eating difficulties. Case studies derived from people's lived experience of eating difficulties have depicted feelings of increased emotional expression, expression of identity, improved self-esteem, connection, and feelings of empowerment through music therapy participation.

This chapter will describe the role of music and music therapy in recovery as well as best-practice music therapy approaches, using the latest international research and voices of people with lived experience. These approaches are in no way representative of all the ways music can be used to promote wellbeing, nor the extent of the methods that music therapists use across their work. Instead, they provide some interesting insights for those with eating difficulties and a way to begin reflecting on your own use of music for wellbeing.

Acknowledgements

The content of this chapter is influenced by my experience of working in the Australian healthcare system for over ten years, in hospital and community-based contexts. I have had the privilege of collaborating with people experiencing eating difficulties by using music. As someone without lived experience of eating difficulties myself, I acknowledge that the content in this chapter has been informed by people brave enough to share their lived experience with me (and you). I hope to share their stories with sensitivity and respect. All case studies have been shared with written consent.

Music therapy research

Music therapy is an evidence-based allied health profession in which university-trained music therapists use targeted techniques to improve quality of life, health and wellbeing. Music therapy methods can be used in group or individual contexts and include structured and unstructured (active) live musical activities such as music improvisation, song writing and therapeutic singing techniques; or receptive methods such as lyric analysis and music-supported counselling. For example, a music therapist may use receptive methods like music listening to help someone develop a coping playlist for regulating their mood during challenging times. Or they could use active methods like singing and playing guitar or piano to adapt live musical elements in the moment with that person, changing the volume, speed, texture of the music to suit their physical and emotional needs.

Research supports the use of music therapy in the treatment of eating difficulties and has been shown to significantly reduce anxiety related to mealtimes (Bibb *et al*, 2019; Bibb *et al*, 2015), increase motivation for treatment and improve mood (Hilliard, 2001), improve self-esteem and feelings of empowerment (McFerran *et al*, 2006; Pavlakou, 2009) and increase connection with peers (Bibb *et al*, 2016).

It is important to note that there are different levels of music engagement for health. Many people can use music to promote their wellbeing without the need for a music therapist. Music is often suggested by mental health professionals as a way for people with eating difficulties to support their mood management, provide a means of distraction, or facilitate relaxation. Input from a music therapist can be necessary if a person has difficulty processing and/or communicating their emotions or experiences verbally, and/or if they need to learn in more detail how to use music to manage their mood effectively. Experience and skill in music is not necessary to participate in music therapy, but people may find their interest or previous experience in music acts as a motivator.

Before you continue reading, take a moment to think about your own experiences with music.

Learning point 1

- Think of an image in your head (or you can draw/paint it) that reflects your most positive memory of engaging with music – this could be listening to, playing, singing or writing music. Why was it a positive experience?
- How would you describe your relationship with music? Has your relationship with music changed over time?
- If you or your loved one is experiencing eating difficulties, does your/their relationship with music change in response to these? How so?

Music listening for healthy coping

An important role for music therapists supporting people with eating difficulties is helping them to understand and use the potential of music outside of therapy. For people already strongly engaged with music, it can be an important tool to modulate their emotional states, and cope with distress or anxiety. One client I worked with described coping with sad feelings by putting negative or sad emotions 'into' the music they were listening to and feeling a sense of relief. In this way, music can be used to self-medicate, regulate emotion, and manage one's mood in everyday life.

Research shows, however, that people who already have difficulty regulating their emotions may use music in ways that are not always helpful and can negatively impact their mood and mental state (McFerran & Saarikallio, 2014; McFerran *et al*, 2014). For example, one person I worked with described to me that they knew a certain song could bring up negative emotions for them, but they would listen to it anyway when they were feeling unwell. Unfortunately, in some cases, people using music in this way are unaware of the choices they make in that moment. Music therapists can therefore support people to develop awareness of how and when to use music as a healthy and helpful strategy for coping, and how to recognize the need to change songs or playlists.

Learning point 2

Before reading further, you may like to consider the following questions or ask them of your loved one living with eating difficulties.

- Do you listen to music to support your wellbeing?
- Have you ever made specific playlists to help you to feel a certain way, such as music for relaxing, music for feeling positive? Have these been helpful or unhelpful?

Sharing stories through songwriting

Writing songs about life experiences can be helpful whether it is done alone, in a group, or with a supporting person. In music therapy, we use songwriting as a way to help clarify people's thoughts and feelings, identify their sense of self, share a story and find meaning in their experiences (among many other things) (Baker *et al*, 2008; Baker & Wigram, 2005; Baker, 2015). Figure 39.1 is an excerpt of a song written by a group of women living with eating difficulties who were participating in outpatient therapy and attending music therapy with me. They wanted to write a song about their experience of recovery – not just the positive elements, but the negative aspects too. With my facilitation and gentle questioning of their experience, we worked on creating lyrics over a few sessions and then composed the music in the next few sessions. Then we sang the song together using my guitar to play the melody, and recorded it onto a CD.

There are endless possibilities as we choose to tread this path
But the road is new and colourful, new strength in the aftermath
Of course it's not so easy, we have been fighting to get this far
Confronting all our demons, in this daily mental war

Recovery is re-discovery
Recovery is re-discovery
Recovery is uncomfortable, not the myths you hear online

In this fight you must be willing to take the first step out,
To find your path away from just existing in this doubt
Pulling out the weeds, within us finding hope,
We are warriors fighting every day, learning to cope

Figure 39.1. Excerpt from 'Recovery song'

You can see from the lyrics of this song that there is a depiction of the challenges of recovery, but also of strength and hope for the future. Writing a song about one's experience of eating difficulties can help to explore thoughts and feelings in a different and sometimes deeper way than can be achieved in verbal therapies. Songs can also be a form of communication, providing a representation of one's experiences which can be shared with loved ones or healthcare professionals. This can be especially useful if the person is unable to talk verbally about elements of their experience.

Learning point 3

Take a moment to reflect on how you relate to songs.

- Is there a special song or poem you connect strongly to?
- Is there a song that holds a special memory for you? How does that song make you feel?

Music-making and creativity

When reflecting on your most positive experience with music earlier in this chapter, you may have identified a time when you made music yourself in some way, for example by singing, playing in a band, or playing an instrument. There are certainly health benefits associated with making music, and this is especially the case when making music in groups. Playing music is commonly used by music therapists to support people to explore a part of themselves or their identity that eating difficulties may have 'closed off'.

However, it is important to acknowledge the potential for engaging with music to be anxiety-provoking and uncomfortable for people with eating difficulties. Playing music without technical proficiency or with very little experience requires a certain level of vulnerability. It may evoke a fear of 'feeling' or 'sitting with' emotions that clients do not want to be or are not ready to be confronted with (Eschen, 2002). There may be a feeling of resistance towards being creative due to this need to be vulnerable or facing the unknown that being creative may represent. This may be particularly relevant for people with eating difficulties if they have experiences of feeling emotionally 'numb' (Schmidt & Treasure, 2006).

I have noticed the intensity that singing can bring to music therapy sessions with clients. Our voices are an expression of our identity which makes it difficult to hide ourselves or our imperfections. In a group setting, singing can be a genuine gesture of authenticity and sharing a part of yourself. This gesture has the potential to accelerate and deepen the therapeutic relationship and can sometimes lead clients to express their thoughts and feelings with others for the first time. Or, if the client is not ready to experience this kind of intimacy, it can create further resistance and space between us.

One young person once told me that hearing me sing was uncomfortable for her as it felt "too real", "too exposing" and "too close". She had spent many years avoiding her emotions and intimate relationships. She expressed a fear of singing in sessions, despite having sung in choirs when she was a child. She described an intense sense of fear and shame around expressing herself this way and believed she wasn't 'good enough' to be heard by others. We later explored that this was tied to her belief that her body was also not good enough to be seen. Seeing and hearing others express themselves and show their vulnerability through creativity was scary and uncomfortable for her, as it showed her what she was not able to confront in herself. Over time, she was able at first to sit with the discomfort of sharing a space with someone who was expressing their creativity, and then slowly reveal a little more of her own creativity by humming with me, then singing with me, and then singing alone while I played guitar.

Learning point 4

Take a moment to reflect on your own beliefs around being creative.

- Are you comfortable with making music, even if this is something you are not skilled in?
- Do you remember a time when you did feel comfortable making music? What did that feel like?
- What would it be like to feel uncomfortable and try a new way of being creative? Would there be anything to gain?

Closing thoughts

This chapter has explored the role of music and music therapy during treatment for and recovery from eating difficulties. We learnt that listening to music can be an important tool for modulating emotional states, and coping with distress and anxiety. In some cases, it is important that listening to music is supported and carefully guided to ensure it is always a healthy strategy. The chapter also explored songwriting and how it can help people to explore their thoughts and feelings in a different way. Last, we explored the potentials of making music, and the challenges of being vulnerable through creativity for people experiencing eating difficulties. The potentials for music in supporting health and wellbeing are far-reaching and certainly more diverse than we have explored in this chapter, but I encourage you to continue reflecting on your own experiences with music and the role it plays in your life.

Key resources

www.austmta.org.au/journal – Australian Journal of Music Therapy is a freely available Australian online academic journal

www.voices.no – Voices: A World Forum for Music Therapy is a freely available international online academic journal

www.tuneyourmood.com – A music based e-platform supporting young people to use music to tune their mood

www.rmtschangelives.com.au/case-studies - Case studies/videos of music therapy

References

Baker F (2015) *Therapeutic Songwriting: Developments in Theory, Methods and Practice*. New York: Palgrave Macmillan.

Baker F & Wigram T (Eds) (2005) *Song writing: Methods, Techniques and Clinical Applications for Music Therapy Clinicians, Educators and Students*. London: Jessica Kingsley Publishers.

Baker F, Wigram T, Stott D & McFerran K (2008) Therapeutic songwriting in music therapy: Part I: Who are the therapists, who are the clients, and why is songwriting used? *Nordic Journal of Music Therapy* **17** (2) 105-123.

Bibb J, Castle D & Newton R (2015) The role of music therapy in reducing post meal related anxiety for patients with anorexia nervosa. *Journal of Eating Disorders* **3** DOI:10.1186/s40337-015-0088-5.

Bibb J, Castle D & Newton R (2016) 'Circuit breaking' the anxiety: Experiences of group music therapy during supported post-meal time for adults with anorexia nervosa. *Australian Journal of Music Therapy* **27** 1–11.

Bibb J, Castle D & Skewes McFerran K (2019) Reducing anxiety through music therapy at an outpatient eating disorder recovery service. *Journal of Creativity in Mental Health*. Online first. DOI:10.1080/15401383.2019.1595804.

Eschen J Th (Ed) (2002) *Analytical Music Therapy*. London: Jessica Kingsley Publishers.

Grocke D, Bloch S & Castle D (2009) The effect of group music therapy on quality of life for participants living with a severe and enduring mental illness. *Journal of Music Therapy* **46** (2) 90-104.

Hilliard RE (2001) The use of cognitive-behavioral music therapy in the treatment of women with eating disorders. *Music Therapy Perspectives* **19** (2) 109–113. DOI:10.1093/mtp/19.2.109

Kooij CV (2009) Recovery themes in songs written by adults living with serious mental illnesses. *Canadian Journal of Music Therapy* **15** (1) 37-58.

McFerran K, Baker F, Patton GC & Sawyer S (2006) A retrospective lyrical analysis of songs written by adolescent with anorexia nervosa. *European Eating Disorders Review* **14** 397–403. DOI:10.1002/erv.746

McFerran KS, Garrido S, O'Grady L, Grocke D & Sawyer SM (2014) Examining the relationship between self-reported mood management and music preferences of Australian teenagers. *Nordic Journal of Music Therapy* **24** (3) 187-203.

McFerran KS & Saarikallio S (2014) Depending on music to feel better: Being conscious of responsibility when appropriating the power of music. *Arts in Psychotherapy* **41** (1) 89–97. DOI:10.1016/j.aip.2013.11.007

Pavlakou M (2009) Benefits of group singing for people with eating disorders: Preliminary findings from a non-clinical study. *Approaches* **1** (1) 30–48.

Schmidt U & Treasure J (2006) Anorexia nervosa: Valued and visible. A cognitive-interpersonal maintenance model and its implications for research and practice. *British Journal of Clinical Psychology* **45** 343– 366.

Silverman MJ (2013) Effects of group song writing on depression and quality of life in acute psychiatric inpatients: A randomized three group effectiveness study. *Nordic Journal of Music Therapy* **22** (2) 131-148.

Silverman MJ (2019a) Comparing educational music therapy Interventions via stages of recovery with adults in an acute care mental health setting: A cluster-randomized pilot effectiveness study. *Community Mental Health Journal* **55** (4) 624-630.

Silverman MJ (2019b) Music therapy for coping self-efficacy in an acute mental health setting: A randomized pilot study. *Community Mental Health Journal* **55** (4) 615-623.

40. Being creative: Art and recovery from eating difficulties

By Lorna Collins

Summary

This chapter explores how art and expression can help people experiencing eating difficulties. I start with my own example. I spent nearly 20 years of my life detained in compulsory admissions at various psychiatric hospitals with a severe and enduring eating disorder. The breakthrough moment came when I began to paint how I was feeling. Painting became my go-to coping mechanism. In this chapter, I describe how art helped me during my struggle and gave me the tools to imagine, build and sustain a new life for myself. I also suggest ways in which the reader can express themselves through art to help them with their eating difficulties. The chapter ends with a practical 'mandala' exercise so, as a reader, you can experiment with your own creativities.

My story

When I was 18 years old I fell off a horse and had a severe traumatic brain injury. I was unresponsive, in a coma, and awoke with total amnesia. I had no concept or memory of who I (or anyone else) was. I developed an eating disorder in my efforts to try and take back some kind of control in a life that had become pure pain and chaos. I became very ill and went on to spend nearly 20 years of my life detained in compulsory admissions at various psychiatric hospitals across the UK and France.

I remember the moment when I began to paint my feelings. This happened spontaneously when suddenly I began to splash paint around my room on large pieces of paper placed on the floor. It was very messy but incredibly cathartic and therapeutic. I began, thus, to interpret my pain and torture: creating dashing, blurred, abstract compositions or wonky self-portraits. There seemed to be a metaphysical transition from my emotional struggles to the painting. I was never very good at drawing objects or people accurately, yet these works seemed to directly and precisely express my experience.

During this time, I would compulsively create, painting terrifying red and black images and writing reams and reams of tiny, scrawled nonsense; sometimes backwards in pidgin French, or Latin. The doctors called this 'hypographia', meaning when a person compulsively writes or makes art. I felt was the only way I could stay alive (just).

In hospital, painting eased the wounds because it allowed me to concentrate on something other than my struggles. It set me free. The abstract images I created embodied my feelings and gave me a voice.

Learning point 1

Offering art activities in in-patient and out-patient settings provides both something outside of the struggle to focus on and an outlet for emotional pain.

Sometimes, the medical team took my artworks very seriously, using them for the diagnosis and treatment of my illness. On my formal care plan, under the list of prescribed medications, the doctor simply put 'painting'. In this way, art-making was directly prescribed as medicine. When I was feeling upset or unsafe, painting was my go-to coping mechanism and support. It calmed me down. Painting gave me a voice. It enabled me to express what I couldn't put into words.

Despite the catharsis art afforded me, I remained locked within a cycle of being the 'Revolving Door Patient'. The only guarantee seemed to be relapse. The illness was a comfort. It was easier to be detained and locked up inside the hospital bubble than to 'live in the real world' (whatever that is). I became institutionalized, caught inside the yo-yo of discharge, relapse, restriction, self-harming, dramatic weight loss, suicide attempts, sectioning, admissions to acute psychiatric wards, refusal of food/water/medication (everything), rapid physical deterioration, admissions to eating disorders units for four to five months at a time, putting on a paltry amount of weight, continuing to self-harm (they made it a policy to ignore my self-harm), being discharged (disturbed and disturbingly underweight): and then the whole circuit went round again.

Finally, I learned that I did not have to be locked and detained inside this eternal, institutionalized cycle. There was a way out – not to die, but to make a new life for myself by entering a revolutionary new spectrum called recovery, which I had never dreamed of existing before.

I believe I found recovery because my art opened doors: I was able to imagine, then create, new options for myself. Difference. Eventually, after so many years of relapse, I was admitted to Cotswold House Specialist Eating Disorders Ward in Oxford. Here, I found the CBT-ED model of care: an innovative, evidence-based model of inpatient treatment which was radically different, in a positive sense, to any other treatment I had ever been exposed to. The CBT-ED model of care was inclusive and holistic; it incorporated and relieved all aspects of my eating struggles (Fairburn, 2008; Fairburn, 2013; Ayton *et al*, 2021).

In Oxford, my psychologist molded and nuanced the CBT-ED model around my individual needs, strengths and weaknesses. Interactions with members of the multi-disciplinary team and attending groups enabled me to use my art, painting and poetry to express my most difficult issues related to trauma, abuse, dissociation and amnesia. In this way it felt as though I was guiding and informing my own recovery.

Learning point 2

The CBT-ED model of care appears to work best when sensitively molded around a person's particular needs and strengths; while taking into account their creative proclivities and propensities.

The ward created a unique and extraordinary difference to my experience of being hospitalized for an eating disorder. I look back on my admission as a 'special' time: not as an experience of being ill but of learning about how to be well. I feel this was down to the team who saved me. Or, rather, they supported me and showed me how I might begin to save myself. I will always be grateful.

During this time, the butterfly became my creative symbol of hope. It helped me to have a sense that I could move from a cumbersome caterpillar, to a cramped, dark, cocoon; to a colourful, brilliant being with wings who could fly wherever she wished. My creativity gave me the motor to facilitate this remarkable transition. During treatment, the butterfly came to represent my 'survivor identity'. The butterfly then symbolised and led my whole recovery. Even now, a few years later, the butterfly still fires up my positive transformation and epitomizes the new life I lead.

These days, I use my art – painting, poetry and film – to express both my most difficult issues and also to celebrate my passion for being well and being alive. I engage creativity to manufacture a crucial coping mechanism with which I can express myself (the good bits and the bad bits). When I paint, thoughts stop and I can simply 'be' in a pure, silent moment.

Exploring our creativity

Readers may be thinking: *How can I be creative? I am not an artist. I can't paint. How does this relate to me?* I strongly advocate the fact that we are *all* artists and believe we can all access our creativities and feel the benefits of doing so. Creativity is the structure of humanity (McNiff, 2004).

> **Learning point 3**
>
> All human beings are artists. We can all access our creativities and experience the benefits of doing so.

Artmaking does not have to be about painting a Renaissance masterpiece. I, for one, have never been any good at drawing. I love art because it is not about comparing 'ability' or being 'good'. Art is the antithesis of judgement. No one can take your creativity away from you, or change it. It is *your* experience.

A good way to begin to express yourself is to keep a journal. I enjoy making collages in my journal, finding words from newspapers and making sentences or phrases I find meaningful. I enjoy writing poems, which often don't make any sense to anyone but myself. I love cooking and making up new recipes; which sometimes work, but often don't! I also often narrate my everyday life in a story, written just for me. I pretend that I am a journalist, writing a story about my experience in the present tense. I love slow, stretchy yoga (nothing too taxing). I spend a lot of time sloshing water onto pieces of paper, then sprinkling coloured pigments on top. They disperse into magical rainbows of hue, capturing my delight. These are just a few examples of my expression, my creativity, my nourishment. There are limitless ways to be creative: to feed us, to sustain us, to set us free.

> **Learning point 4**
>
> Keeping a daily creative journal is a helpful way to begin engaging in the artistic process.

When we simply express ourselves, the creative experience gives us a space to iterate, be released from and transform our struggles. This can be as simple as drawing a circle and expressing ourselves inside the boundary.

Mandala exercise

'Mandala' is the Sanskrit word for a circle. It is an ancient, sacred symbol of perfection (Tucci, 2012). The mandala can be seen in stone age cave paintings and in different cultures across the world including South Africa, Scandinavia, North America, Australia, Tibet and India. The exercise of drawing mandalas is to let our imaginations run wild and find out what happens inside of them. Working with whatever art or writing materials we can find, we simply create; using the circle as a boundary line or stimulus for our expression (Scelzo, 2018).

Materials needed: paper, round pot/cup, pencil, pen, colours (e.g. felt tips, paint, coloured pencils).

Mandalas can open geometric or organic forms. They can be a space for scribbling, colouring in, drawing a scene, or experimenting with different materials. The exercise carries meaning for the person who creates it since mandalas are said to represent the connection between our inner worlds and outer reality.

Designing your own mandala can be inspirational and therapeutic. The creation of your mandala is an echo of your soul. Psychoanalyst Carl Jung once described mandalas as "cryptograms concerning the state of the self which were presented to me anew each day. In them I saw the self – that is, my whole being – actively at work" (Jung, 1961, p239). Mandalas can be used to access and express the deeper self. The process of creating mandalas can be meditative and provide the opportunity to pause and reflect on your situation.

Here is my example of creating a mandala. You can use this as a template to create your own expressions, which can take any form (within the circle). Firstly, I draw a circle. I can do this free-hand, or with a round pot.

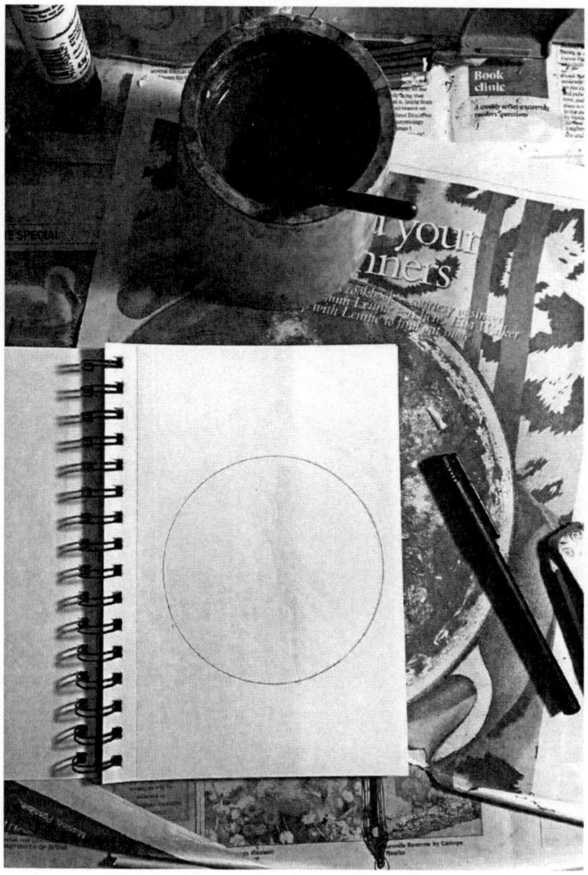

Here is my circle. Now I am going to draw something inside of it. I am not sure what this is going to look like. I choose a pencil, sharpen it, and start drawing some lines. Without intention, I let whatever appears find its way through my fingers.

I have now created a rough, basic shape. I can see I have drawn my hands, some light, a heart. It is as though light and love are flowing out of my arms and fingers. I am not sure what this means. I feel like adding colours.

I engage in some colouring in with watercolour pencils. It's still rough and not very exact. But the bold colours are sustained by my bare fingers. I enjoy the interconnection. I feel the need to add some lines and make it a bit more cohesive.

I add some ink. I am still not sure what exactly my mandala means. But I find it very relaxing to simply create in this way. I enjoy working with the materials. I enjoy the not-knowing. I have trust that whatever this picture is, it is nourishing me while I create it.

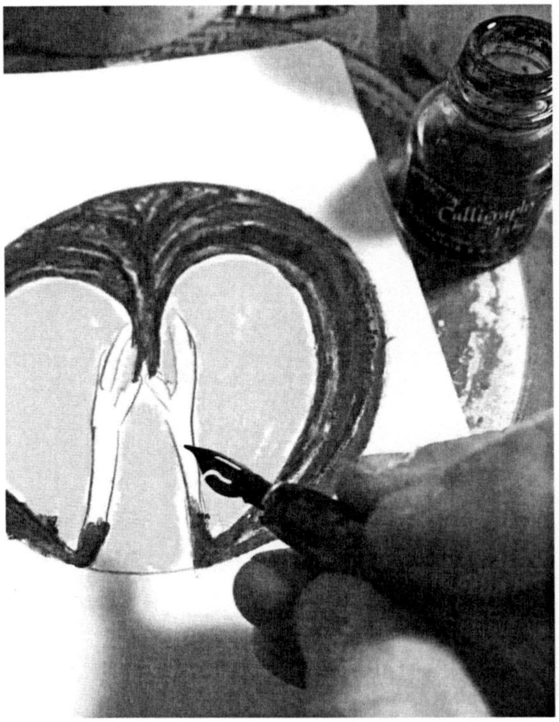

My finished mandala is still pretty rough and I still don't know what it means! But I can see something gentle and energized, connected and loved. This is what I want to be.

I am left feeling contented and uplifted. I make several more mandalas, using watercolour paints. The process of creating these pieces boosts me and sets me up for the day.

I have a 'mandala manuscript' in which I draw a circle and see what happens therein each and every day. Often, my thoughts, feelings or sensations exceed the circle and become something else. But the circle provides the starting point, the stimulus for my expression.

What next?

Being creative can provide a nourishing practice in and beyond recovery from eating difficulties (Heiderscheit, 2015; Malchiodo, 2006). Certainly, my own creativity has become the most important and valued part of my life. It has allowed me to think differently and to consider alternative ways of being. Life has become a positive, intriguing experiment which I express and narrate along my way (Collins, 2017).

Let us keep being creative! You might like to think about how you can do this. I have given several examples in this chapter. Now you can choose your own medium and style. Why not get a piece of paper and begin this process now? What first comes to mind? You could even scribble around the words and pictures in the margins of this chapter. Here is your opportunity to express yourself and find that free space. It's yours for the taking.

References

Ayton, A., Viljoen, D., Ryan, S., Ibrahim, A., & Ford, D. (2021). Risk, demand, capacity and outcomes in adult specialist eating disorder services in South-East of England before and since COVID-19. *BJPsych Bulletin*, 1-7. Available at: https://www.cambridge.org/core/journals/bjpsych-bulletin/article/risk-demand-capacity-and-outcomes-in-adult-specialist-eating-disorder-services-in-southeast-of-england-before-and-since-covid19/67D521312A8B00A9C79B846FC38103F6/share/708e4a3e167b1b35420061f8d4bf78970eb6df23 (Accessed September, 2021).

Collins L.: www.be1ngcreative.com

Collins L. (2014) *Making Sense: Art practice and transformative therapeutics*. London: Bloomsbury.

Collins L., Ayton A. & Viljoen D. (2020) Treatment for eating disorders during and after covid-19. *The British Medical Journal*. Available at: https://blogs.bmj.com/bmj/2020/08/04/treatment-for-eating-disorders-during-and-after-covid-19/ (accessed August 2021).

Fairburn C. (2008) *Cognitive Behavior Therapy and Eating Disorders*. New York: The Guilford Press.

Fairburn C. (2013) *Overcoming Binge Eating: The proven program to learn why you binge and how you can stop*. New York: The Guilford Press.

Heiderscheit A. (ed.) (2015) *Creative Arts Therapies and Clients With Eating Disorders*. London: Jessica Kingsley Publishers.

Jung C. (ed. A. Jaffé) (1961) *Memories, Dreams, Reflections*. Penguin: Vintage books.

Malchiodo C. (2006) *Art Therapy Sourcebook*. New York: McGraw Hill.

McNiff S. (2004) *Art Heals: How creativity cures the soul*. Boston: Shambhala Publishing Ltd.

Scelzo A. (2018) The Use of Mandala in the Treatment of Eating Disorders: The Journey of the Soul from the Symptom to the Symbol. *Eating Disorders Resource Catalogue*. Available at: www.edcatalogue.com/use-mandala-treatment-eating-disorders-journey-soul-symptom-symbol/ (accessed August 2021).

Tucci G. (2012) *The Theory and Practice of the Mandala*. New York: Dover Publications.

41. Writing because the page listens: Therapeutic writing to support the recovery journey

By Dr Nicole Schnackenberg

Summary

We each engage in the sense-making of our emotions and experiences in a multiplicity of ways. There are numerous potential approaches to therapeutic writing for those struggling with eating difficulties, and each is in some way embedded in the narrative therapy paradigm. In this chapter we will explore therapeutic letter writing, diary/journal writing, poetry and stories in particular, including practical approaches for insight, growth and healing.

Narrative therapy: underlying tenets

Therapeutic writing is based on the work of social workers Michael White and David Epston, the fathers of narrative therapy (Epston, 1989a; 1989b; 1991; White & Epston, 1990). A core basic assumption is that people make sense of their lives through stories, particularly the stories they tell themselves about themselves. Within the narrative therapy approach, mental health struggles are not viewed as intrinsic or essential attributes of people or relationships. Rather, mental health labels and diagnoses are seen to be part of a wider pathologising discourse or narrative, which maintain rather than resolve struggles of living.

A relationship can be drawn here between the narrative therapy approach and the recent 'Power Threat Meaning Framework' (Johnstone *et al*, 2018), which asserts that mental health struggles, including eating difficulties, are a sane response to an insane reality (Laing, 2010) based on:

- How power has operated in a person's life.
- What threat this power has posed to them.
- What meaning they have made of this threat.

When considering eating difficulties, therefore, it is vital to explore how and where the client has experienced oppression, for example through developmental trauma, abuse and/or bullying experiences. One could argue, and indeed I would, that eating difficulties are a desperate bid for survival. To understand this, we are invited to appreciate what the person is surviving against and for, including the meaning they have made of the threats posed by oppressive power differentials in their past and current experience.

Learning point 1

Consider the ways in which you and/or your client has experienced a powerful differential in your/their history i.e. through a relationship with a parent/carer, teacher, faith leader, mental health professional etc.

- What threats has this power posed to you/them?
- What meaning have you/they made of these threats?
- How may this have impacted on the narrative you/they hold about yourself/themselves?

Within a narrative frame, human struggles are viewed as arising from, and being maintained by, oppressive stories which dominate the person's life. Thus, the way the person's life is storied by themselves and others may be different, potentially leading to a confused and fragmented identity; a key aspect of eating difficulties. Therapeutic writing approaches serve to thicken the thin, oppressive narrative which has been assimilated into the person's felt sense of identity and offer fresh, rich perspectives both on their struggles and on their felt sense of self.

Examples of therapeutic writing approaches

Therapeutic letter writing

Classically, therapeutic letters are written from the therapist to the client after a therapeutic session, beginning with detailing the client's strengths and wisdom before moving onto conceptualising and reflecting on the client's situation through a non-pathologising lens. The client can be an editor in the process if wished, pointing out any aspects of the letter which do not resonate, or they would like to be altered. Thus, the letter is co-produced and the power differential reduced. Ideally, the client's words and metaphors are used within the letter to stay as close to the client's narrative as possible. The letter might contain elements of externalization (White, 2001). Externalization describes the process of viewing and therefore languaging the difficulty as outside of and separate to oneself in order to put distance between the felt sense of self and the struggle, e.g. 'when the urge to starve comes to visit' rather than 'when you starve yourself'.

Using the term coined by Lev Vygotsky, Rombach (2003) conceives of the therapeutic letter as a 'scaffold' that emerges from the client's experience and offers possible ways of moving forwards. Some therapists might focus on a 'star resource' within their letter: a particular strength of the client including scaffolding suggestions about how to potentially utilize this resource for healing. Reflective questions might be employed to support the client's thinking (and feeling) about how their inner wisdom and resources can be drawn upon to the advancement of their recovery journey, e.g. 'I wonder how you could use your capacity for compassion for others to explore possibilities for demonstrating increased compassion for yourself?' Reflective questions such as these create a space for the client to assess their inner dialogue and any underlying beliefs (Rombach, 2003), particularly beliefs about the self. Thus, the therapeutic letter can provide a means of establishing a new perspective through which to view one's experience.

Clients may choose to write a letter back to the therapist, to verbalise their response or not to make any direct response at all. A powerful aspect of the therapeutic letter is that it can be kept and re-read time and again when desired or needed, thus providing a message of strength and hope that doesn't get lost in memory in the way the spoken word may. As Rasmussen and Tomm (1992) note, "there is no other system of psychotherapy (aside from therapeutic letter writing) in which the client has so much more control over the rate, depth, and intensity of his or her personal therapeutic work" (cited in Nau, 1997, p4).

Learning point 2

Consider how you might make all aspects of the therapeutic letter process invitational, supporting the client to be an editor in the process, for example by:

- Asking the client whether therapeutic letter writing is a modality they would like to explore.
- Seeking the client's preferred way of sharing letters e.g. written, via email, and whether written letters will be received by hand, posted etc.
- Prompting clients to suggest edits to letters and welcoming any edits with openness and acceptance.
- Inviting clients to make the decision about whether they would like to reply to any letters without any sense of preference on your part or obligation.

Therapeutic letters can be used for numerous means including to reflect, summArise, validate, invite, encourage, elucidate and impassion. It would seem that the written word can be more digestible than the spoken word for some clients experiencing eating difficulties, particularly in the early stages of the struggle when inhibitions, resistance to change, shyness and trauma-related mistrust (i.e. struggling to trust others due to being chronically hurt/let down/ having to defend themselves in the past) can make absorbing the spoken word strenuous and challenging. In a world and experience that feels fraught with uncertainty, there is also something reassuring, and subtly empowering, about words on a page which tangibly exist and can be returned to, or indeed destroyed, at any moment of choosing.

Clients can also be encouraged to write their own letters for therapeutic benefit. This may include writing letters to and from a body part; writing a letter to an attachment figure; writing a letter to the self as though from an attachment figure; writing to the current self from an older, wiser self; writing to the self from the heart of one who loves them, and so on. These letters most typically remain unsent and may or may not be shared with the therapist.

One might like to consider therapeutic letters as transitional objects (Winnicott, 1953). As such, the letter supports the client in appreciating the distinction between supposition and reality, as well as separating out their sense of self from the suffering they are experiencing (O'Keefe & Berk, 2009). These letters can provide the soothing and exposition required to make emotional and experiential leaps from a felt sense of helplessness and reliance to an experience of increased independence and safety.

Diary/journal writing

Therapeutic diary writing is diametrically different to the oft-employed practice in eating difficulties treatment of keeping a food diary or similar. It provides a safe and private (if so wished) space for the person to express their emotions and emerging experience and knowledge of others and the self. The journal or diary may be written in sporadically, weekly, daily or even multiple times a day. This can offer a sense of agency: paced to the person's unique needs and desires, rather than to the needs and schedule of anyone else, such as a weekly time slot given by a therapist.

When a diary is written in regularly, it can assist the writer in developing reflective processes including reflection upon memories, frustrations, fears, anxieties and hopes (Utley & Garza, 2011). Given their personal nature, diaries allow the person the freedom to explore feelings and impressions in a safe (and typically private) place, facilitating both reflection and contemplation and acting as a 'mirror for the mind' (Utley & Garza, 2011). Pattern finding and inner analysis may emerge as part of the process.

Thus, keeping a diary or journal is a meaning-making process. It allows one to take a step back and assume the simultaneous position of observer and participant in one's life. From the observer perspective it is possible to notice rising and departing emotions, thus asserting the truth of the temporality of all experience. Charting the ebbs and flows of one's emotional experience allows the writer to gain a fresh and more distanced perspective, offering hope that disturbing emotional states can, and always somehow eventually are, moved beyond.

It may be that selected diary entries are desired to be shared with the therapist, who can then take up the role of validating the client's feelings and other inner and outer processes while supporting them to reflect upon, and possibly also re-frame, their beliefs, actions and assumptions. Self-reflexivity of the therapist is key here, encompassing the awareness of the therapist of their own life story and how this may interact with and inform any suppositions and bias they may have towards the client's journey, relationships and experiences.

Learning point 3

Self-reflexivity of the therapist is a key tenet in therapeutic writing approaches. If you are a therapist, you might like to consider:

- How you have made sense of key events in your life and what has helped you to do so.
- How your life's journey currently informs your approach as a therapist/counsellor etc.
- How your values impact on your views of, and approach to, therapeutic writing.

A criticism levelled at using approaches such as therapeutic diary writing is that of situating the client's struggles 'within person', and thereby reducing social issues to the sphere of the individual. However, many diarists have beautifully demonstrated how diaries can be successfully used as a coping tool in the face of systemic adversity (while at the same time highlighting social/political etc. aspects), which Anne Frank's (1952) mesmeric diary of hiding from the Nazis, to use just one famous example, attests to.

Poetry

Poetry has a special place in the history of healing. As Geri Geibel Chavis (2011), author of *Poetry and Story Therapy* reminds us, the shamans and medicine men and women of ancient civilizations chanted poems as part of their healing rituals, treatments and ceremonies.

When selecting poems for therapeutic purposes, Chavis (2011) suggests it is useful to ask oneself:

- What qualities does this poem have?
- What do you imagine is this poem's potential as a therapeutic tool or catalyst?

It is recommended to avoid clichéd poems which, while they can offer comfort, do not tend to provide the same insights and revelations ignited by original metaphors: that '*aha*' moment of falling into a poem's underlying landscape of experience and meaning. Avoiding poems which are solely hopeless and/or which invite ruminations is prudent also. It makes sense to select poems which are congruent with therapeutic goals, considering also the *isoprinciple*[1] (Chavis, 2011) concerned with selecting poems which match with a client's mood and inner experience. However, there will also be times when it will be necessary and therapeutically ethical and beneficial to select poems which are tangentially or indirectly related to the client's struggle or situation.

It is helpful to ask open, rather than closed 'yes or no' questions to elicit the client's thoughts and feelings in response to the poem. Avoiding 'why' questions can be helpful, e.g. 'Why did that poem make you feel angry?', as this may elicit a defensive reaction. To support the process of healing and change, the client can be encouraged to move beyond simply exploring the poem(s) towards incorporating any insights into their life situation and applying what they have assimilated.

Intrinsic to the medium of poetry is that of metaphor. "Metaphor," writes Paivio, "is a solar eclipse. It hides the object of study and at the same time reveals some of its most salient and interesting characteristics when viewed through the right telescope" (Huckins, 1992, p232). Through poetry, therapists encourage clients to use metaphors to communicate with them about the depth of their lived experience. Leavitt and Pill (1995) observe that metaphor in expressive writing, "facilitates rapid access of innermost thoughts, often in disguised form, thus making them easier to approach and ultimately confront" (p139).

Full poems can be used as therapeutic and/or expressive writing prompts, or sections of lengthier poems. Clients can also be invited to write their own free-expressive poems without using the work of other poets as prompts.

---

1 The isoprinciple was first introduced in the late 1940s within the field of music therapy as a method of mood management in which the music therapist provides music that matches their client's mood, then gradually changes the music to help the client shift to a different emotional state.

Story

Like poetry, telling stories has long been embedded in our human evolution and experience, serving both a personal and a community function. Both the reading and writing of stories can be employed in the therapeutic space for insight and healing.

Readers typically take an active role in absorbing written stories, vicariously experiencing within their own bodies the characters' journeys and emotions. The reader, thus, is an active participant, exploring and finding new dimensions of themselves through the characters and plot. While we identify with, and feel alongside, the characters in the stories we read, we also experience a detachment of our own struggles; viewing them as an observer thus allowing us to assess our situation more objectively.

Stories used therapeutically can include myths, fairy tales, fables, allegorical tales, picture books, literary short stories and short story collections, memoirs and vignettes, and full-length novels. Selections can be matched to areas of struggle, areas of growth and therapeutic goals. They can be read aloud to or by the client, sent as an audio file (it can be lovely for the client to have a story read to them by their therapist) or provided in written form for them to read in or in-between sessions. Stories can also be shared in group therapeutic contexts. It may also be that the client supplies their own story or stories following an invitation from the therapist, e.g. to bring along a fairy tale which is memorable to them or had personal significance to them in childhood.

Learning point 4

Stories of personal significance, especially from childhood, can be particularly beneficial in the therapeutic space. Take a moment to ask yourself:

- Do any stories from your childhood spring to mind as having particular significance?
- Which emotions arise when you remember these stories and why do you think this might be?
- What characters did/do you identify with from these stories? What might this tell you about your core values and sense of self?

Chavis (2011) suggests that the first objective is to address and explore elaborations on the various identifications and projections elicited by elements of the story. Asking sensitively selected open questions invites personal engagement with the story, for example, '*What is your reaction to the story?*' and '*What were you experiencing as the story unfolded?*' (Chavis, 2011, p.141). Other useful avenues to explore include which characters the client was drawn to and why; what this character's perceived hopes and motives are within the story; differences and similarities between the client and this character; reflections on communication patterns between characters; and how the client hoped the story would end.

Once some level of personal engagement with the story has been achieved, the client can be supported to further delve into emotional and cognitive responses. 'What', 'How' and 'When' questions can be valuable here, e.g. 'How would you have responded to the character's mother when she…?'

If desired, stories (particularly short stories of various forms or passages from longer stories) can be used as prompts for therapeutic story writing of the client's own.

Taking therapeutic reading and writing forward

Exploring therapeutic reading and writing with clients experiencing eating struggles can be beneficial and enriching in a multitude of ways. There are few other therapeutic mediums that can be so easily and inexpensively accessed. Indeed, a book or the pen and paper are available to the client any time, day or night, unlike a therapist or psychiatrist. Therapeutic writing can be engaged in at the client's pace without fear that once words leave their mouths they cannot be retracted. Rather, written revelations can be kept private; re-read and revised before sharing; and even destroyed. Clients can be assured that they cannot write the wrong thing and that writing is a gentle process therapeutically; the pen does not reveal more than the client is ready to hear and address. This can facilitate a process which feels both safe and empowering.

References

Campbell J (2008) *The hero with a thousand faces* (Vol. 17). New World Library.

Chavis GG (2011) *Poetry and story therapy: The healing power of creative expression*. Jessica Kingsley Publishers.

Epston D (1992) *Experience, contradiction, narrative & imagination: selected papers of David Epston & Michael White*, 1989-1991. Adelaide: Dulwich Centre Publications.

Frost R (1972) Poetry and Prose, ed. Edward Connery Lathem and Lawrance Thompson. *New York: Holt, Rinehart & Winston, 1072*, 304.

Huckins BA (1992) Metaphor, psychotherapy, and transformative experiences: Exploring relationships. *Smith College Studies in Social Work* **62** (3) 229-243.

Laing R (2010) *The divided self: An existential study in sanity and madness*. Penguin UK.

Leavitt RS & Pill CJ (1995) Composing a self through writing: The ego and the ink. *Smith College Studies in Social Work* **65** (2) 137-149.

Nau DS (1997) Andy writes to his amputated leg: Utilizing letter writing as an interventive technique in brief family therapy. *Journal of Family Psychotherapy* **8** (1) 1-12.

O'Keefe P & Berk M (2009) Writing letters to patients. *Acta Neuropsychiatrica* **21** (6) 314-316.

Pennebaker JW (1997) Writing about emotional experiences as a therapeutic process. *Psychological science* **8** (3) 162-166.

Progoff I (1977) *At a journal workshop: The basic text and guide for using the Intensive Journal.* Dialogue House Library.

Progoff I (1992) *At a journal workshop: Writing to access the power of the unconscious and evoke creative ability*. TarcherPerigee.

Rasmussen, P. T., & Tomm, K. (1992). Guided letter writing: A long brief therapy method whereby clients carry out their own treatment. *Journal of Strategic and Systemic Therapies*, **11**(4), 1-18.

Rombach, M. A. M. (2003). An invitation to therapeutic letter writing. *Journal of Systemic Therapies*, **22**(1), 15-32.

Utley, A., & Garza, Y. (2011). The therapeutic use of journaling with adolescents. *Journal of Creativity in Mental Health*, **6**(1), 29-41.

White, M. (2001). Narrative practice and the unpacking of identity conclusions. *Gecko: A journal of deconstruction and narrative ideas in therapeutic practice*, **1**, 28-55.

Winnicott, D. W. (1953). Transitional objects and transitional phenomena—a study of the first not-me possession. *International journal of psycho-analysis*, **34**, 89-97.

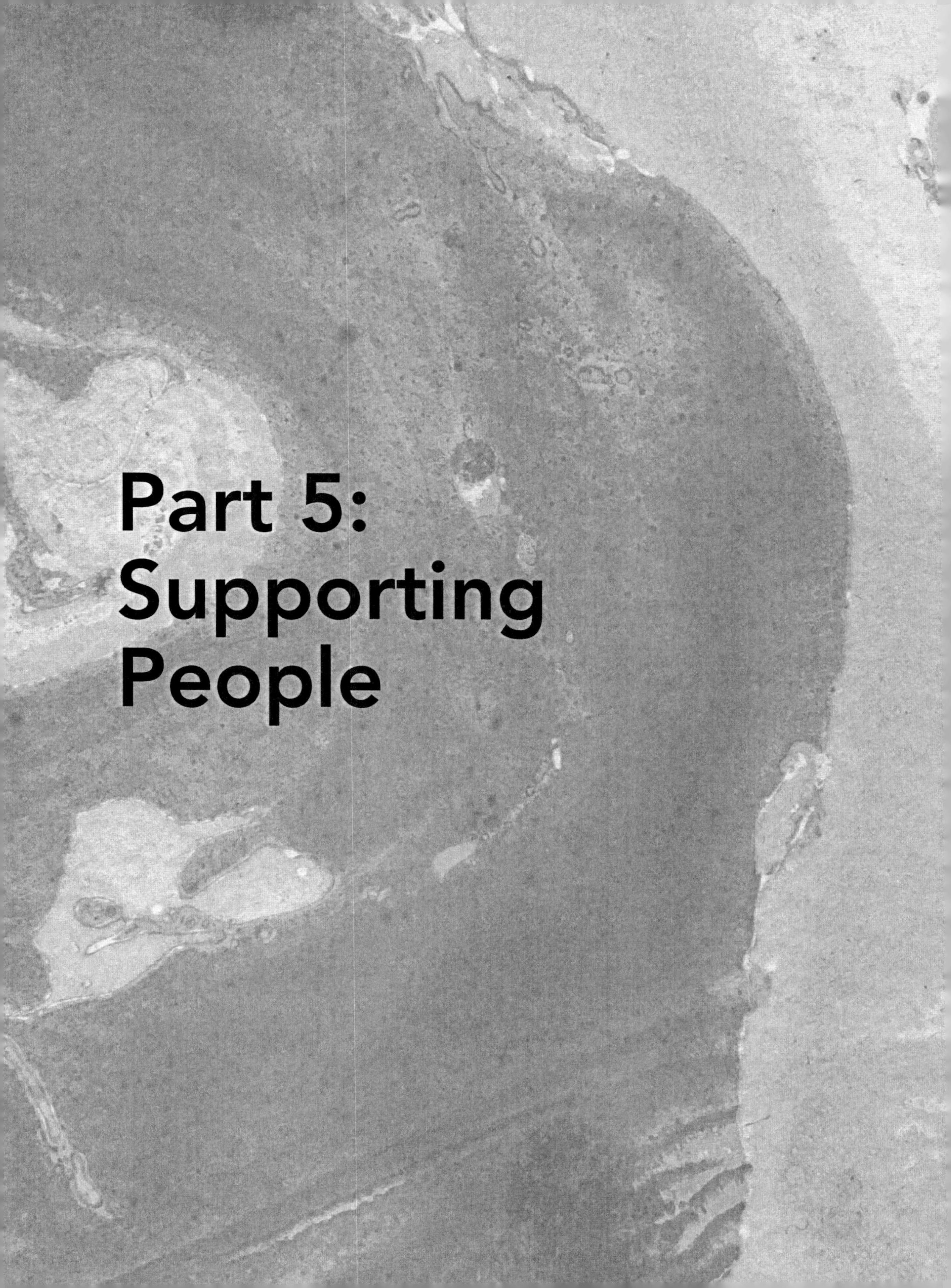

Part 5: Supporting People

42. Caring for a child diagnosed with anorexia nervosa: a parent's perspective

By Frances Grey

Summary

In this chapter I hope to give some description of our experience of anorexia nervosa as a family, including ideas and supportive aspects that have helped us to manage. However, I have come to realise that if you know one person diagnosed with anorexia, you know one person diagnosed with anorexia. From my experience, anorexia is a complex biopsychosocial interaction between genes, epigenetic events, environmental factors and personality. No two recovery paths are therefore the same.

Some background

In the Summer of 2016 my son, then aged 13, became anxious and reluctant to eat food he considered unhealthy. At the time, he was a keen basketball and football player and I supported him in eating so-called 'healthier' foods, thinking this was related to his interest in sport. As time went on, my son's resistance to eating and his obsession with exercise became increasingly marked.

> **Learning point 1**
>
> Be aware of the early warning signs, such as your child cutting foods or food groups out of their diet or beginning to exercise excessively.

During a holiday in Florida in January 2017, my son struggled to eat with the family and I found him running along the beach at 5am. I referred him via email to the Emotional Wellbeing and Mental Health Service (EWMHS) (called the Child and Adolescent Mental Health Service (CAMHS) in some geographical areas).

His first assessment appointment was on 25th January. The conclusion was that my son may be struggling with anorexia. From this point onwards, my son sadly deteriorated to the stage where it took him hours to eat a single meal.

On the 9th February, my son got to the point where could not eat or drink at all. I took him to the Children's Assessment Unit at our local hospital. He was worryingly thin and his eyes appeared completely empty and hollow. He was admitted to the hospital due to bradycardia (slow heart rate) and electrolyte imbalances. A nasogastric feeding tube was inserted on the same day and remained in place for two weeks.

Learning point 2

It is important to make sure that medical professionals check your child's heart and electrolytes, not only their weight and height.

My son's mood was changeable. Sometimes he was full of anxiety and hatred and sometimes he was affectionate and loving. He was very ill physically and required a wheelchair if we went outside. After he fainted in the shower, I always had to be there with him. Seeing his naked body was shocking; it was hard to bear the sharp jutting of his shoulder blades and hipbones. While my son was in hospital, he ate only two small pieces of broccoli. I took him to an inpatient facility on the 27th February of this same year.

Treatment

At the pre-visit to the inpatient facility, the psychiatrist told me I could change my mind about admission if I wanted. However, I was acutely aware that my son was dangerously ill, thus every day and every hour were important in this race against anorexia taking a tighter, more malevolent hold.

I was reassured by the ward manager that my son would be fine; she later phoned me to say he had had eaten a sandwich. By this time, I understood more about the relentless bullying of the anorexic 'voice' and knew eating this sandwich must have come at a huge emotional cost to my son. My son did not eat anything else for some days and once again had a nasogastric tube fitted. However, in the unit the feeding tubes were inserted and removed before and after every meal as each of the three meals and three snacks represented an opportunity for him to eat orally. The constant reinsertion of tubes caused sores and painful discomfort around his septum and throat.

Each day we had a 6pm phone call with our son, which became progressively more abrupt and challenging over time. Our son would accuse us of not understanding and of being rubbish parents. This phone call became a moment of each day that I dreaded. As part of the treatment, there was also a programme of weekly family visits followed by family meals. My daughter was studying for her GCSEs at the time and my ex-partner became frustrated at my son's non-compliance during family therapy (he would leave after five minutes or not come in at all) and also during family meals. Therefore, it seemed like the right thing to do to continue these visits alone as, at the time, my relationship with my son seemed to me to be the strongest.

Learning point 3

Family therapy is often offered as part of treatment. You may find that some family members are resistant to this. While not ideal, family therapy can still go ahead and indeed be beneficial if only some members of the family are present.

As part of his treatment, my son and I struggled through various picnics and restaurant meals out. After each meal I had to check my son's mouth, clothes and the floor for signs of food or excessive crumbs. I remember being close to tears after one such meal having been called names and insulted for two hours. During a walk following that meal, my son stood still and mumbled that he was sorry and then hugged me and burst into tears. He said he did not know what had happened to him or why he kept saying everything he said. It was one of few moments during that time when I caught a glimpse of him as he had been before the anorexia had taken hold.

Despite the many difficulties and frustrations, including one failed return home where my son ran away and was so violent and unpredictable he had to be driven back to hospital by both myself and my husband, I would say that his time in hospital may well have saved his life.

After hospital

In my experience, there is always a tension between pushing your child and appeasing the anorexia. If you push for more calories or insist on no exercise, you know that your child will likely be bullied by the anorexic 'voice' resulting in an outburst and distress. If you appease the anorexia to keep the peace, on the other hand, you are strengthening the hold the illness has on your child.

While my son was in hospital he was not supposed to do any exercise, which was extraordinarily difficult to enforce during family outings. My son would shout irrationally at me if I missed a turning or was not sure where to pay for parking: he was so relentlessly focused on walking as far and for as long as possible that he could not tolerate any delay. He adopted a strange walking style, due to attempting to do around four exercises as he walked. When walking it was hard to stop my son trotting, energetically moving his arms or suddenly stopping to do lunges. Once I was very close to calling the police: after an altercation about exercise, my son ran away from me, sat on an old tree trunk in the middle of a lake and would not come back. Many visits involved some form of extreme challenging behaviour: trying to exit a moving car, running away from me, and kicking the car violently while I was driving. Each time I would discuss this with the staff and the result was that my son's return home was delayed; his four-month stay ended up lasting seven months.

Learning point 4

Compulsive exercise can be part of the experience of anorexia for many young people. It helps as a parent to have clear boundaries around this and to communicate these boundaries with clarity to your child, enlisting the support of professionals, if available.

The tension continued at home. Although it was frightening and resulted in verbal abuse and occasional violent outbursts, I learned it was necessary to stand up to the anorexia in order to make progress. We followed a strict meal plan from the hospital which, after reading various books and articles about the importance for full brain recovery of high calories and fats, I realised was too low in calories (Lobera & Rios, 2009; Troscianko, 2020). I then set about adding extra calories in the form of proteins and fats to the existing meal plan.

As in hospital, so it was at home: my son would either eat, or he wouldn't. My daughter and I prepared for his return home by watching the New Maudsley Success DVD[1] (5) and tried our best not to be a Rhinoceros (me) or a Jellyfish (her), but rather the patient, ever-resourceful Dolphin or St Bernard's dog (Treasure *et al*, 2016). My son commented that he found us to be very helpful when we used this approach. When he didn't eat, I used a letter I had asked for from the EWMHS team authorising the general hospital to administer a nasogastric feed. Thankfully, I only had to use this letter twice. When distraction in the form of games stopped being effective, we adopted a business-like approach whereby my son had half an hour to eat dinner and pudding. In reality, it never took this long.

Signs of hope

By the end of November 2017, my son was thankfully back at school full time. Although many teachers were extremely kind and supportive, when my son told me he was ready to stop having lunch in the car with me, I was told that staff were too busy to sit and have lunch with him. I made a written complaint in order for this decision to be overruled and for my son and his friend to have lunch overlooked by a member of school staff.

---

1 https://newmaudsleycarers-kent.co.uk/the-succeed-dvd/ (accessed November 2021).

Learning point 5

As a parent of a child struggling with anorexia, you may need to be their advocate including in their educational setting, laying out what reasonable adjustments need to be made to support their recovery.

Around Christmas 2017, I noticed that my son had began to relax. It was as if a cold, black and white outline was slowly being filled with warm colour. He became loving and affectionate. I began to find his socks on the sofa where he had been lying and relaxing. He told me that he knew that I had fought the illness as hard as he had and thanked me for all my patience, which he hoped someday to repay.

Ongoing treatment

Our EWMHS support after the hospital admission was limited. Over the summer of 2018, I had really struggled with my son who was (I felt) actively avoiding meals when he could. In September 2018, the CBT-E therapist agreed with my son that he could 'free flow' and manage his own snacks and lunches. Horrified, I kept a food diary which detailed multiple occasions where my son didn't eat or drink for 12-hour stretches. At times, he lost 2kg in a single week.

In January 2019, the therapist admitted that the anorexia seemed to have returned and discussed the possibility of re-admission to inpatient treatment. I decided to take back control and told my son he would not be able to do his GCSEs unless he returned to the meal plan as I would remove him from school. I adopted a full 'Life Stops Until You Eat' (Lock & Le Grange, 2001) approach including removal of computers and phones. Luckily, my son took this seriously and within two weeks he was back on the meal plan, albeit with huge resentment and anger towards me.

My son has a very high metabolism and I initially returned to the hospital goal of 100% weight-for-height restoration. It remained difficult for my son to gain or maintain this higher weight. It is important to note that my son is a tall child who had always been at the 60th or 70th percentiles for weight and height. I questioned why his goal weight was calculated using 100% weight-for-height measures (to understand this, see Eva Musby (2020). In the end I used the weight chart from his Red Book (a Personal Child Health Record, given to all parents in the UK with full height and weight charts provided up to age twenty) to ascertain what weight my son should be. I understand this is now considered best practice (Gaudiani, 2020; Muhlheim & Collins, 2018; Muhlheim, 2020).

Why did my son experience anorexia?

Anorexia is a devastating, often long-lasting chronic illness with a high mortality rate. Inevitably parents will question themselves, as indeed I did: was it because I had split up from my son's father? Because I had moved counties to live with his step-father? Because of the family history of depression and anxiety? Because my son was bullied the year before he got ill? No one will ever know, but all these factors very likely played their part. It is not helpful or productive for parents and families to blame themselves, particularly as they wouldn't blame themselves for their child developing cancer or another physical illness. My son having anorexia has changed us all, but I hope that someday my son will be a stronger person for his experiences (Rosen, 2013; for a YouTube video, see also www.youtube.com/watch?v=wE3fyQV_chI (accessed November 2021).

Accessing support

If you are very isolated with an ill child it is easy to feel resentful when scrolling through other people's seemingly perfect lives on Facebook. No one brings you casseroles if your child has anorexia. Only one parent of my son's friends ever made contact with me, despite the fact that he was out of school for nine months. The flip side of social media is that it is quite easy to find online Carer's Groups for eating disorders, for example on Facebook and those run by Beat or FEAST. The exchange of TED talks, articles and experiences can be invaluable in the difficult early stages.

Once (you think) your child is weight-restored, gaining support can be more complex. At this point we have to develop our own intuition and judgement as parents, hopefully forming a team with our child. As I mentioned at the beginning of this chapter, recovery paths are all different. Some of my son's contemporaries from hospital have relapsed several times with multiple admissions, while a few only needed to go to hospital once and were motivated to return home; they were in and out of the illness quickly. I remember feeling at the beginning that I could make this illness go away within months; that we would be one of the lucky ones.

The reality has been much more complicated. My son has not needed to return to hospital, but keeping to his meal plan has required commitment and hard work, made more complicated by his physical growth to 183cm, meaning that his target weight was constantly changing. We still maintain three meals and snacks, all prepared by him apart from dinner. Although my son appears able to eat everything without difficulty, usually without being reminded, he has not fully recovered cognitively or behaviourally despite his physical weight gain. He sometimes voices concerns that he has binge eating disorder or asks when he can eat less food. This tells me that my son is not fully recovered, has limited insight and as such is still vulnerable to relapse.

As my son is nearly 18, the 'Life Stops Until you Eat' approach is now less appropriate and we talk about how he will manage when he is independent and if he goes to university. He has appeared to recognize that underlying the development of anorexia was his social anxiety and has finally accepted that he needs help for this, which gives me hope for the future. Unfortunately, parenting a child with anorexia nervosa is usually a marathon and not a sprint. It requires determination, the ability to take the long view and to rejoice in small successes. Statistically, 46% of all those with anorexia will fully recover (Beat, 2020) and the prognosis is particularly good for adolescents who are in treatment early.

So, what does it take to parent a child with anorexia?

1. The ability not to give up: unless you perfect your Dolphin or St Bernard's dog (from the Maudsley Approach) you will make mistakes, lose your temper or appease the anorexia. Tomorrow is always a new day with the opportunity of a different approach.
2. A thick skin: you may be sworn at and your child may well be violent towards you. The anorexia will find your weak spots and exploit them. Thus, you have to learn not to take what your child does or says personally.
3. The capacity to apologise: if you mess things up, explain why you made a mistake.
4. Focus on separating the child from the anorexia: it can be hard not to retreat in the face of relentless aggression but somewhere beneath all the difficult behaviour and negativity your child is in there, suffering terribly.
5. Make time for self-care: take time out, see friends, have meals out. Talk about it, try not to feel ashamed – anorexia loves isolation and secrecy.
6. Share the load: ask friends to eat with your child sometimes, and/or their friends if you trust them. Make school professionals aware of your child's difficulties and enlist their support also.

References

Treasure J, Smith G & Crane A (2016) Skills-Based Learning for Caring for a Loved One With an Eating Disorder The New Maudsley Method. Maudsley Hospital: London, England.

Le Grange D & Lock J (2001) *Treatment Manual for Anorexia Nervosa: A family based approach*. Guilford Press.

Rosen M (2013) The anorexic brain: Neuroimaging improves understanding of eating disorder. *Science News* **184** (

Musby E (2020) *What do BMI and Weight for Height Mean?* [online]. Available at: https://anorexiafamily.com/bmi-weight-for-height-wfh/?v=79cba1185463 (accessed August 2021).

Muhlheim L (2020) *Children Paediatric Growth Charts and eating disorders* [online]. www.verywellmind.com/chart-prevent-eating-disorder-1138306 (accessed August 2021).

Gaudiani JL (202) *Weight Goals in Anorexia Nervosa Treatment* (online). Available at: www.gaudianiclinic.com/gaudiani-clinic-blog/2020/4/22/weight-goals-in-anorexia-nervosa?fbclid=IwAR2O2DLQsVmOm-FqXp7Ti8rDTJ0PajC41jq8iUWxEgLaxL-wo_NUzw176hk (accessed August 2021).

Muhlheim L & Collins L (2018) *When Your Teen Has an Eating Disorder: Practical Strategies to Help Your Teen Recover from Anorexia, Bulimia, and Binge Eating*. New Harbinger.

Lobera IJ & Ríos PB (2009) Choice of diet in patients with anorexia nervosa. *Nutricion Hospitalaria* **24** (6) 682-687.

Accurso EC, Sim L, Muhlheim L & Lebow J (2020) Parents know best: Caregiver perspectives on eating disorder recovery. *International Journal of Eating Disorders* **53** 1252– 1260.

Troscianko E (2020) *Anorexia and Dietary Fat: Brain function, hunger and satiety* (online). *Psychology Today*. Available at: www.psychologytoday.com/gb/blog/hunger-artist/202003/anorexia-and-dietary-fat-brain-function-hunger-and-satiety (accessed August 2021).

Support groups and resources

www.feast-ed.org/
www.facebook.com/EDPS-354398417918769/

43. How schools can support pupils with eating difficulties and their families: findings from a combined-methods study

By Bethany Elms and Andrea Higgins

Chapter summary

This chapter will focus on school and family systems to consider how schools could more effectively support individuals with eating difficulties (EDs). School staff and parents of children and young people (CYP) with EDs from across the UK were surveyed to explore what schools currently provide. We asked about areas such as staff knowledge and awareness of EDs; the effectiveness of practice; support available for CYP, families and involved school staff; strategies and interventions being offered; and links with other professionals (Elms, 2020). The chapter will outline the findings and consider the implications for practice and how families and professionals could work together to improve outcomes for pupils. This study demonstrated that steps could be taken by schools at three different levels: A) supporting those who are receiving treatment; B) identifying and acting proactively in the emergent stages of difficulties; and finally C) looking at wider school factors necessary for schools to become more eating-difficulty friendly. We will conclude with discussion on the importance of collaborative working between all those supporting this vulnerable group.

Support for children and young people with eating difficulties in the school system: an overview

In the UK, therapeutic support for CYP with EDs is typically provided by specialist services (Knightsmith, 2015). Nevertheless, continuing challenges are evident, such as poorer outcomes for individuals with anorexia (Murray *et al*, 2018), moderately high drop-out rates (Hilbert *et al*, 2012), and systemic factors influencing access to treatment e.g., long waiting periods (BEAT, 2017). This suggests that an enhanced approach to supporting the recovery of CYP with EDs could be required. Therefore, understanding how key systems surrounding these individuals could meet their needs may be pertinent.

Following increases in mental health (MH) needs amongst CYP, in 2017 the government released the document *Transforming Children and Young People's Mental Health Provision: A green paper* (Department for Education & Department of Health and Social Care, 2017). This set out plans for the improvement of MH support in British schools with the creation of Mental Health Support Teams (MHSTs), who would deliver "group-based interventions engaging participants in critiquing the 'thin ideal', which can be effective in reducing eating difficulty symptoms and body image concerns, when targeted toward high-risk adolescent girls" (Department for Education and Department for Health and Social Care, 2017, p22). However, guidance on how to implement this proposal appears to have been lacking from consequent MHST competence frameworks and manuals.

Research suggests that sociocultural influences play a role in the aetiology of EDs (Culbert *et al*, 2015). Bronfenbrenner (1979; see Figure 43.1) identified the two systems closest to CYP as their school and home. Therefore, consideration of the support in school systems, and how it integrates with the family may be beneficial. It could be argued that when CYP have difficulties that result in significant involvement of healthcare professionals, diagnosis and treatment become the primary focus, and the school particularly (and often the family) may be slightly marginalized. The aim of this chapter is to look at how these systems can take an active part in supporting CYP, firstly exploring how the family can work collaboratively with schools, and then focusing on the school.

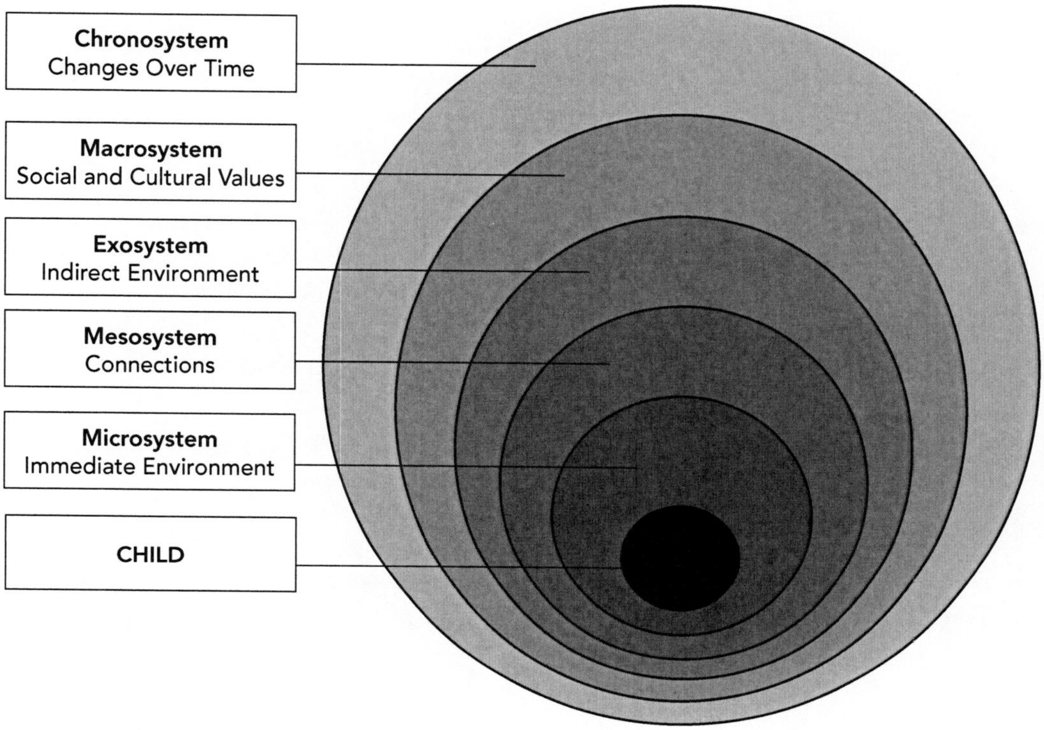

Figure 43.1: Bronfenbrenner's Ecological Systems Theory (1979).

The Family System

Supporting CYP with EDs places stress on all family members including parents and siblings, adversely affecting their psychological wellbeing, mental health, relationships and causing problems with employment (McCormack & McCann, 2015; Jungbauer *et al*, 2016). Therefore, family involvement and support should be an important consideration in the management of EDs, from the earliest points of identification through to full and lasting recovery. Sadly, many families report feeling excluded or marginalized by both services and schools, and that their voices are not heard.

What families have told us

Findings highlighted that parents had strong feelings that schools are not effectively meeting the needs of their children, providing rich information about why this was and what more they felt should be done. Some key findings are presented in Box 43.1.

Box 43.1: Results from a survey of parents – The headlines

- **93%** of parents were not provided with information about EDs by their child's school.
- **77%** of parents did not think that schools are currently providing adequate support for pupils with EDs.
- **93%** felt that it was important for schools to support families of CYP with EDs, yet **86%** felt that the support they received was less than effective.
- **Half** of parents felt that they could/should have received better support from their child's school.
- **87%** of parents believed that siblings of CYP with EDs should receive support themselves.
- **52%** of parents did not believe their child's school actively tried to prevent the onset of EDs.
- Only **13%** felt that staff in their child's school were knowledgeable about EDs or that the school had effectively provided support for them or their family.
- **74%** felt that staff were concerned for their child's wellbeing.
- **63%** of families reported that school staff **never** attended multi-disciplinary meeting about their child.

Parents discussed the improvements they would like to see. These included suggestions for: wider school systems and practices; preventative measures; thoughts about the curriculum; and how their child could have been better supported in school, during treatment, and post-treatment. Their ideas have been incorporated the discussion below on 'What schools can do for parents/families' on page 408.

The school system

From the age of five, CYP can spend at least 25 hours a week at school. It is where they learn, socialise, develop their personalities, and are supported to become capable, healthy, well-rounded individuals. Furthermore, their key support systems may lie here, in the form of friends and other significant adults. Thus, it is argued that the role of the school should be considered in supporting EDs, including prevention and management.

What is happening in schools currently?

There is little research in the UK exploring school practice. Key findings include:

- School staff have a limited understanding and knowledge about EDs, and do not feel comfortable discussing the issues with pupils (Knightsmith *et al*, 2013).

- Literature that evidences the impact and outcomes of school-based interventions and development of practice is limited and ambiguous.
- Clear policies in schools can be beneficial. In the UK, new policy initiatives surrounding mandatory personal social and health (PSHE) education have been implemented, which reference body image and EDs in the curriculum guidance (Department for Education, 2020).
- Effective procedures for CYP who are reintegrating back into school (having had an extended absence due to treatment for their EDs), are essential.
- Successful reintegration is more likely when using a staged approach with a multi-disciplinary team, which is person-centred.

One study from the US highlighted the benefits of school-based interventions for EDs (Schiele, 2016). Findings showed that CYP with EDs and many of their parents were pleased with the support offered by schools, which included consultations, forums to educate students, referral to medical professionals for assessment, social support, and individual therapies. Although the data may not be fully generalisable to UK schools, it highlights the potential that school systems can effectively meet the needs of pupils with EDs and their families.

What schools told us?

As with parents, we sought the views of school staff to survey what support was available to pupils with EDs. Participants were from across the UK, worked in a range of educational sectors, and held a variety of roles/positions in schools. In Box 43.2 we have shared some of the results.

Box 43.2: Results from a survey of school staff – The headlines

- **76%** of staff were aware of a pupil in their school who currently/previously had an ED, yet fewer than **50%** of staff felt that the support provided was effective.
- **All** staff felt it was important for school staff to understand EDs, and that it was part of the school's role to support pupils with EDs; however, not all felt that every member of staff was sympathetic.
- **60%** of staff had received no training but **all** participants indicated that it would be useful.
- **96%** of school staff felt that those working closely with a CYP with an ED should receive support, such as ongoing supervision and continual professional development (CPD).
- **78%** felt that siblings should receive support.

- **60%** had undertaken **'a little'** preventative work around EDs. Nevertheless, **all** believed that educating pupils about EDs would 'possibly' or 'definitely' be beneficial as a preventative measure.
- **85%** of schools were not currently running intervention programmes around EDs.
- Only **18%** noted that their school organised individual therapy sessions for CYP with EDs.
- **55%** reported that their school had policies that address the needs of CYP with an ED such as attendance and wellbeing, and **50%** of this group felt these were effective.
- **54%** reported that their school had effectively supported the reintegration of pupils with EDs who had been absent for an extended period of time.
- **81%** of staff felt confident discussing concerns about EDs with parents, and **all** felt it was important to work collaboratively with parents to support pupils.

Learning point 1

What do these findings tell you? What would be top of your list for actions?

Working successfully with the school and the family: What could schools do?

School effectiveness is dependent on addressing all parts of the system in an integrated and embedded way. Figure 43.2 below illustrates the three levels of school interventions which have been found to be essential in enhancing practice.

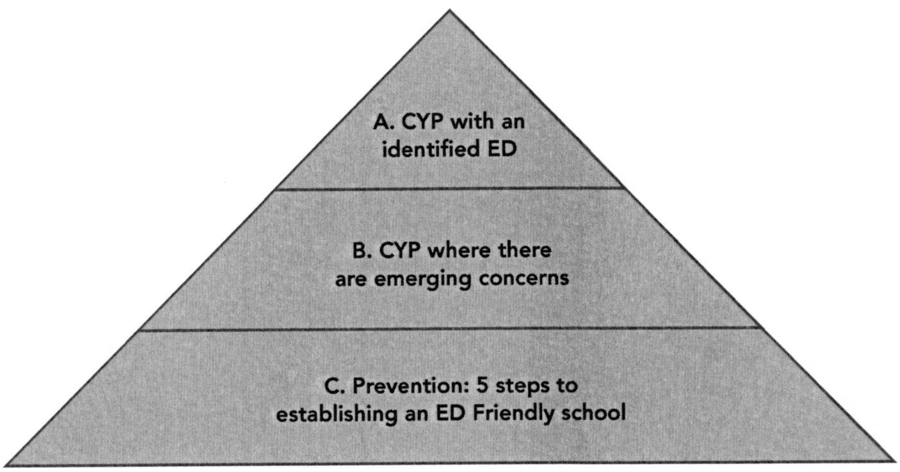

Figure 43.2: Opportunities for prevention aligned with the public health model

A. Supporting those with an identified ED: Suggestions for educational staff

1. **Be flexible and bespoke** – every student in a school is an individual and this applies to those with EDs. Thus, use a person-centred and tailored approach which will look different for every student and could include a range of different elements such as modifications to daily routines, timetables and curriculum.
2. Ensure there is a **clear and achievable plan, agreed with the pupil and their family**, with details of the support that will be provided, by whom, and where the student can go when they need some help.
3. Have an **identified key person** who the student, parents and other staff know is taking on this responsibility and can **develop a positive, supportive relationship with the pupil**. Furthermore, ensure they are both supported and effectively supervised in this role.
4. **Consider siblings** – what support do they need? How can this be offered? Sometimes a 'listening ear' is enough.
5. **Work collaboratively with external agencies** – seek assistance and advice. Most schools will have an Educational Psychologist (EP) who is assigned to them.
6. **Liaise closely with settings that a CYP may need to attend temporarily**– provide work that can be done to avoid students falling behind with schoolwork.
7. Actively **address the challenges for students in reintegrating into school** – Meet with parents, the student, representatives from the treatment centre and Educational Psychologists (EPs). What is needed to support continued recovery? How this can be implemented? What are the concerns of everyone involved (particularly the student)? Agree on a plan, monitor, review and amend as necessary.

'Offer time out and support for a sibling to talk about how the ED is affecting them and the family.'

B. Suggestions for working effectively with those CYP where there are emerging concerns

1. **Involve the young person**

One factor that students may give for their eating patterns is a desire for control. For a complexity of reasons, they may feel powerless in different areas of their lives and eating is a way of them trying to address this power imbalance. Thus, if professionals and parents ignore the voice of the student this powerless feeling is further reinforced.

Involve the students in everything- planning strategies, meetings, and sharing information with others. Ensure they are the focus point for the management of their own ED.

2. **Work with parents** – more on this is outlined in the section below. The key message is that the family and the school are the two primary systems involved so it is essential that they **work in partnership**.

3. **Work with peers – Remember:**
   - **Peer negativity** can be an influencing factor in the development of EDs.
   - **Educate pupils about EDs:**
     - They may be able to help identify early signs of EDs and raise this with school staff, which is crucial in providing support for recovery.
     - An awareness of EDs could help increase empathy and reduce weight-related bullying.

> **'Support with bullying which led to anxiety and the eating disorder'**

4. **Include friends of the CYP with the ED;** they could be a key part of the support system, so help them to feel able to do this (e.g. by providing scripts on what to say if the CYP mentions their weight).

> **'How could they [peers] be involved in part with the sort of support and care plan, maybe from a few selected trusted friends, for instance?'**

5. **Key messages for staff:**
   - **Talk to students and express your concern** – the sooner a problem is addressed, the quicker the recovery will likely be.
   - **Be empathetic** – understand that acknowledging that they have a difficulty may be challenging for many reasons.
   - **Avoid talking specifically about food and weight** – instead, try to discuss how they are feeling, listen carefully and respectfully to what they have to say, encourage them to seek help, and express concerns with the family.
   - **Develop a range of appropriate interventions** that are tailored to the individual's needs, e.g. learning, anxiety, or social relationships.

> **'...would comment on and ask her about her lowest weight... Triggered her to relapse countless times.'**

C. Prevention: 5 steps to establishing an ED-friendly school

1. **Identify a 'Designated Senior Lead for Mental Health'**
   The government Green Paper (Department for Education and Department of Health and Social Care, 2017), suggested that schools should have a member of their leadership team take on this role so that they can:
   - Support the development of a whole-school approach.
   - Establish effective pastoral support systems.
   - Ensure early identification.
   - Develop strong links with (and knowledge of) mental health services.

- Overview interventions being implemented.
- Consider staff support and wellbeing.

2. **Ensure there is a school policy for mental health and wellbeing**
   All schools need to have and maintain a mental health and wellbeing policy, which is reviewed regularly and addresses evolving needs, e.g., added pressures and changing circumstances during the 2020 pandemic. It should be concise, developed in partnership with stakeholders (students, families, staff, governors and partner agencies) with clear and accessible messages in providing appropriate guidance. Both this, and wider school policies (e.g. those relating to bullying, discrimination, behaviour management, and school exclusion), should be reviewed by students with experience of EDs to make sure they are fit for the purpose. The best policies will include a statement about providing a body-image friendly environment and celebrating diversity.

3. **Create a caring and supportive ethos**
   All young people need to know that they are part of a school that is welcoming and caring so that they feel that they belong. Pupils (particularly those with mental health needs) must feel safe, supported and able to develop trusting relationships with staff. Furthermore, they should feel that they are being listened to and not judged, dismissed or ignored.

   Everyone has a role to play in nurturing a caring school ethos, always modelling a positive body-image message and acceptance of diversity.

   For pupils, there must be a consistent message of zero tolerance of appearance-related teasing, including cyber-bullying.

4. **Train and support all staff to develop and embed an understanding of EDs**
   In accordance with the proposals of the Green Paper, noted previously, everyone working with students should be well-equipped to provide the right environment for learning and wellbeing. It is important that all staff are informed about the early signs of an ED. As well as training, staff require access to literature/information about EDs and the role they can play in supporting students. Interactions at school (including between) should be body-friendly. This could be supported by MHSTs through workshops and staff training to upskill them to be able to deliver group-based body image interventions and ED preventative programmes.

   'Train teachers to understand what is involved and how they can help.'

5. **Enhance the knowledge and understanding of young people about all aspects of EDs**
   Peer groups can have both a positive and negative influence on CYP's eating attitudes and behaviour. Parents and staff were clear about the importance of both increasing CYPs awareness and understanding of Eds, and responding quickly if negative attitudes emerge.

But beware...

Heathy eating is now included in the statutory guidance relating to PSHE, however it is worth noting the potential dangers of education and over emphasis on Healthy Eating education, as one parent told us:

> **'My 10-year-old daughter has recently been diagnosed with anorexia. This started following a healthy eating talk at school... I have heard a lot of children who have been triggered by the same talks or similar.'**

Think about the messages being shared, e.g. avoid the concept of 'good' and 'bad' foods.

What schools can do for parents/families?

> **'Reassurance that the school are working with us to help my child.'**

1. **Work closely and collaboratively with parents** – alerting them at the earliest point; organising regular meetings; sharing information, and ensuring they are fully informed.
2. **Listen to parents and take their concerns seriously** – 'Space to be heard' is how one participant expressed this.
3. **Be sensitive to parents' needs** – try to place them at ease; avoid judging them; and ensure they are happy with decisions.
4. **Help them to access information and advice** – for example local support networks and national charities (e.g. BEAT).
5. **Be aware that this will be difficult for families** – there may be some tough conversations; try to remain neutral, offer reassurance to manage their emotions, and defuse any conflict that may emerge.
6. **Ensure parents have a named member of staff** who knows their child well, with whom they can build a positive working relationship. To parents, schools can be anonymous places with many staff; they may not know who they can talk to and get fed-up with having to repeat their 'story' to new people.

Learning point 2

Imagine that you are the parent of a CYP with an ED, what would be the most important thing you would like the school to do?

Support for schools

Development of practice in schools is something that will not be easily achieved without specialist support. One profession that could take a role with this are EPs. Most schools will have a named EP who works closely with them. EPs are already involved in improving support and addressing the needs of students with a broad range of mental health difficulties and have much to offer. Interviews completed with eight EPs identified many ways in which their work could be tailored to the needs of this specific group. For example through providing consultation, support for staff and parents, completion of holistic assessments, offering parent workshops, and providing training and supervision for key staff. Figure 43.3 illustrates this:

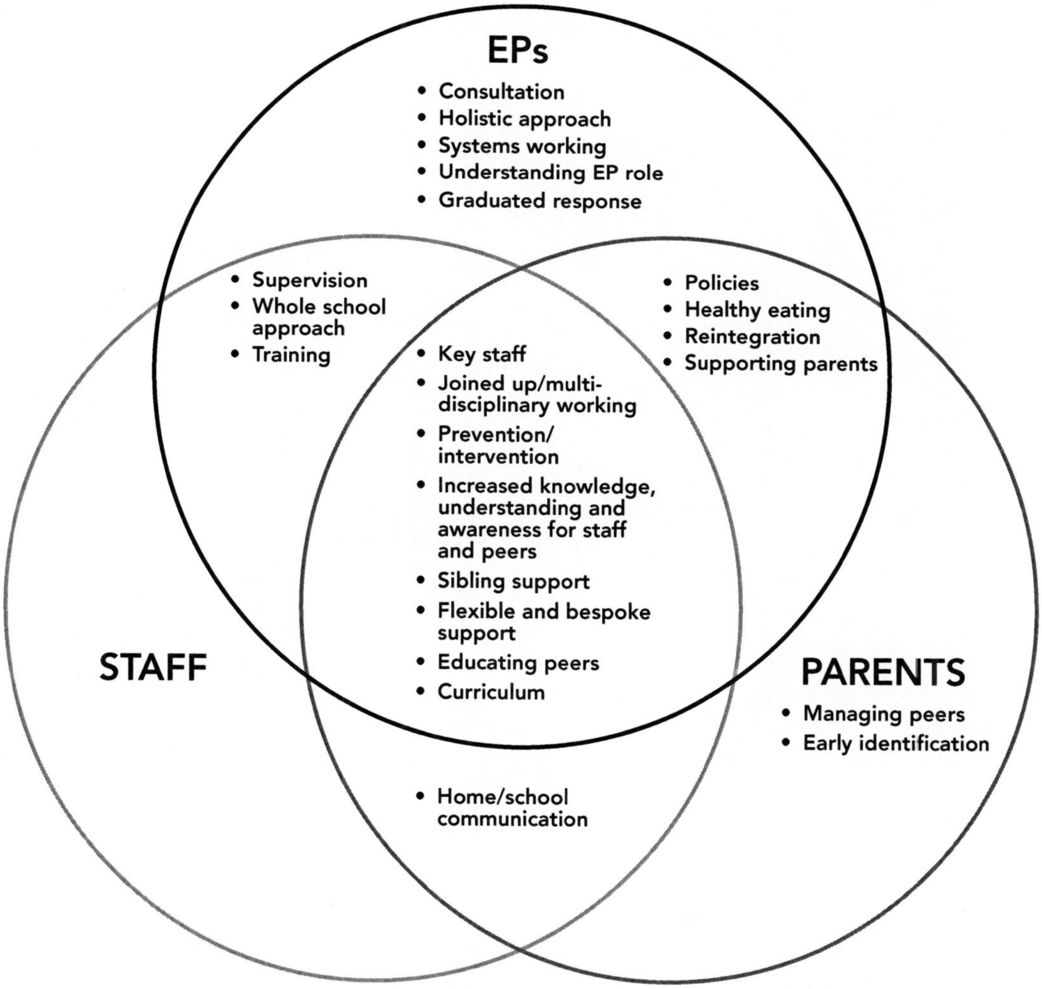

Figure 43.3: Venn diagram showing ways school staff, parents and EPs felt the support for CYP with EDs could be provided.

Working with others

The government's mental health Green Paper (Department for Education & Department of Health and Social Care, 2017) identified the need to increase communication and joined-up working between schools and health services to provide earlier support to CYP in schools. This will impact upon those with EDs who will gradually gather around them a complex network of 'supporters' (see Figure 43.4).

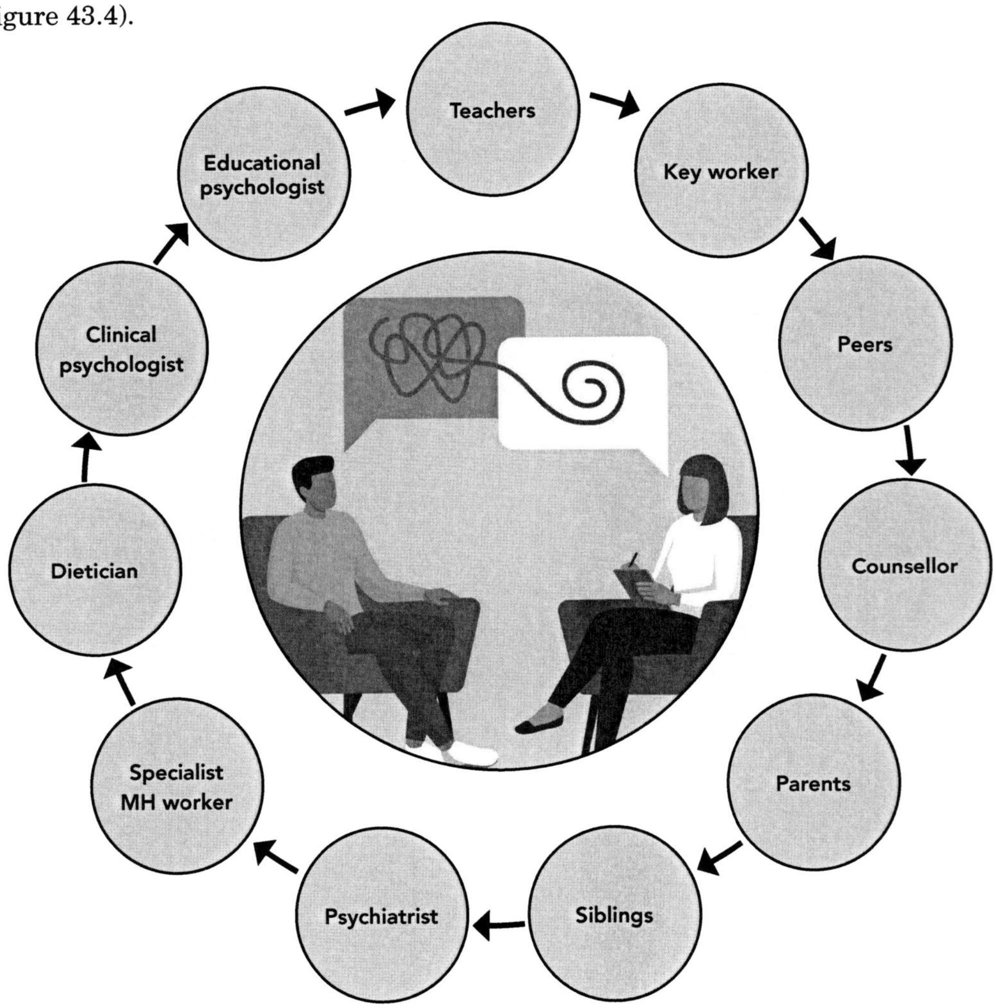

Figure 43.4: A network of supporters

For these professionals to provide effective support, what is needed is close communication, coherence of approaches and partnership working. This was highlighted as an area for development in this study, e.g. the majority of parents reported that schools never attended multidisciplinary meetings for their child, yet school staff said that they would welcome more support from other agencies and identified a need for more collaborative working and communication between key people.

Learning point 3

Think about your role – how could you enhance collaboration with other professionals?

In summary, it is clear the parents and school staff believe that support for pupils with EDs in schools should be enhanced. This chapter has discussed a range of strategies that could be implemented, and how key adults and professionals can work together to support the needs of this vulnerable group of CYP.

Suggestions for further reading and information

Knightsmith P (2015) *Self-Harm and Eating Disorders in Schools: A guide to whole-school strategies and practical support.* London: Jessica Kingsley Publishers.

For schools in the UK, one potentially very useful resource is this book by Pooky Knightsmith. It identifies many positive strategies schools could implement, including how to increase staff competency through training, and it provides strategies and practical ideas. There is discussion about the value of clear policies and the implementation of evidence-based programmes in UK schools.

Beat Eating Disorders (BEAT)
https://www.beateatingdisorders.org.uk/about-us
Beat is the UK's eating disorder charity. The website is not only rich in information and resources for CYP, families, friends and schools, but also has a helpline and an online peer support network.

National Eating Disorder Collaboration, Australia
https://nedc.com.au/assets/NEDC-Resources/NEDC-Resource-Schools.pdf
A valuable resource on addressing EDs in schools, which covers prevention, early identification and response.

References

BEAT (2017) *Three-and-a-half-year delay for eating disorder treatment worsens illness and cost to the NHS* [online]. Available at: (https://www.beateatingdisorders.org.uk/news/beat-news/three-half-year-delay-eating-disorder-treatment/ accessed October 2021).

Bronfenbrenner U (1979) *The Ecology of Human Development: Experiments by nature and design*. USA: Harvard University Press.

Culbert KM, Racine SE & Klump KL (2015) Research Review: What we have learned about the causes of eating disorders–a synthesis of sociocultural, psychological, and biological research. *Journal of Child Psychology and Psychiatry* **56** (11) 1141-1164.

Department for Education (2020) *Relationships and sex education (RSE) and health education: Statutory guidance for governing bodies, proprietors, head teachers, principals, senior leadership teams, teachers* [online]. Available at: https://assets.publishing.service.gov.uk/government/uploads/system/uploads/attachment_data/file/908013/Relationships_Education__Relationships_and_Sex_Education__RSE__and_Health_Education.pdf (accessed August 2021).

Department for Education & Department of Health and Social Care (2017) *Transforming Children and Young People's Mental Health Provision: a Green Paper* [online]. Available at: https://assets.publishing.service.gov.uk/government/uploads/system/uploads/attachment_data/file/664855/Transforming_children_and_young_people_s_mental_health_provision.pdf (accessed August 2021).

Elms B (2020) *An Exploration of Practice in Schools When Working with Young People with Eating Disorders, and Their Families: The potential role for educational psychologists*. DEdPsy Thesis, Cardiff University.

Hilbert A, Bishop ME, Stein RI, Tanofsky-Kraff M, Swenson AK, Welch RR & Wilfley DE (2012) Long-term efficacy of psychological treatments for binge eating disorder. *The British Journal of Psychiatry*, **200** (3) 232-237.

Jungbauer J, Heibach J & Urban K (2016) Experiences, burdens, and support needs in siblings of girls and women with anorexia nervosa: Results from a qualitative interview study. *Clinical Social Work Journal* **44** (1) 78-86.

Knightsmith P, Treasure J & Schmidt U (2013) Spotting and supporting eating disorders in school: recommendations from school staff. *Health Education Research* **28** (6) 1004-1013.

McCormack C & McCann E (2015) Caring for an adolescent with anorexia nervosa: parent's views and experiences. *Archives of Psychiatric Nursing* **29** (3) 143-147.

Murray SB, Quintana DS, Loeb KL, Griffiths S & Le Grange D (2018) Treatment outcomes for anorexia nervosa: a systematic review and meta-analysis of randomized controlled trials. *Psychological Medicine* 1-10.

Schiele BE (2016) *Promoting Progress to Assist Youth with Disordered Eating in School Mental Health*. PhD Psychology Thesis, University of South Carolina.

44. Experiencing eating and body image difficulties in the context of higher education: challenges and potential solutions

By Hannah Lewis

Summary

Written from a lived experience perspective, this chapter will discuss the various transitions within higher education, and the triggers which may catalyse eating difficulties. This chapter discusses the impact of living independently, 'drinking culture', academic pressures, as well as Disabled Students Allowance (DSA) and mitigating circumstances. This chapter will also include a specialist service case study, alongside a lived experience case study.

Introduction

The mental health of university students has risen up the agenda in recent years, with an increasing awareness and demand for appropriate services. Eating difficulty prevalence among the student population remains high, and transitions to university present a unique set of circumstances which can accelerate body image disturbance and eating difficulties.

The student environment and potential risk factors

Moving away from home to university can be unsettling. Usual routines, habits and pre-existing support networks, including friends, family or healthcare services in one's hometown, are disrupted and academic pressures alongside a lack of accountability while navigating new experiences can create a perfect storm for the onset or relapse into eating difficulties.

Underlying traits, such as perfectionism and a drive for high attainment, are commonly seen in eating difficulties. Partnered with external pressures for academic achievement, stress related to studies can often trigger the need for control, leading to unhelpful coping mechanisms including eating difficulties, such as restricting, bingeing and purging.

New-found independence and autonomy, paired with a loss of accountability around meal preparation and exercise could also potentially lead to eating difficulties, and while university is often seen to be a time of socialising and meeting new friends, for some it can be an overwhelming period leading to isolation, enabling the secrecy that eating disorders thrive on.

Furthermore, 'university culture' is often synonymous with a drinking culture, which many young adults may experience for the first time when they move away from home. Drinking alcohol at university can interact with eating difficulties in different ways, for example restricting food to compensate for calories in alcohol; drinking alcohol to engage in bingeing; or drinking alcohol to disguise purging (FREED, 2021b).

In addition, financial independence can be a novel experience for many students. Managing a student loan can be anxiety provoking and thus lead to issues with budgeting where food and grocery shopping may not be prioritised in favour of other activities. Meal choices which cost less and have lower nutritional value may be chosen with ulterior motives of low calorific content.

Learning point 1

Are you or a loved one planning on transitioning to university soon? What do you anticipate could be the main risk factors for increased stress or eating difficulties?

Managing risk factors

To mitigate risk factors, self-management techniques could prove helpful. Disclosing your feelings to trusted friends and family is crucial, as we know eating difficulties thrive in secrecy. We know that disclosure can be a particularly difficult task, however by sharing what you are experiencing with a trusted family member, friend or member of academic staff, you could find help and prevent eating difficulties from escalating. Please refer to the next chapter for further information about disclosing eating difficulties in higher education and the legislation that can support you.

Recognising that isolation maybe a trigger could be an important protective factor before going to university. Researching which societies you think might interest you and whether there are any clubs which can help you maintain your hobbies and meet new people with common interests could be helpful. Scheduling video calls with friends and family so that you've got a strong support network can also be a good way to know you will always have an opportunity to catch-up and check-in with your loved ones who support you.

If you suspect that you may struggle to adhere to a meal plan, then advanced planning could be integral for you. Before leaving home, spend some time establishing your preferred meals and practise these at home. Accommodating for the costs of your favourite meals by managing your student budget and prioritising food shopping can be an important factor in maintaining healthy food intake while at university.

Furthermore, if you know that alcohol may be a trigger for your eating difficulties, be mindful of this prior to going to university. While many social events may revolve around alcohol, have confidence in alternating alcoholic drinks with soft drinks, or choosing single measures of spirits or half pints. Planning what you are going to eat the day after drinking and ensuring you have a substantial meal before you start drinking may also prevent bingeing.

While these self-management techniques may be helpful for some people, further professional support may also be useful or necessary in some cases.

Learning point 2

How do you think you could mitigate the risk factors when you or a loved one transition to university? For example, is there professional support or local support groups that you could access? Can you organise regular catch-ups via video call with your friends or family? Would having meal plans or shopping lists be helpful to prepare ahead of time?

Accessing professional support

While the provision of mental health and eating disorder support services may vary across universities, it is expected that each university will host an internal advice, wellbeing or support service. Student support services can help you with practical issues, such as applying for 'extenuating circumstances', which can allow you to extend deadlines for coursework or postpone examinations.

Counselling services are often included in the offer of support services. These services can often offer short-term, one-to-one counselling, as well as wellbeing groups and workshops. While this support is often appropriate for people with mild to moderate mental health or eating difficulties, it could act as a useful source of support in the interim period of waiting for specialist eating disorder support.

Universities may also have student medical practices embedded in their student support services. This can be a good opportunity to inform a GP about your eating difficulties and access physical health monitoring, as well as accessing referrals to more specialist services.

Finally, peer-led support groups and societies have become increasingly popular sources of support in recent years. Charities such as Beat and Student Minds have worked with mental health societies to facilitate some student-led support groups.

Learning point 3

- Have you researched your university's service provision?
- Could you make contact early so things are in place before you move?

Specialist service case study: eating disorders in student services (EDISS)

This is a case study of how a third sector organization worked to become embedded into a university's support service to offer specialist peer support for eating difficulties.

Eating Disorders in Students Services (EDISS) was a pilot study based on the First Steps Eating Disorder Early Intervention and Prevention Model (2015), which aims to 'catch' students and offer support before they fall into the grips of an eating difficulty.

The success of the pilot has led to a roll-out of the service across eight universities and colleges across the East Midlands.

The aims of the service were two-fold: to provide an effective and targeted service for students presenting with mild to moderate eating difficulties; and to work alongside internal and external services in a local area/university to embed EDISS in the university environment – all in a way that was 'flexible, holistic, and easily accessible'.

Central to accessing the service were 'robust; consistent; and outcome-measured' assessments, within an ambitious five-day target from the time of referral. All of the treatment options – which were commenced within a further five-day target from the time of assessment – had peer support from experts-by-experience at the fore. Treatment options ranged from one-to-one face to face, or online peer support; online befriending; or self-help workshops.

The outcomes from this specialist student service pilot were wholly positive, with a reduction in eating disorder symptomology measured by the EDE-Q (Global) scale.

> *"Absolutely essential service which kept me going this year. NHS services are harder and harder to access, and this fills a massive gap."* (EDISS service-user)

The pilot study and consequent roll-out of the service demonstrates that "provision of a 'bundled package' of specialist support for eating difficulties among university students appears to be helpful in addressing an unmet need and is received by users."

This case study also demonstrates how collaboration with the third sector can be a vital element of service provision, especially in terms of providing peer support for people with eating difficulties. It also provides the blueprint for a scalable model to be implemented across UK universities, where support for eating difficulties is embedded across all health and wellbeing services.

Learning point 4

How do you think a student could benefit from specialist or peer support which is embedded into their university's support offering? For example, how do you think it would feel to know that other students were experiencing similar difficulties? Could this raise awareness of the local statutory services?

Transfer of care

For people who have a pre-existing eating difficulty or who have previously accessed treatment in their hometown, a smooth transition of care is crucial to maintain recovery and prevent relapse. However, we know that due to local variation in provision of services, this can often be quite difficult to achieve.

The tragic case of Averil Hart demonstrates the profound consequences of a lack of joined-up support for people transitioning to university. Averil tragically passed away at the age of 19 following missed opportunities from NHS services to appropriately support her in recovering from her eating difficulty as she moved away from home to attend university.

Following an inquiry into this case, it was concluded that "inadequate coordination and planning of Averil's care during a particularly vulnerable time in her life, when she was leaving home to go to university", led to her being failed by services.

However, service models such as 'First episode and Rapid Early intervention for Eating Disorders' (FREED) recognize and prioritise how co-ordination and continuity of care can be crucial, and have adapted service provision to accommodate for emerging adults who may be transitioning to university by using telemedicine and remote consultations. Aligned with the NHS's priorities for increasing service provision for adults with eating disorders, 18 new FREED pilot sites were funded in November 2020.

Learning point 5

- What is the referral process for the eating disorder service in your university town?
- Is there a way your hometown service can refer you before you leave?
- Is your university town one of – or near to – the 18 new FREED pilot sites?

Disabled Students Allowance (DSA)

Disabled Students Allowance[1] (DSA) is an additional, non-repayable financial support to help students in higher education to access all areas of student life. This financial support can contribute towards disability-related living costs, such as extra travel, specialist equipment and non-medical helpers.

Non-medical helpers can be a useful resource to support you both emotionally and academically. Below is a case study of a student with body image and eating difficulties who received support from a non-medical helper.

1 Help if you're a student with a learning difficulty, health problem or disability can be found at https://www.gov.uk/disabled-students-allowance-dsa (accessed November 2021).

Lived-experience case study: non-medical helpers to support a student with body dysmorphic disorder and bulimia nervosa

"I had always been preoccupied with my appearance, especially with my weight and shape. I had engaged with fad diets in the past, and as a dancer was constantly pressured to have a slimmer frame.

I moved into university halls in 2012 and started experiencing more anxiety about my weight and appearance and stopped attending my lectures, meaning I fell behind with my work. I started to engage in some disordered eating behaviours, such as restrictive diets, use of calorie tracking apps, and occasionally using laxatives. I would then have episodes of binge-eating after excessively drinking alcohol.

At first, I was unsure how to deal with my mental health difficulties, and so I would avoid dealing with them. However, things got a lot better once I spoke to the GP at my student medical practice. I described what I was experiencing and was referred to a psychologist for an assessment. It was then that I was diagnosed with body dysmorphic disorder (BDD) and was referred for psychological therapy.

Having a diagnosis was helpful for communicating my issues with the university. I was able to apply for extenuating circumstances which meant that my coursework deadlines could be extended, and I was able to have extra time and my own room for written examinations. In my second and third year, I had started engaging with restriction, purging and bingeing, and my low mood and anxiety were unmanageable, leading to a period of time where I was severely unwell and unable to attend lectures and fell behind with my coursework.

This time, I applied for DSA and qualified for a non-medical helper. I started seeing a study mentor who helped me to manage my time efficiently while in recovery and I got back on track with writing my dissertation.

This was so helpful that it encouraged me to apply for DSAs once again when I relocated to another university to do my master's degree. The relocation and stress from my postgraduate studies triggered disordered eating behaviours again with restriction, bingeing and purging with vomiting and compulsive exercise. My study mentor once again supported me in navigating my studies and time management skills, while supporting me with a referral to a specialist eating disorder outpatient service where I received treatment for bulimia nervosa.

This has led to me continuing to study at a doctoral level, to research prevention strategies for the very issues I have experienced. While I have received great support from university, I do regret not being aware of my issues beforehand and waiting until things got really bad instead of intervening earlier. Hopefully others will learn from my mistakes."

Learning point 6

- How do you think a student could benefit from DSAs, such as a non-medical helper?
- If you think you or a loved one could benefit, don't forget to apply for DSAs alongside your Student Finance application.

Conclusion

While this chapter has highlighted some of the potential risk factors for eating difficulties and body image concerns in the transition to the university, it has also provided suggestions as to how these risks can be mitigated – both from a self-management perspective and by illustrating the types of services available.

University can be a challenging yet rewarding experience for people with – or at risk of developing – an eating difficulty. It is important that both statutory and third sector services prioritise both continuity of care and early intervention.

References

Beat (2021) *Fundraising at University* [online]. Available at: www.beateatingdisorders.org.uk/get-involved/universities (accessed August 2021).

First Steps ED (2021) *Eating Disorders in Student Services* [online]. Available at: www.firststepsed.co.uk (accessed August 2021).

FREED (2021a) *Fitness to Study* [online]. Available at: www.freedfromed.co.uk/guides/1/fitness-to-study (accessed August 2021).

FREED (2021b) *Preparing for University* [online]. Available at: www.freedfromed.co.uk/img/guides/Preparing_For_University-FREED.pdf (accessed August 2021).

HM Government (2021) *Help if you're a student with a learning difficulty, health problem or disability* [online]. Available at: https://www.gov.uk/disabled-students-allowance-dsa (accessed August 2021).

Hambly E & Byrom N (2021) *University Challenge: Integrating care for eating disorders at home and at university* [online]. Available at: www.studentminds.org.uk/uploads/3/7/8/4/3784584/university_challenge.pdf (accessed August 2021).

NHS England (2020) *Hundreds of young people with eating disorders to benefit from 'gold standard' NHS treatment* [online]. Available at: www.england.nhs.uk/2020/11/hundreds-of-young-people-with-eating-disorders-to-benefit-from-gold-standard-nhs-treatment/ (accessed August 2021).

Webb H & Schmidt U (2021) Facilitators and barriers to supporting young people with eating disorders during their transition to, and time at, university: An exploration of clinicians' perspectives. *Eur Eat Disorders Rev.* https://doi.org/10.1002/erv.2795

Royal College of Psychiatrists (2011) *Mental health of students in higher education* [online]. Available at: www.rcpsych.ac.uk/docs/default-source/improving-care/better-mh-policy/college-reports/college-report-cr166.pdf?sfvrsn=d5fa2c24_2 (accessed August 2021).

45. Disclosure and reasonable adjustments in the workplace

By Hannah Lewis, Isla Parker, James Downs and Caroline Moughton

Summary

This chapter will discuss key processes in the workplace and educational setting which could support a disclosure of an eating difficulty – such as how the Equality Act 2010 can protect people with eating difficulties from discrimination in the workplace – as well as highlighting other useful processes to support disclosure, reasonable adjustments, and care surrounding a potential long-term absence. Using a case study methodology, this chapter will also explore the experiences of two individuals who have been diagnosed with an eating difficulty and are in full-time employment. It will highlight the employment practices and 'reasonable adjustments' that can support a person with an eating difficulty to continue employment and also address complexities in doing so. The chapter will also explore how employees with eating difficulties may manage transitions between jobs, the transition to maternity leave or paternity leave, as well as a gradual return to work, to maintain wellbeing and quality of life.

Introduction

The secrecy and ambivalence which surround eating difficulties and recovery from them make disclosures particularly difficult, despite research showing that self-disclosures increase motivation to recover. People may be discouraged from disclosing an eating difficulty for a number of different reasons. For example, disclosing an eating difficulty breaks its concealment and so makes public the physical health risks associated. Disclosing an eating difficulty may have to be faced in a number of different circumstances, including in educational settings (such as schools and universities) and to employers.

'Reasonable adjustments' – which are aligned with the Equality Act 2010 – may reduce stress in the workplace (such as business lunches, unsocial working hours, pressure from unmanageable targets), and provide help and support for people with eating difficulties. Line managers also play an important role in supporting their employees and students with eating difficulties.

The Equality Act 2010

The Equality Act 2010 is a key piece of legislation that protects people who live, learn and work in the UK from discrimination against certain 'protected characteristics'. Currently, there are nine protected characteristics: age, disability (including mental health difficulties), gender reassignment, marriage and civil partnership, pregnancy and maternity, race, religion or belief, sex, and sexual orientation.

People who disclose a mental health difficulty in work – including an eating difficulty or disordered eating – are protected by the Equality Act 2010 under the protected characteristic of 'disability'. While some people with an eating difficulty may not personally identify with the term 'disability', this legislation defines being disabled as experiencing "a physical or mental impairment that has a 'substantial' and 'long-term' negative effect on your ability to do normal daily activities". For many people with an eating difficulty, this definition may be relevant.

Protection under the Equality Act 2010 means that people experiencing an eating difficulty or disordered eating have the right to request 'reasonable adjustments' or 'adjustments' in different areas of public life, including in the workplace and in educational settings. Reasonable adjustments or adjustments can be defined as actions which make sure workers or learner with disabilities, including physical or mental health conditions, are not substantially disadvantaged when doing their jobs. Reasonable adjustments can include flexible working hours or more regular supervisions. If your employer believes that your reasonable adjustments may require more resources, then you may be eligible for further support services through the Access to Work scheme.

The Equality Act 2010 applies to England, Wales and Scotland, although some areas of the legislation may be slightly different. However, there are significant gaps in equality legislation between Northern Ireland and the rest of the UK. The Equality and Human Rights Commission (EHRC) and the Equality Commission for Northern Ireland (ECNI) detail the variation in different pieces of legislation.

Learning point 1

- Are you, or a person that you work with, *substantially affected* by eating difficulties? If so, you/they may be protected by the Equality Act 2010.
- Depending on where you are in the UK, would this protection be different?

Disclosing an eating difficulty

In order to benefit from the protections discussed above, people need to first make the disclosure of their eating difficulty to their line manager at work. Making a disclosure can be a difficult process, so it is important that you prepare what you are going to disclose as well as how this affects your ability to work or learn. You may also already have an idea of what kind of reasonable adjustments you would find helpful, or this can be a collaborative decision between you and your employer.

A Wellness Recovery Action Plan (WRAP) is a widely used tool which has been found useful in making disclosures to employers about a person's mental health concerns. Devised by Dr Mary Copeland in the late 1990s, the tool can be used to guide a conversation in which you have to share your needs and how they can be met. A WRAP is commonly split into the following sections: Daily Maintenance; Triggers; Early Warning Signs; Breaking Down; and Crisis Plan. These sections can be used to express what a person needs to keep them well, to prevent them from becoming unwell, and how to recover from a potential crisis.

Learning point 2

- If you were to disclose an eating difficulty to an employer, what environment would make this as comfortable as possible for you?
- If you were to construct a WRAP, what would be included in your Daily Maintenance; Triggers; Early Warning Signs; Breaking Down; and Crisis Plan? Use the template in the bibliography to complete.

Occupational health

Occupational health is a medical service which is used for supporting both employers and employees to achieve health and wellbeing in the workplace. They are a useful function to conduct assessments and produce recommendations for reasonable adjustments, long-term absences, and returns to work. Occupational health services can either be outsourced or serve as part of a wider Human Resources (HR) function. Employers and line managers may wish to seek advice and support from occupational health if they are managing someone with an eating difficulty, or an employee may wish to speak with their occupational health service to seek guidance on implementing reasonable adjustments in the workplace.

Employee Assistance Programs

Most larger employers are likely to offer an Employee Assistance Program (EAP) – a service that provides certain benefits for their employees. Many EAPs offer short-term counselling or psychotherapy services, which may be useful for someone who is struggling with disordered eating in the workplace. Whilst the type of counselling or psychotherapy available from an EAP may not be the recommended type or length of treatment for an eating difficulty, it could be a useful tool for managing how your eating difficulty affects you in the workplace, while you are waiting to receive the recommended treatment for an eating difficulty.

Long-term absences

For some people with an eating difficulty, a long-term absence from work may be necessary in order to take time to recover or to engage with inpatient or intensive day treatment.

Each employer has local policies regarding long-term absence, so it is important to check these. However, the statutory sick pay (SSP) means that you won't receive less than £95.85 per week. During a long-term absence from work, you are eligible to claim SSP for up to 28 weeks, from the third day of absence. Following this, other welfare benefits such as Employment and Support Allowance (ESA), Universal Credit (UC), or Personal Independent Payment (PIP) may be able to support you financially during your long-term absence. Applying for welfare benefits can often take a long time, so if you think you will be absent for longer than 28 weeks, it is a good idea to submit an application as soon as possible. If you take a long-term absence from education you have the option to defer your studies until you feel well enough to continue, although different education providers may have varying policies.

Following a long-term absence, it is important to make sure your return to work is as safe and sustainable as possible. This is often managed through a 'phased return to work'. This means that instead of returning at a full-time capacity, you may prefer to return to reduced hours and lighter or different duties.

Learning point 3

- If you were to return to work or education after a long-term absence, what would help you make this return as successful as possible?
- If someone you managed was to take a long-term absence, how could you keep in touch in a way that was supportive and meaningful?

What is a reasonable adjustment?

In considering whether an adjustment is 'reasonable' or not, various factors need to be taken into account. These include whether the adjustment is likely to be effective in overcoming the barrier posed by the policy, criterion or practice; whether it would be practical; whether it would be affordable (taking into account the resources of the whole organization) and how disruptive it would be. Possible alternatives would be considered. Ultimately, the decision on whether a particular adjustment is 'reasonable' would be decided in a court of law.

Reasonable adjustments should have the effect of enabling the person with an eating difficulty to perform the role for which they have the relevant skills and for which they were recruited. The line manager and individual should discuss what support the individual might find helpful at work. They may not know in advance what would be helpful, so this is likely to require experimentation and review. Areas to think about include:

- **Canteen or work kitchen:** Offer a range of balanced, healthy foods (including fresh fruit and vegetables), so that people with eating difficulties can follow eating plans recommended to them by their dietitians and psychiatrists/GPs.
- **Work lunches:** Some people with eating difficulties may struggle to eat with colleagues present. They may benefit from a separate room or break-out space where they can eat alone or with a friend or particular colleague.
- **Work social events:** People with eating difficulties may struggle to attend work social events where the focus is on eating a meal. It may help to change the focus by offering some kind of activity or entertainment as well, or hosting the social event in a museum or art gallery. You may also choose to give the employee options for what type of food is offered (such as Thai, or Indian).
- **Bathroom:** Ensure that in the bathroom toilets flush properly, and an air freshener is provided, in case the employee ever experiences bulimia while at work.
- **Working pattern:** when someone is unwell, they may prefer part-time to full-time working to allow time to attend self-care activities such as therapy groups, although obviously this has financial implications. Someone may work five days a week, but be paid for four days a week (so they have some flexibility). If the person does not take much time off, they could be given a week's extra leave at the end of the year. This builds in the acknowledgement that the person may need to take some time off work at times, but does not leave their employer or colleagues feeling short-changed.
- **Working hours:** different start or finish times may suit the individual better, enabling them to travel at less busy times. Also, if medication (such as antidepressants) is prescribed, this may make some times of day difficult.
- **Regular work shifts:** to support an employee in maintaining regular mealtimes, avoiding the additional disruption of night working.
- **Extra time for travel to work:** for example, to attend conferences.

- **Review meetings:** for the first year of the person's employment, there could be regular meetings each three to four months with the person's line manager and HR department. These review meetings could continue for another year of the person's employment.
- **Induction:** adjustments to the standard induction programme, such as a phased introduction of tasks.
- **A point of contact for any questions:** this may be the manager or a designated work colleague. Make it easy for the individual to ask questions, so that anxiety levels don't build up.
- **More frequent contact with manager:** some people find it helpful to meet briefly at the end of the day or first thing in the morning to review work. This also provides an opportunity to raise and address any problems early and for the manager to give specific feedback on progress.
- **Time off for medical appointments:** permission to attend medical appointments (such as appointments with a GP or dietitian) when these cannot be arranged outside working hours within a reasonable period of time. Some organisations ask the individual to make up the time, but it would be good practice to be generous about this, especially if the individual is unwell and is struggling to remain in work.

Support at work for people who experience eating difficulties forms part of a bigger picture of support for the wellbeing of all employees, including those with diagnosed mental health conditions, and there are few suggestions here that are specific to people who experience eating difficulties alone.

Learning point 4

- Do you think that the above 'adjustments' would be 'reasonable' in your workplace or educational setting?
- Have you asked your line manager for any 'reasonable adjustments'? Did s/he agree to your request?

Recognising early warning signs

Triggers and early warning signs that a person is becoming less well should be discussed. These might include loss of weight and changes in behaviour, such as appearing restless and tense, avoiding meals in the workplace, taking long trips to the bathroom, becoming easily upset and overwhelmed, finding it difficult to make decisions and struggling to meet deadlines.

The employee's eating difficulty may be worse in a place associated with stress or trauma. When the individual feels stressed (which might be due to something at work or outside work) they may eat less or restrict what type of foods they eat. When it is harder for the individual to eat they may avoid certain places or situations and may feel that their thoughts are dominated by food, their weight, and exercise.

It is helpful for the line manager and employee to agree in advance what support is needed if someone appears to be becoming less well. It may be sufficient to remind the person with the eating difficulty of their usual strategies, such as following a meal plan. For some people, early warning signs may be an indication that they need to take a day or two off work to rest. In some organizations this can be done as 'disability leave'.

As a next step, the person with an eating difficulty may agree to the line manager contacting a close family member or another agreed contact to alert them to the situation. Clearly this is something that should have been agreed in advance.

Case study: James

I didn't disclose my eating difficulty when I started working in a hospital setting, hoping that I would have a fresh start and maybe that my new job would help my recovery – which has often been an appealing idea for me when starting something new. Sadly, when my health got worse, I realised that I wasn't able to cope with work as well as I would like and ended up disclosing to my employer after having to take time off with hospital admissions for suspected cardiac problems relating to anorexia.

Initially my employer told me that it would be a disciplinary matter and that I should have disclosed my condition on my occupational health clearance before starting my role. But I was worried that the job might have been withdrawn as this had happened in the past when I had been open about my mental health. After some discussion, my manager became extremely supportive once she could understand how to help. I explained that it would really help me to be able to attend appointments during the workday, so I worked the same hours in a different pattern in order to do so. I asked for longer breaks to manage eating lunch without having to rush and we drew up a plan for what to do and who to talk to if I felt like I was getting worse or needed additional support.

In hindsight, I wish I hadn't pushed myself so far without asking for help, and think that with the right support at the right time – in the form of small changes to my work schedule, breaks and someone to talk to if I was worried about work – I could have managed my work better and not become so unwell as I struggled in silence.

Case study: Roz

I stayed quiet about my eating difficulty when I worked as an English tutor, hoping that I wouldn't be discovered. Sometimes when I was under pressure, I would buy crisps or chocolate, and then discreetly vomit in the staff loo and spray air freshener afterwards.

Things improved when I was able to confide in another teacher who worked in one of the schools where I tutored English. A few of her students had eating difficulties, such as anorexia, and she admitted that often she felt out of depth dealing with supervising lunches, and contacting parents afterwards, as she found it extremely difficult to get the girls to eat all of their lunches. She asked me if I could make a list of 'reasonable adjustments', as this would help her with supporting the girls with their eating.

I found that several 'reasonable adjustments' helped me to cope with giving individual tuition, and travelling between schools and students' homes. First of all, I ate lightly and often in the day – snacks such as Ryvitas and fruits, so that I didn't become hungry. Secondly, I paced myself with work-tasks, so that there was not a big build up of pressure. I also listened to mindfulness exercises when I was travelling on buses or trains between locations where I was working. I found that mindfulness helped me to live more in the moment, and worry less about my bulimia. I also wore clothes that were not tight-fitting, so that I spent less time worrying about my size and shape, than if I had worn tight trousers or a tight skirt. Finally, I read a book by Dr Christopher Fairburn called *Overcoming Binge Eating*, which helped me to learn more practical strategies for managing my bulimia, such as not restricting my intake of food, as this itself could trigger a binge. I found it helpful to work as a tutor, and enjoyed the work: this itself gave me a focus that took me away from my bulimia, so that I could have income and a sense of purpose.

Conclusion

To conclude, this chapter provides the UK policy context for the Equality Act, and demonstrates how this could be implemented in the workplace to protect the rights of those living with eating difficulties or an eating difficulty by giving examples of reasonable adjustments. Illustrated by case studies, this chapter also demonstrates the potential barriers to implementation and areas of improvement for employers.

References

ACAS (2021) *Using occupational health at work* [online]. London: ACAS. See: www.acas.co.uk.

ACAS (2021) *Supporting mental health in the workplace* [online]. London: ACAS. See: www.acas.co.uk.

Copeland ME (1997) *Wellness Recovery Action Plan* [online] See: www.combined.nhs.uk.

Equality and Human Rights Commission (2014) *Your Rights to Equality at Work: When you apply for a job* [online]. London: EHRC. See: www.equalityhumanrights.com.

Equality and Human Rights Commission (2014) *Your Rights to Equality at Work: Working hours, flexible working and time off* [online]. London: EHRC. See: www.equalityhumanrights.com.

Equality and Human Rights Commission (2014) *What equality law means for you as an education provider – further and higher education* [online]. London: EHRC. See: www.equalityhumanrights.com

Equality and Human Rights Commission (2014) *Your Rights to Equality at Work: Pay and Benefits* [online]. London: EHRC. See: www.equalityhumanrights.com.

Equality Commission for Northern Ireland (2021). *Disability discrimination laws* [online]. See: www.equalityni.org

Fairburn, Christopher (2013) *Overcoming Binge Eating*. New York City: Guildford Publications.

HM Government (2015) *Equality Act 2010: guidance* [online]. London. See: www.gov.uk.

Mind (2021) *Disability discrimination* [online]. London. See: www.mind.co.uk

46. Navigating recovery when body dysmorphic disorder (BDD) and eating difficulties interact

By Dr Nicole Schnackenberg

Introduction

Body Dysmorphic Disorder (BDD) is a clinical diagnosis within which a person experiences a distressing preoccupation with a perceived defect or defects in their appearance that are either not visible to the outside eye or are perceived by the outside eye as part of normal human variation. Some of the most common perceived defects are related to the skin, hair and nose. However, any body part or parts can be the focus of distress. The preoccupation has a significantly detrimental impact on the person's activities of daily living, perhaps rendering them unable to go to school, work or to socialise (Albertini & Phillips, 1999; Phillips, 2007). Some people struggle to leave their house or even their bedroom for weeks, months or years (Phillips, 2005).

BDD is estimated to affect around 2.2% of the population (e.g. Veale *et al*, 2016) and has one of the highest suicide rates of any mental health diagnosis (Phillips & Menard, 2006; Phillips, 2007). Muscle dysmorphia appears in the Diagnostic and Statistical Manual (DSM-V) as a sub-type of this diagnosis (APA, 2013).

This chapter considers BDD in the context of eating difficulties. It will explore how these diagnostic categories can overlap and conflate and possible directions for support.

Overlaps between BDD and eating difficulties

In many ways, BDD and body-image focused eating difficulties are two sides of the same coin. Both are typically fuelled by pervasive feelings of low self-worth, shame and a felt sense of unlovability that are projected (pinned) onto the appearance with the hope that once the appearance is altered or 'fixed' in some way, the person will feel lovable, safe and whole. People who project the hoped-for resolution of their distress and low self-worth onto their weight may receive an eating disorder diagnosis, while those who pin their pain onto a specific body part, without a focus on the overall weight or shape of the body, may receive a diagnosis of BDD. Of course, life is not as clear-cut as putting manifestations of suffering into the discreet diagnostic boxes that the Diagnostic and Statistical Manual and the International Classification of Diseases prescribe. In reality, BDD and eating difficulties intersect in a myriad of ways.

The outward manifestation of distress of each person will depend on the body part this distress has been projected onto. Regrettably, few screening questionnaires and first port-of-call professionals like GPs appear to ask curious, open, 'why' questions about the behaviours engaged in and their origins: assumptions are often made (for a list of the most commonly used screening questionnaires which are available for BDD, please see the Resources section at the end of the chapter). If, for example, a person is distressed by the shape of their face and believes that losing weight may alter their face-shape, they may engage in calorie restriction, excessive exercise and so on. However, their aim may not be to lower the overall weight of their body, but rather to change their face's shape and contours. If the person is not asked why they are extensively restricting their diet, they may receive an eating disorder diagnosis rather than a BDD diagnosis. This is important because the diagnosis a person receives, in the current medical model context and climate, will determine the sort of treatment and support that they are offered (e.g. Johnstone *et al*, 2018).

Learning point 1

It is important to ask open, curious questions when a loved one or client tells you they are experiencing eating difficulties and a distressing preoccupation with a perceived defect in their appearance. Pause here to consider what questions you might ask. They may include questions like:

- I wonder if you might feel able to talk to me about which body part or parts are causing you distress.
- How many minutes or hours a day would you say you are feeling preoccupied with this/these body part(s)?
- How is the distress you are experiencing about this/these body part(s) impacting on your eating? Is it impacting on other areas of your life i.e. socialising, work/education, hobbies etc.?

Muscle dysmorphia

Muscle dysmorphia (MD) is a sub-type of BDD in which a person is distressed by the notion that they are insufficiently muscular and appear 'puny'. Distinct and both psychologically and physically damaging eating practices go alongside this experience, such as reducing or removing carbohydrates from the diet and scheduling one's day around the ingestion of protein. Indeed, some researchers and specialists in this area have argued that MD would be more suitably placed in the DSM as an eating disorder diagnosis. Excessive exercise is an intrinsic aspect of MD, with people spending hours in the gym every day, including when they are acutely fatigued or even seriously injured.

Difficulties with diagnoses

It is more common than previously thought or understood for people with an eating disorder diagnosis to later go on to receive a BDD diagnosis and vice versa (Ruffolo *et al*, 2006). In essence, the focus of the distress has 'moved', for example from the weight to the skin; or the hair to the weight and so on. Of course, the focus of distress can move within each diagnosis also.

It is vital that people presenting with eating difficulties are *always* asked, with genuine curiosity, about the particular focus or foci of their distress and the reasons for their presenting behaviour. It is beneficial to ask the person what they are hoping to change/alter/fix/achieve specifically by engaging in excessive exercise, self-induced vomiting, calorie restriction, laxative consumption and so on.

Sincerely curious questioning is especially important as shame may prevent open sharing without prompting of this kind. Likewise, if a person is presenting with a distressing preoccupation with a body part aside from the overall weight of the body, it is important to ask if they have ever, or are currently, engaging in any eating behaviours which may be emotionally and physically detrimental. Physical ramifications of unhealthful eating behaviours can, and sadly do, occur at any weight. Thus, it is important that weight is *never* the measure of possible damage or detriment in either diagnosis.

Insight in eating difficulties and BDD

A key aspect where BDD and eating difficulties overlap is poor insight. While the outside eye may see that the person is underweight, for example, the person struggling with a diagnosis like anorexia may see areas of fat on their body and perceive the need for further weight loss. Similarly, where a person struggling with body dysmorphia may perceive large, dark circles under their eyes, the outsider may either not see these circles or view them simply as part of normal human variation. Thus, the physical self as perceived by the person is qualitatively different to the reality perceived by others. This can lead to conflict, such as the person believing that what they require is a diet, a cosmetic surgeon, a dentist, a dermatologist etc. while their loved ones believe they require access to psychological help. This can leave the person feeling misunderstood, isolated and even lied to by those they love.

The CBT-based idea of Theory A / Theory B, often used in treatment for BDD, can be helpful here.

Theory A	Theory B
I have a physical defect and therefore require a diet/cosmetic surgeon/dentist/dermatologist etc.	I am struggling with an issue of an emotional/psychological nature and therefore require psychosocial support.

Learning point 2

The CBT approach of Theory A / Theory B can be supportive when BDD and eating difficulties overlap. Important considerations as part of this approach include:

- Putting a pause on tackling the struggle from a Theory A perspective, as far as possible, for an agreed period of time.
- Focusing on Theory B accordant treatments i.e. psychosocial treatments as opposed to cosmetic surgery, dermatology, dentistry etc.

Within this approach, the person is encouraged to lay aside the theory that their perceived 'problem' is physical in nature for an agreed amount of time, and to treat the difficulty 'as if' it is emotional and psychological in nature. The clinician suggests the client lays aside approaching their distress by trying to lose weight, clear up their skin, seek cosmetic surgery etc. for a set period of time and attend psychotherapeutic appointments to address their needs from an emotional and psychological perspective. People experiencing eating difficulties themselves can adopt this approach outside of any treatment being offered, for example by setting a date in the diary, making a pledge to oneself to address the distress from an emotional perspective, and laying aside endeavours to change or 'fix' the physical appearance until the decided date. To provide accountability, it can be extremely helpful to share the commitment with a trusted person who can be checked-in with regularly.

The next step is then to create a plan in alignment with a psychological perspective in collaboration with a mental health professional(s) if such support has been sought and secured. Many people find it reassuring to know they can return to Theory A, including any related plans, after the decided time frame is over. For example, one may postpone scheduling a cosmetic surgery consultation or an appointment with the dermatologist until the 12 weeks of working from the premise of Theory B are up. In many cases, with a concerted effort focused on the emotional aspects of distress, the desire for surgery, dermatology etc. can gradually diminish. Many people say that while it was comforting to know they could return to seeking physical treatments at the end of the decided period, they let go of these plans after receiving support, and supporting themselves, through treatment of a psychosocial nature.

Learning point 3

Reassuring people that they can return to tackling their struggle from a Theory A perspective in the future can be reassuring and negate experiences of hopelessness and despair. Without such an assurance there is the risk of:

- Increased feelings of suicidality.
- Reduced willingness to engage in treatment.
- A decreased sense of feeling understood/felt minimisation.

Below is an example plan based on the Theory A / Theory B approach one might consider adapting.

Theory A actions and behaviours to postpone/ attempt to reduce significantly	Theory B actions to take and behaviours to endeavour to adopt
Seeking of dentistry, cosmetic surgery, dermatology etc.	Seek support of a psychological nature. Focus on finding a therapist who specialises in BDD and/or eating difficulties. Delete related social media accounts. Place blocks on phone/laptop etc.
Restriction of diet and/or dietary practices which are potentially physically and/or emotionally detrimental.	Enlist the support of a registered dietician, if possible, to create a realistic and healthy meal plan and/or explore intuitive eating approaches or similar. Choose foods based on their functionality (how the foods make the body feel and the sustained energy they provide) rather than on form (how one believes they will make the body look). Delete social media accounts related to diets and associated practices. Place blocks on phone etc. Refrain from watching documentaries, reading magazines and books etc. on weight loss and diets. Refrain from weighing oneself.

Theory A actions and behaviours to postpone/ attempt to reduce significantly	Theory B actions to take and behaviours to endeavour to adopt
Excessive exercise	Schedule reasonable amounts of enjoyed exercise. Exercise with a trusted person to keep one accountable if possible and appropriate. If seeking a personal trainer etc. find someone whose focus and associated instructions privilege the function of the body over the form.
Purging behaviours such as self-induced vomiting, laxative abuse etc.	Seek psychological support for refrainment from purging behaviours. Identify 'touch points' in the day/week when one is more likely to purge and structure phone-calls with loved ones, enjoyed activities etc. at these times. Engage in arts/crafts and other creative pursuits for at least half an hour after meals and snacks; set a timer.
Checking one's appearance numerous times within short time frames and/or spending long periods of time in front of the mirror scrutinising one's appearance.	Place a clock near the mirror and/or set a timer for getting ready in the morning, for, say, five or ten minutes. Leave the mirror when the timer goes off. Relinquish any small hand-held mirrors in pockets, handbags etc. Count to 20 when the urge to check in the mirror is noticed before checking; taking long deep breaths. Gradually increase this time.
Repetitive reassurance-seeking from others about aspects of physical appearance.	Notice the urge to seek reassurance about the appearance and extend self-compassion to the underlying distress. Seek closeness and reassurance from loved ones in relation to emotional and psychological wellbeing; for example, asking for a hug, a chat, a cup of tea etc.

Outlining a sample plan such as the one above is by no means to simplify the complexity of eating difficulties or BDD, or to suggest that moving forwards in one's recovery is as easy as writing down and following a few steps. It is respectfully recognized that amending one's mindset and associated behaviours takes tremendous commitment, often considerable time, and extensive emotional outlay. Such a plan should certainly not be used to berate oneself with if there are blips in sticking with the Theory B rather than the Theory A behaviours. This would be detrimental and counterproductive. Rather, such a plan can be a starting point to make a commitment to approaching one's struggle from an emotional, rather than a physical perspective for a set amount of time.

Feelings of shame in eating difficulties and BDD

Shame is a hidden and secretive emotion by its very nature. It is wholly different from guilt, with guilt being the sense of '*I have done something bad*' and shame being the sense of '*I am bad*'. A pervasive sense of shame typically underpins the experience both of eating difficulties and of BDD (e.g. Fuchs, 2002; Schnackenberg, 2021).

The sense of the self as 'bad' and shameful can come to be projected or pinned onto the weight or another aspect of the physical appearance with the hope that, once the appearance is improved, the feeling of the self as shameful and bad will fall away. Of course, the master plan fails to deliver as no number of physical alterations to the body ultimately changes how the person feels about themselves inside. Thus, one appearance project becomes another, and the person can find themselves caught in a conveyor-belt of appearance-focused distress.

Shameful narratives about the self, emergent within the operation of threat and power, can eclipse a person's true self (Winnicott, 1960). A false self (Winnicott, 1960) may then take centre-stage. In the context of eating difficulties and BDD, this could be a self which is only felt to be worthy and lovable if one is without appearance defects/flaws, is thin enough, is toned enough etc. One focus of therapy is to challenge these dominant, oppressive narratives and to thicken thin and marginalized narratives about the person's self and experiences. Therapeutic letters, as outlined in more detail in Chapter 41 may be an element of such an approach.

It can be helpful to support clients to view their sense of shame as a vulnerable and frightened aspect of the self; seeking to have its story told and to transmute into its naturally valuable state. In this way, the messages shame appears to be communicating under the guise of eating difficulties and body dysmorphia may be transformed. Here are some possible transformations, based on clinical work with clients experiencing these struggles:

Message from shame in its fear state	Message from shame in its naturally valuable state
You are a bad/unlovable person.	You have been treated by others at times as though you are bad/unlovable.
You are not good enough.	You have internalised the message from others that you are not good enough.
You are ugly/fat/disgusting/hideous.	You have projected your sense of unlovability onto your physical appearance based on the messages you have been exposed to.
You do not deserve a place in this world or anything good.	You have deducted, based on some of the ways you have been treated, that you are undeserving of life's greatest treasures like connection and love.

In closing

It is hoped that this chapter has prompted you to reflect upon how BDD and eating difficulties can, and often do, overlap, and that it has offered some ways of understanding and working with this conflation. It has highlighted the importance of openness and curiosity in place of minimization and judgment, and suggested the CBT Theory A/Theory B approach as a helpful starting point for working with this client group alongside a deeper exploration of the aspects of shame and sense of self in particular.

In summary, the invitation is to work with the person's lived experience – their story – rather than focusing on diagnostic labels and any assumptions arising from these.

Screening questionnaires for BDD

Cosmetic Procedure Screening questionnaire (COPS) (Veale *et al*, 2012).

Appearance Anxiety Inventory (Veale *et al*, 2014).

Both available on the BDD Foundation website: https://bddfoundation.org/helping-you/questionnaires/

References

Albertini RS & Phillips, K. A. (1999). Thirty-three cases of body dysmorphic disorder in children and adolescents. *Journal of the American Academy of Child & Adolescent Psychiatry* **38** (4) 453-459.

American Psychiatric Association (2013) *Diagnostic and statistical manual of mental disorders* (DSM-5®). American Psychiatric Publications.

Fuchs T (2002) The phenomenology of shame, guilt and the body in body dysmorphic disorder and depression. *Journal of Phenomenological Psychology* **33** (2) 223-243.

Johnstone L, Boyle M, Cromby J, Dillon J, Harper D, Kinderman P, Longden E, Pilgrim D & Read J (2018) *The Power Threat Meaning Framework: Towards the identification of patterns in emotional distress, unusual experiences and troubled or troubling behavior, as an alternative to functional psychiatric diagnosis*. Leicester, England: British Psychological Society.

Phillips KA (2005) *The Broken Mirror: Understanding and treating body dysmorphic disorder.* Oxford University Press, USA.

Phillips KA (2007) Suicidality in body dysmorphic disorder. *Primary Psychiatry* **14** (12) 58.

Phillips KA & Menard W & Fay C (2006) Gender similarities and differences in 200 individuals with body dysmorphic disorder. *Comprehensive Psychiatry* **47** (2) 77-87.

Ruffolo J, Phillips KA, Menard W, Fay C & Weisberg RB (2006) Comorbidity of body dysmorphic disorder and eating disorders: severity of psychopathology and body image disturbance. *International Journal of Eating Disorders* **39** (1) 11-19.

Schnackenberg N (2021) Young people's experiences of body dysmorphic disorder in education settings: a grounded theory. *Educational Psychology in Practice*. DOI: 10.1080/02667363.2021.1895079

Veale D, Ellison N, Werner TG, Dodhia R, Serfaty MA & Clarke A (2012) Development of a cosmetic procedure screening questionnaire (COPS) for body dysmorphic disorder. *Journal of plastic, reconstructive & aesthetic surgery* **65** (4) 530-532.

Veale D, Eshkevari E, Kanakam N, Ellison N, Costa A & Werner T (2014) The Appearance Anxiety Inventory: Validation of a process measure in the treatment of body dysmorphic disorder. *Behavioural and Cognitive Psychotherapy* **42** (5) 605-616.

Veale D, Gledhill LJ, Christodoulou P & Hodsoll J (2016) Body dysmorphic disorder in different settings: A systematic review and estimated weighted prevalence. *Body Image* **18** 168-186.

Winnicott DW (1960) Ego distortion in terms of true and false self. *1965 The Maturational Processes and the Facilitating Environment.*

47. The role of peer support in helping people with eating difficulties to recover

By Georgie Lazzari and Antonia Lagou

Summary

Peer support is a process that occurs when people use their own experiences to help each other through life's challenges. The common aims are to unite people with shared experiences to support each other and provide outlets where they each feel accepted, understood and comfortable to express their emotions in a safe and non-judgmental environment.

In this chapter we will explore the role of peer support in eating difficulty recovery and how this relationship traditionally differs from the typical therapeutic one. We will use a case study to demonstrate the impact of receiving support from others with lived experience and the positive influence this can have on the recovery journey. We will also evaluate the methods of peer support delivery, the versatile nature of this form of care provision and the widespread benefits to the service user as a result.

Defining peer support

In the mental health setting, a peer is defined as a person with 'lived experience of mental illness', and the peer support process is viewed as 'an established intervention in which peers offer support to others with mental illness' (Puschner *et al*, 2019).

It is common for the peer support relationship to feature two or more individuals who have undergone a similar condition to share their first-hand experiences for the benefit of one another. It is often provided 'independent of conventional mental healthcare with formal partnerships' in many cases, but movements are shifting to encourage collaborations between 'ex-patients/users, mental health professionals and researchers to co-produce training programmes for 'experts by experience' (Mahlkea *et al*, 2014).

Peer support promotes a wellness model that focuses on the positive aspects of people and their ability to function effectively and supportively, rather than an illness model, which places more emphasis on symptoms and problems of individuals (Carter, 2000).

O'Hagan *et al* (2009) identify three primary values: equal power relationships, reciprocal roles of helping and learning and a 'whole of life' approach. This identifies peer support as typically following a person-centred method which can positively impact a patient and contrasts other types of more formal therapy.

In eating disorder services, peer support and mentoring has been used primarily as a prevention initiative that assists with increasing self-esteem and improving body image (Lippi, 2000).

Fogarty *et al* (2016) also stated in their review that other benefits included 'lower post-intervention levels of bingeing, purging, emotional eating and dieting behaviours and an increase in feminist identity, quality of life in the domains of education/vocation, family and close relationships, future outlook, psychological, emotional, values and beliefs and physical domains.'

Learning point 1

Have you or somebody you care for engaged in a peer supported environment or conversation as part of your or their recovery journey?

Modes of delivery

The Mental Health Foundation defines the different methods of peer support delivery as including mentoring, education, listening, mediation and tutoring.

Chinman *et al* (2014) stated that: "historically, peer support began in the form of peer groups, in which participants with similar difficulties met to provide mutual support, discuss their problems, and receive empathy and suggestions from other members on the basis of shared experiences."

What originated in a group setting has now progressed to environments including one-to-one sessions, telephone and email communications, social media channels and through complimentary therapies such as meditation and art. In the eating disorder setting, some organizations offer peer supported activities such as eating meals together, food preparation and appropriate exercise sessions to assist with normalising such tasks and raising the confidence of both parties.

Elements of these services have adapted to be delivered both in-person and digitally, with online befriending support services becoming more readily available now than ever before.

Peer support roles have progressed noticeably from voluntary to paid during the last ten years, and an online search returns a host of employment opportunities in this area. Chinman *et al* (2014) also discuss this in their journal and identify the differences between 'individuals who fill designated unique peer positions' and 'peers who are hired into traditional mental health positions.'

They believe the latter can create an 'asymmetrical relationship' as 'the peer provider and the recipient are not at the same level of skills or degree of recovery, and both parties are not expected to receive mutual benefit'. This highlights the main difference between the role of voluntary and paid peer support positions.

Learning point 2

Before reading on, why not question whether you have experienced peer support in a group or individual setting? How did it benefit you? Was the support offered from an individual or a professional and did the two approaches differ?

Case study

The following testimonial is from a service user of First Steps ED, an eating disorder and mental health charitable organization in the Midlands. A case study of their Eating Disorders In Student Services (EDISS) is available in Chapter 44.

> "I have benefitted from almost seven years in a peer support environment, helping me with an eating disorder, anxiety and low mood.
>
> I have accessed this through First Steps ED, in the form of one-to-one counselling, group support and online befriending. In each setting I was assisted by an individual that had experienced similar mental health difficulties and was either engaged in their own recovery or at a point whereby they felt they had progressed enough to no longer require services.
>
> Whatever the setting, the peer support model had a hugely positive impact on my recovery. I felt safe, understood and empathised with which made such a difference. There was nowhere quite like it for meeting like-minded people.

I remember when I walked in to my first support group at First Steps ED and even though I was anxious and unsure what to expect, I felt instantly understood. It was the first time I'd been in a room surrounded by people who knew exactly what I was going through and could offer guidance from first-hand experience.

In 2015, I spent nine months having 1-2-1 counselling sessions with an ex-sufferer who was training to be a therapist. She had an understanding perspective and her advice came from a place of both personal experience and professional and academic knowledge. She assisted me with setting goals and focusing on the associated mental health difficulties that accompanied my eating disorder such as anxiety and low self-confidence.

Similarly, I now receive weekly emails from an online befriender who has been in eating disorder recovery for around five years. She is helping me to tackle the biggest challenges I have including body image, discomfort after meals and building recovery goals to prevent relapses. This is proving to be invaluable advice and I am truly benefitting from hearing it from someone that has experienced the exact same struggles herself. I have altered the way I view my body and normalised uncomfortable feelings such as fullness and bloating. I feel no-one else could offer such an exclusive insight to both reassure me that I'm not alone and help me view things differently.

I have a great relationship with my therapist in the NHS Eating Disorder Service I am under and feel completely supported. In the three years I have been attending appointments we have created a great level of mutual trust and understanding and I have progressed slowly but surely as a result. What cannot be achieved in that environment though, is conversing with somebody with first-hand experience of the problem. Doctors are highly qualified and thoroughly knowledgeable, but as they have typically never 'been there' themselves, it is hard to replicate the uniqueness of the peer to peer setting."

Learning point 3

Is there anything in particular about this testimony that stands out to you? Can you spot the clear differences between peer support and therapeutic support?

Evaluation of peer support

Evidence-based research in the field of peer support is steadily growing, as it becomes a part of the UK's mental health support system offer (Gillard, 2019). A number of benefits and drawbacks are indicated below.

Benefits of peer support

Easily accessible and often readily available

One of the main benefits of peer support is that it appears to be easier to access than traditional therapies, with a flexibility in regard to how an individual actively participates. For instance, research has found that peer support delivered via technology has been well received by a diverse range of individuals (O'Leary *et al*, 2017; 2018).

For many, a simple search online for local support groups can bring up a whole range of options – often accessible without rigid criteria or waiting list. It has recently been stated that peer support addresses the 'treatment gap' between the size of population and the size of the economy (Puschner, 2018).

Flexible approach: peer support can be guided or unguided in a way that is person-centred

Helen Cowie (2020) states: 'Peer support is not one particular program or method that can be applied in any context'. Whether peer support is defined in a guided way that suits the individual receiving/delivering the support or developed in a way that is less structured, the flexibility in regard to content and discussion, two-way communication and goal setting is unquestionable in comparison to more traditional therapy.

Many participants described the importance of feeling 'normal' and being able to express their feelings without judgment when involved in the mentoring relationship.

Mentees found support from 'staying motivated and committed to doing the hard work of recovery' (Perez *et al*, 2014, p8).

Drawbacks of peer support

Inconsistencies in quality of peer support being delivered

It has been argued that the distinctiveness of peer support is 'attributable to a values-base grounded in naturally occurring, real-world interactions between people supporting each other with their emotional distress' (Mead & Macneil, 2006).

With this is in mind, there is no way of guaranteeing a positive and fulfilling peer support experience, due to the subjectiveness and discrepancies that are so clear to individual experience of the real-world.

Not always appropriate for an individual with an eating difficulty

Eating difficulties are known to be a mental health issue, but there is a very clear level of physical risk to the individual suffering, particularly on the severe end of the spectrum (Solmi *et al*, 2020). For this reason, it can often be the case that the individual requires a more medical intervention as the priority. Peer support may sometimes compliment the medical support, but this would be assessed on an individual basis.

Ineffective for some areas of recovery

Fogarty *et al* (2016) noted in their Eating Behaviours review that many mentees stated there was no change in their motivation levels, energy and confidence towards recovery and psychological distress, objectified body consciousness and self-esteem. While initial positive changes were found in social physique anxiety, drive for thinness and body dissatisfaction, these changes were not maintained at a one-year follow-up.

Learning point 4

Can you think of any other benefits or drawbacks to delivering/receiving peer support in an eating difficulty context?

Conclusion

Considering the information this chapter has discussed, we will now evaluate the role of peer support in helping people with eating difficulties to recover.

It is undoubtable that, for an individual with a mild to moderate eating difficulty (that is to say, an individual that carries a small level of physical risk), the unique and varied nature of peer support may prove useful. Eating difficulties can often be experienced on a very personal and individual level, and therefore a flexible and person-centred peer support approach could offer an opportunity for many experiences and stressors to be discussed.

Sharing experiences with others that are going through a similar issue has also been shown to increase an individual's level of hope and connectedness (Chinman *et al*, 2014).

It would seem that the mode of peer support (one-to-one, group, online) might also play a critical role in the effectiveness of the intervention. For some individuals, online support may allow a certain level of anonymity and therefore create a willingness to speak more freely. For others however, a sense of community can be an important factor in recovery and therefore being able to speak to someone in person, one-to-one or in a group, might be better suited.

It is important to note that literature shows that peer support is still developing. Fogarty *et al* (2016) believed the mentoring partnership 'has potential benefits for both mentors and mentees and should not be underestimated, but rather further harnessed and explored in future studies.'

Peer support poses many challenges if it is delivered without thorough training, supervision and management (Repper & Carter, 2011). It is therefore advised that an individual enters peer support with an open mind, and an understanding that peer support has no universal model and thus every experience will be subjective.

References

Carter ML (2000) Social support systems as factors of academic persistence for African American, lower-income, first-year college students and high school graduates not attending college. *Dissertation Abstracts International* **61** (5) 2061.

Chinman M, George P, Dougherty RH, Daniels AS, Ghose SS, Swift A & Delphin-Rittmon ME (2014) Peer Support Services for Individuals With Serious Mental Illnesses: Assessing the Evidence [online]. Psychiatric Services Washington D.C. *ResearchGate*. P3. Available at: www.researchgate.net/profile/Matthew_Chinman/publication/260252813_Peer_Support_Services_for_Individuals_With_Serious_Mental_Illnesses_Assessing_the_Evidence/links/02e7e53206e87b88df000000/Peer-Support-Services-for-Individuals-With-Serious-Mental-Illnesses-Assessing-the-Evidence.pdf P3-4 (accessed August 2021).

Cowie H (2021) Peer Support. In The Encyclopaedia of Child and Adolescent Development (eds S Hupp and J Jewell). https://doi.org/10.1002/9781119171492.wecad285

Julie Repper & Tim Carter (2011) A review of the literature on peer support in mental health services. *Journal of Mental Health* **20** (4) 392-411. DOI: 10.3109/09638237.2011.583947

Fogarty S, Ramjan L & Hay S (2016) A systematic review and meta-synthesis of the effects and experience of mentoring in eating disorders and disordered eating. *Eating Behaviors* **21** pp66-75.

Lippi DE (2000) The impact of the mentoring relationship upon women in the process of recovering from eating disorders. (Doctor of Philosophy) Temple University, Bell & Howell Information and Learning Company (UMI Microform 9969913).

Mahlke C , Kraemer UM, Becker T & Bock T (2014) Peer Support in Mental Health Services [online]. 27 Number 4. *ResearchGate*. P276. Available at: https://www.researchgate.net/publication/262580200_Peer_support_in_mental_health_services (accessed August 2021).

Mead S & MacNeil C (2006) Peer support: What makes it unique. *International Journal of Psychosocial Rehabilitation* **10** (2) 29-37.

O'Hagan M, McKee H & Priest R (2009) Consumer survivor initiatives in Ontario: Building for an equitable future. Toronto: Ontario Federation of Community Mental Health & Addiction Programs.

O'Leary K, Bhattacharya A, Munson SA, Wobbrock JO & Pratt W (2017) Design opportunities for mental health peer support technologies. In: *Proceedings of the 2017 ACM conference on computer supported cooperative work and social computing* (pp1470-1484).

O'Leary K, Schueller SM, Wobbrock JO & Pratt W (2018) "Suddenly, we got to become therapists for each other." Designing Peer Support Chats for Mental Health. In: *Proceedings of the 2018 CHI conference on human factors in computing systems* (pp. 1-14).

Perez M, Kroon Van Diest A & Cutts S (2014) Preliminaray examination of a mentorbased program for eating disorders. *Journal of Eating Disorders* **2** (24).

Puschner B (2018) Peer support and global mental health. *Epidemiology and psychiatric sciences* **27** (5) 413-414.

Puschner B, Repper J, Mahlke C, Nixdorf R, Basangwa D, Nakku J, Ryan G, Baillie D, Shamba D, Ramesh M, Moran G, Lachmann M, Kalha J, Pathare S, Müller-Stierlin A & Slade M (2019) Using Peer Support in Developing Empowering Mental Health Services (UPSIDES): Background, Rationale and Methodology. Abstract, Background [online]. *Annuals of Global Health*. Available at: www.ncbi.nlm.nih.gov/pmc/articles/PMC6634474/#:~:text=Background%3A,mental%20illness%20receive%20no%20care (accessed August 2021).

Solmi M, Radua J, Stubbs B, Ricca V, Moretti D, Busatta D & Castellini G (2020) Risk factors for eating disorders: an umbrella review of published meta-analyses. *Brazilian Journal of Psychiatry* (AHEAD).

Steve Gillard (2019) Peer support in mental health services: where is the research taking us, and do we want to go there? *Journal of Mental Health* **28** 4 341-344, DOI: 10.1080/09638237.2019.1608935

The Mental Health Foundation (2020) Peer Support webpage (online). Available at: www.mentalhealth.org.uk/a-to-z/p/peer-support (accessed December 2020)

Afterword

By Dasha Nicholls

This handbook of eating difficulties is not like the textbooks I encountered in medical school. It contains some of the same material – for example, a chapter on medical complications of eating difficulties, one on cognitive behavioural models, one on the role of the dental practitioner and one on the healthcare systems that support treatment and recovery. Yet, interspersed among these chapters, and sometimes within them, are personal narratives, ideas, new ways of thinking and real life, practical suggestions and strategies for action. As a textbook, it represents a coalescence of professional and lived experiences in a field which has often been quite fragmented. Some chapters are written by leading clinical authorities in the field, extolling the science (a paediatrician, a clinical psychologist, a dietitian, a psychiatrist); others by experienced practitioners in creative therapies who write from experience (an equine therapist, music therapist, and practitioners who use art and writing in the recovery process). Many chapters are written or co-written by people with lived experience of an eating difficulty or caring for or living with someone with this experience. And some embody multiple perspectives – those with lived experience who have become professionals in the field, and professionals using their personal experiences to help others. This book exemplifies the move away from rigid boundaries between distinct roles – the patient, the carer; the clinician, the researcher – to a position where all perspectives in promoting recovery are valued and where the voice of experience shines through, regardless of how that experience was gained.

The holistic approach of this handbook provides a narrative that will interest readers approaching the topic from a range of backgrounds. This is a book designed to make the reader think, not just to learn and understand. Each chapter is peppered with learning points and prompts for reflection. This handbook is easy to read but not simplistic, reflecting the full complexity of the struggles and opportunities eating difficulties present, debunking reductionist myths and stigma in the process. It encompasses the seldom heard voices of men with experience of eating difficulties and those of the LGBTQ+ community, as well as the sadly too common and heart-breaking experiences of parents and siblings.

Despite narrating topics that can make for difficult reading, this book is ultimately infused with hope. It empowers through raising understanding of issues fundamental to those living with or managing the challenges of an eating difficulty. Examples include what is reasonable to expect in the workplace; the challenge of living with perfectionism; and the role that schools and social media, both positive and negative, can play. The chapters cover the range of disciplines, care settings and diagnoses, from prevention through primary care to inpatient treatment.

Not everything we know about eating difficulties is contained herein. Scientific knowledge of epidemiology; genetics; the why, when and when-not of family-based treatment approaches; the relationship between higher weight, weight stigma and eating difficulties; and the neuroscience-informed thinking around difficulties in emotional processing, reward processing and social/interpersonal problems, have taken a back seat to the personal stories of a father, a sibling, and a person on their route to recovery. The aim, and effect, is to engage the reader and humanise a topic that has for so long been trivialised and, at times, provoked negativity and even hostility.

There is much more to know and learn about eating difficulties, including in the context of a global pandemic, the burning question of why there has been such as specific surge in presentations in young people. We can speculate about the role of social isolation and loss of peer support, of food insecurity, of a life lived through social media, and of personal loss and existential fear. Yet at a population level, the same question that applies in an individual person's journey needs to be asked: with all the pressures that could impact on mental health and wellbeing the pandemic has presented, how did it so often become about food, weight and shape? It is hard to imagine a global pandemic that could have brought into sharper relief the prioritization and value of exercise and the fear of obesity, whilst simultaneously disconnecting people from all that brings them joy, balance and hope. From a life event that affected everyone, we may learn more about the modifiable factors that can turn risk into reality, and also look for clues about resilience – who was not affected and why?

This book is an important step in a journey towards knowledge, understanding and acceptance, making state of the art ideas and real-world experiences accessible to a wide audience. The field is changing fast – eating difficulties have expanded in scope, with binge eating disorder and avoidant restrictive food intake disorder (ARFID) added to the fold of diagnoses in the Diagnostic and Statistical Manual (DSM-5). Alongside this, the demographic of those affected has widened, and what were once seemingly rare experiences infrequently encountered in clinical practice outside specialist services, are now a public health concern prompting policy review.

Work on the prevention of eating difficulties, once a largely academic endeavour, has become a national priority. The stigma and shame that once surrounded eating struggles in their various forms is beginning to erode, thanks to high profile testimonies and advocacy. Addressing the paucity of funding for research into the array of eating difficulties has become an imperative – we cannot solve an issue that we do not yet fully understand. This research needs to be undertaken fully in partnership with those with lived experience. I commend the editors and authors of this practical handbook for opening up some new perspectives and moving the dialogue forward.

